The Two Sides of Perception

Cognitive Neuroscience
Michael S. Gazzaniga, editor

The Two Sides of Perception

Richard B. Ivry and Lynn C. Robertson

A Bradford Book
The MIT Press
Cambridge, Massachusetts
London, England

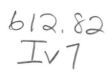
© 1998 Massachusetts Institute of Technology

This book was set in Palatino using Ventura Publisher under Windows 95 by Wellington Graphics and was printed and bound in the United States of America.

Library in Congress Cataloging-in-Publication Data

Ivry, Richard B.
    The two sides of perception / Richard B. Ivry and Lynn C. Robertson.
       p.   cm.—(Cognitive neuroscience)
    "A Bradford Book."
    Includes bibliographical references and index.
    ISBN 0-262-09034-1 (hc : alk. paper)
    1. Cerebral dominance. 2. Laterality. 3. Perception.
I. Robertson, Lynn C. II. Title. III. Series: Cognitive neuroscience series.
    [DNLM: 1. Perception—physiology. 2. Dominance, Cerebral—physiology.
3. Brain—physiology. WL 705 I96t 1997]
QP385.5.I886 1997
612.8'25—dc21
DNLM/DLC
for Library of Congress   96–50975
                                                                           CIP

To our two Steves, Steve Keele and Steve Palmer

Contents

Acknowledgments

We wish to thank the many people who have assisted us in this project. Michael Gazzaniga provided a critical reading of an early manuscript and encouraged us to expand the project into a book for the Cognitive Neuroscience series. We have also been fortunate to have the opportunity to discuss this work with many of our colleagues and students including Lori Bernstein, Asher Cohen, Shai Danziger,Robert Egly, Liz Franz, Stacia Friedman-Hill, Marcia Grabowecky, Erv Hafter, Joseph Hellige, Steve Keele, Nancy Kim, Paul Lebby, Bill Prinzmetal, Michael Posner, Bob Rafal, Susan Ravizza, Ruth Salo, and Anne Treisman. Eliot Hazeltine was instrumental in all of the modeling work and we are grateful to him for allowing us to present this work. Robert Knight and John Walker guided us in interpreting the MRI and neurological reports of the patients.

This work would not have been possible without the many hours of assistance provided by Catherine Lackey in preparing the manuscript and figures. Additional technical assistance was provided by John Lackey, Brent Stansfield, Lisa DiIulio, and Sara Druss. Support for this work has been provided by the National Institute of Mental Health, the National Institute of Neurological Disorders and Stroke, the National Science Foundation, and the Veterans Administration. Finally, we thank our spouses, Brent Robertson and Ann Lacey, for their support and understanding during the writing of this book.

The Two Sides of Perception

1 Introduction and Historical Overview

The asymmetric function of the mammalian brain took hundreds of years to discover. Anatomically, the central nervous system appears remarkably symmetrical. It looks much the same on each side with only minor and inconsistent differences in overall size and orientation of different areas. This symmetry is manifest at all levels of the nervous system, from the relatively simple structures of the spinal cord to the complex and extensively convoluted folds of the cerebral hemispheres (figure 1.1).

Correspondingly, the early writings on the biological basis of behavior tended to assume that function was symmetrically organized (see Finger, 1994; Harrington, 1995). The last 100 years of neurological study, however, have made it clear that the two hemispheres are not identical in function. The consequences of injury to one side of the brain or to the other are not the same: Patients with left hemisphere damage in a particular location can show vastly different symptoms than those shown by patients with right hemisphere damage in an analogous location.

The clinical observations of asymmetric function motivated researchers to ask whether evidence for this asymmetry could also be found in the neurologically intact brain; that is, in the behavior of healthy humans. The results of these investigations have consistently supported the hypothesis that cerebral functions can be represented asymmetrically. Indeed, the lay population has accepted the notion of hemispheric specialization with a passion. Popular books proselytize new techniques that are supposed to allow us to discover and strengthen our unique hemispheric preferences. It is claimed that we can learn how to improve drawing or cooking skills, for example, by releasing the capabilities of the right side of the brain or heighten our analytic abilities by tapping into the left side of the brain.

Scientific arguments are expected to be more conservative. The differences in hemispheric function appear quite subtle, at least when studied by behavioral methods in normal human beings. This means that understanding hemispheric specialization requires that we both acknowledge the similarities between hemispheres and continue to search for more appropriate descriptions of the functional differences between the two

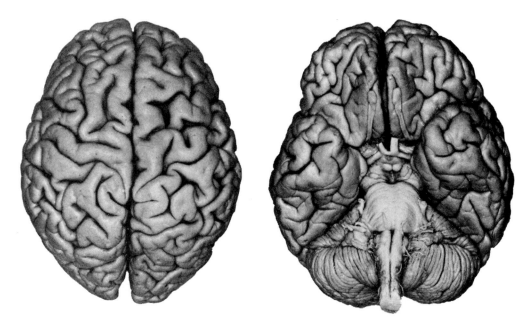

Figure 1.1 Viewed from the top or the bottom, a human brain looks symmetrical. (From DeArmond et al., 1989).

hemispheres. The theory presented in this book is intended to begin to offer such a balance. This work centers on a hypothesis concerning functional asymmetry across perceptual modalities in perceptual processing; the proposed asymmetry, however, begins with an overall similarity between the hemispheres in how information is initially represented and processed. We argue that perceptual asymmetries in performance reflect a difference in strength rather than in kind. There are small but important differences in relatively early stages of information processing. As these small but asymmetric differences interact with higher-order systems, the results may appear as if the hemispheres are qualitatively different, but this may be the result of basic and more subtle asymmetries early in information processing.

Much of the initial work in neuropsychology focused on delineating basic dichotomies that could capture the functional differences between the left and right hemispheres. For example, the right brain has been described as holistic and spatial, the left brain as analytic and verbal. These dichotomies continue to resonate in some current reports, although the focus has shifted to the development of detailed cognitive theories that tend to focus on specific phenomena. Advances in sophistication and detail, however, have also entailed a cost in generalizability and integration.

We introduce this book with a brief history of the study of hemispheric specialization and development in other areas that influenced its popularity. First, we review some of the major clinical findings in the neurological literature that provided the most obvious demonstrations of functional asymmetry in humans. We then discuss how behavioral scientists historically have attempted to incorporate these abnormal patterns of behavior into their general understanding of the human mind. This work has been guided by a strong reliance on methods and concepts derived from cognitive psychology, a field in which the ability to parse component processes and elucidate interactive computations of cognition has been fundamental in developments within neuropsychology and neuroscience.

APHASIA: THE ORIGINAL CASE FOR HEMISPHERIC SPECIALIZATION

The thought of losing the ability to speak is a terrifying prospect. Our social world revolves around verbal communication. Language skills are acquired with seemingly minimal effort and in today's technological world we spend little time without hearing or engaging in some form of linguistic interaction. Yet there are neurological disorders that can transport a normal, communicating person into a world of isolation in which the patient is at a loss to understand speech and is unable to generate spoken or written language. These deficits, classified as aphasias, are typically associated with damage to the left cerebral hemisphere.

It was the dramatic effects of left hemisphere damage on language abilities that first awakened the scientific community to the possibility that the brain could appear to be physically symmetric but function asymmetrically. The evidence for left hemisphere contributions to language has been steadily catalogued in the neurological literature for more than a century. Such insights preceded the advent of modern neuroimaging tools such as computerized tomography (CT) and magnetic resonance imaging (MRI) that have made it possible to more precisely localize brain damage. Indeed, behavioral analysis coupled with crude localization techniques proved sufficient for quite some time. It had long been known that head trauma, perhaps the result of blows to the head or penetration from sharp projectiles, could produce sensory and motor problems on the opposite side of the body (contralateral). This effect on sensory-motor function could also provide a correlational basis for problems in other domains. For instance, language deficits accompany right-sided paralysis more than left-sided paralysis.

In retrospect it seems surprising that it took so long for the scientific community to note the high correlation between right-sided motor or sensory deficits and problems in language. A visit to any neurology ward or rehabilitation center will provide easy confirmation. Nonetheless, it was not until the nineteenth century that the study of human disorders began to firmly adopt the requisite tools to objectively investigate these correlations.

Even as members of the neurological community began to share their observations about the relationship between brain and behavior, the idea of brain localization met with resistance. The late eighteenth century had been a heyday for those favoring a localizationist position. Following Franz Gall's description of the numerous faculties of the human mind, the idea that different functions were associated with localized brain regions gained wide acceptance (figure 1.2). These crude ideas floundered, however, in the face of experimental work by researchers such as Pierre Flourens and others. Lesions of so-called centers of function rarely produced their predicted effects. The zietgeist of localization was replaced by a view of brain function as a holistic process. The brain was seen to be equipotential, with each behavior requiring the interactions of the entire structure.

A telling example of the dominance of this view is given by the reaction, or lack thereof, of the scientific community to an 1836 report linking language deficits and the left hemisphere. Springer and Deutsch describe the scene in terms that are hard to improve upon (1981, p. 1).

Marc Dax, an obscure country doctor, read a short paper at a medical society meeting in Montpellier, France. . . . [He] was struck with what appeared to be an association between the loss of speech and the side of the brain where the damage had occurred. In more than 40 patients with aphasia Dax noticed signs of damage to the left half, or hemisphere, of the brain. He was unable to find a single case that involved damage to the right hemisphere alone. In his paper to the medical society, he sum-

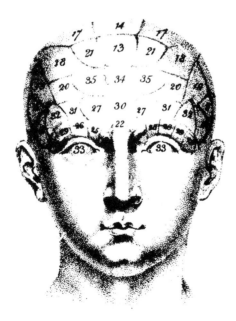

Figure 1.2 An example of phrenology. Each number represents a different proposed brain function. (From Finger, 1994.)

marized these observations and presented his conclusions: each half of the brain controls different functions; speech is controlled by the left half.

The paper was an unqualified flop. It aroused virtually no interest among those who heard it, perhaps because it ran contrary to the dominant view of equipotentiality. Dax died the following year and the paper was soon forgotten.

The possibility of language localization did not resurface for nearly 25 years. At a scientific medical meeting in 1861, Paul Broca, a respected anatomist (as opposed to an obscure country doctor), displayed the brain of a patient who had suffered inarticulate speech following a lesion to his left frontal lobe. Broca reported (1861) that the patient had been able to comprehend what was said to him before his death, but that when he attempted to speak all that could be heard was the nonsensical syllable "tan" repeated over and over. Broca subsequently described a second patient with a milder yet similar speech problem, and from this concluded that articulation deficits in language resulted from damage in the frontal lobe in the area of the third convolution.

It is somewhat ironic that even in this seminal report the emphasis was not on hemispheric specialization. Rather than focus on the left-right dimension, Broca emphasized an anterior-posterior distinction. Initially, he did not appear to be very interested in the significance of his findings for hemispheric differences. In the spirit of the debate of the time, Broca argued that his findings provided strong evidence for localization, and in his early description he placed less importance on the left-sided position of the lesions than on their effects on a specific function.

The significance of Broca's findings for hemispheric specialization began to grow as more reports accumulated ascribing to the left hemisphere a dominant role in language (see De Renzi, 1982). Within a few years, the German neurologist Karl Wernicke (1874) provided another case report enlarging the spectrum of language deficits that could be linked to left hemisphere damage. Whereas Broca had addressed the inarticulate speech that was associated with lesions of the anterior hemisphere (and, as it turned out, on the left), Wernicke described a different language disorder associated with lesions to the posterior regions of the left hemisphere. These lesions created problems in language comprehension. The patients either failed to understand what was said to them or responded in a manner indicating that they had not accurately perceived what was said. Surprising at the time was the fact that the spontaneous speech for patients with Wernicke's aphasia was fluent and articulate. It also tended to be devoid of meaning or semantic consistency, however. These findings led Wernicke to propose a taxonomy of aphasic disorders that were linked to lesions of different parts of the left hemisphere (figure 1.3).

These neuropsychological reports triggered a general excitement concerning the role of the left hemisphere in language, and in particular concerning a division of function within the left hemisphere for different

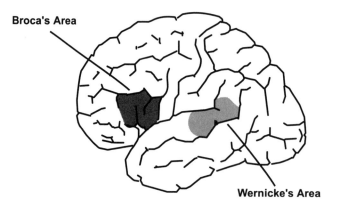

Broca's Area

Wernicke's Area

Figure 1.3 Classical Wernicke's and Broca's areas of the left hemisphere.

linguistic processes (for additional historical details, see Harrington, 1995; Springer & Deutsch, 1981). By the end of the nineteenth century the left hemisphere began to be frequently described as the "dominant" or "major" hemisphere, a designation still prevalent in some scientific journals today. These designations are increasingly challenged by the explosion of data from contemporary cognitive neuroscience investigations.

Early accounts treated the right hemisphere like a poor stepsister to the left. The right hemisphere was called the "minor" hemisphere, and there was a general lack of interest in its functions. Researchers who may have wanted their work to meet a better fate than Dax's focused on the left hemisphere and its capabilities. Indeed, hemispheric specialization in these early days was almost exclusively domain driven.

Of course, there were exceptions to this pattern. Hughlings Jackson in 1876 and Jules Badal in 1888 described disorders of spatial representation in patients with right hemisphere lesions. The patients retained their visual capabilities, but they had difficulty navigating in well-known environments. In 1909 Russo Balint described a patient who appeared to see only a single object at a time and who had great difficulty reaching for the object he did see or tracking its position if it moved. In a classic study of head injury patients from World War I, Holmes (1918; Holmes & Horrax, 1919) observed a similar syndrome in a number of patients and named the behavioral constellation "Balint's syndrome."

This syndrome did not bear directly on the issue of hemispheric specialization because the patients almost invariably had bilateral lesions. As other disturbances of spatial representation were reported during this period, however, it became clear that visual-spatial deficits could occur without any accompanying disturbance of language and that they were more often associated with right hemisphere damage. This dissociation provided the foundation for what would become the dominant theme for many decades: that language and spatial processing represented two fundamental cognitive capabilities. Language was associated with the left hemisphere, and visual-spatial representation with the right hemisphere.

UNILATERAL NEGLECT: THE CASE FOR HEMISPHERIC DIFFERENCES IN SPATIAL COGNITION

How might a visual-spatial problem be experienced? Suppose you were to awaken one morning and the left half of the world had disappeared from your awareness. Of course you would not notice because, by definition, you would not be aware that part of the world had disappeared. At first, you might think that things looked normal. You might notice a bird sitting on a branch on the right side of the tree outside your window. You may try to get up but fail, yet you may not care. One of your family members may be the first to notice that the situation is very serious. If this person approaches you from the left, you may not notice. Quite likely you lapse back into unconsciousness. When you wake up sometime later in the emergency room of your local hospital, you may feel that there has been some mistake and fail to appreciate the concerns of the people around you. In other words, not only are you failing to orient to anything on your left side, because you are unaware of its existence, but you may even deny that you are in trouble at all. Such denial is a symptom known as anosognosia that sometimes accompanies the symptoms of unilateral neglect just described.

Scenarios such as this one can occur even following a relatively small stroke in the right hemisphere, if the stroke is located in a strategic place. Surprisingly, not all stroke patients are aware that they have experienced a serious cardiovascular accident. The patients may ignore a paralyzed limb, or if the limp state of their arm is pointed out by an observer, the patient may attribute it to an old war wound or prior surgery. The disappearance of a part of contralesional space from conscious awareness, known as unilateral neglect, is sometimes although not always accompanied by anosognosia. Unilateral neglect is more likely during the first few days after an insult such as a stroke. These symptoms are most often found following right hemisphere damage.

Patients with unilateral neglect either do not respond to objects located in the contralateral side of space or do so only after long pauses or coaxing. When approached from the neglected side, they may not orient appropriately. In severe cases, the patients may ignore their own body, pushing away a contralateral hand or leg as if it were an intruder. These problems can be separated from those associated with a simple sensory deficit. For example, patients with neglect typically detect a bright light flashed in an otherwise dark field regardless of whether the stimulus is shown in a location ipsilateral to the lesion (e.g., on the right side in right hemisphere stroke patients) or contralateral to the lesion (e.g., on the left side in a right hemisphere stroke) (figure 1.4). They may be able to detect the presence or absence of a simple feature such as motion or color on their neglected side. However, they may report that these features are located on the ipsilesional, or good, side rather than on the neglected side. Furthermore, individuals with blindness on the side contralateral to their

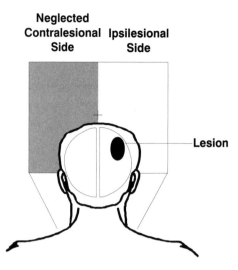

**Neglected
Contralesional Ipsilesional
Side   Side**

Lesion

Figure 1.4 A patient with right hemisphere damage may neglect items in the contralesional side of space (represented by the shadowed area).

lesions who do not suffer neglect will compensate by turning into the direction of their scotoma. Individuals with neglect will not.

As one can imagine, it is nearly impossible to function in everyday situations following the onset of unilateral neglect. Most patients cannot move around a room because they consistently bump into things. Often their eyes and head deviate toward the ipsilesional side. In the acute phase, the patients are confused and lethargic. As days go by, patients with neglect typically become less confused and fatigued, and those who in the acute phase had twisted their body and eyes to one side usually show less and less of these behaviors. Yet they continue to ignore the neglected side, although they often orient to it if told to do so. When attempting to perform simple everyday acts such as dressing or eating they may fail to place their left arm in a shirt sleeve, may comb only one side of their hair, and may restrict their eating to food on the unneglected side of their plate. As noted above, they can be completely undisturbed by the disappearance from their consciousness of one side of a scene. It is as if the world had never appeared any different.

A female patient was seen by one of us in the acute stage of her illness. She was seen at her hospital bed about 5 days after she suffered a right hemisphere stroke. She was alert and friendly. She told us that a visitor had dropped by and put a box of candy in the drawer of her bed stand. The bed stand was located on her left, and she remarked that she couldn't find it. When she was told to look to her left, she followed instructions readily and spotted the table and its drawer. After opening the drawer, she took a piece of candy from the box, politely offering some to us as well. She then turned back toward her right side and shortly thereafter wanted another piece of candy. Again, she couldn't find the bed stand. After a long time spent searching the room (on her right), she said that someone must have stolen the candy. She had not forgotten about the candy or that she had eaten a piece from the box located in the bed stand, but she seemed unable to imagine that there was a part of the room where it was still located.

This patient had suffered a middle cerebral artery infarct (stroke), producing a large lesion in the right hemisphere similar to that shown in figure 1.5. It is unlikely that a comparable lesion in the left hemisphere would produce the same behavioral deficits. Such a lesion would likely produce an aphasia. While it has been argued that neglect in left hemisphere patients is often overlooked because language problems make it difficult to test these patients, large-scale studies have shown that profound neglect is more frequent and more severe than lesions of the right than left hemisphere (Ogden, 1987).

Constructional Apraxia: The Case for Qualitative Hemispheric Differences in Spatial Cognition

Unilateral neglect can be considered one of the more extreme forms of a unilateral deficit in spatial cognition. If we were to just consider the occurrence of this syndrome in assessing the brain mechanisms involved

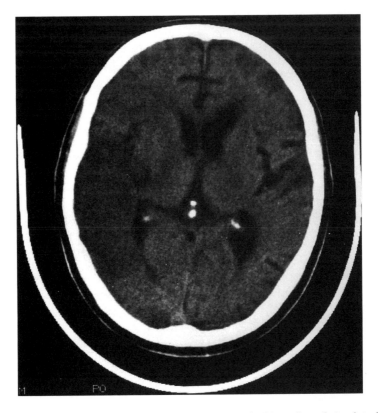

Figure 1.5 CT scan of a patient whose infarct resulted in unilateral visual neglect. Standard coordinates are used in the image—the right hemisphere appears on the left.

in spatial abilities, we would conclude that these processes are related more to the right hemisphere. When we consider more subtle types of spatial deficits, however, it becomes clear that both hemispheres play a role in constructing a representation of spatial information and in moving attention to locations within that space. Indeed, these deficits reveal important insights into the bases of hemispheric specialization.

A standard neuropsychological test that has been used for decades to assess perceptual disturbances is the Rey-Osterrieth test. Patients are presented with the figure shown at the top of figure 1.6 and, after studying it, they attempt to copy the complex drawing while it is present in front of them. After they complete this drawing, the figure is taken away and the patient is asked to make a second production, this time from memory. Representative drawings from two patients are shown at the bottom of figure 1.6. The patient with left hemisphere damage accurately drew the overall shape, but failed to fill in the finer details. In contrast, the patient with right hemisphere damage failed to reproduce the overall pattern, yet was able to draw the individual parts. Thus, both patients demonstrated problems in reproducing accurate spatial relations, but of different sorts.

Historically, this dissociation has been discussed in terms of the representation of parts and wholes for motor planning. Within this framework, the left hemisphere patient was said to have difficulty in reproducing the parts; the right hemisphere patient had difficulty in reproducing the whole because the proper motor plans could not be carried out.

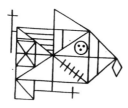

Left Hemisphere
Damage

Right Hemisphere
Damage

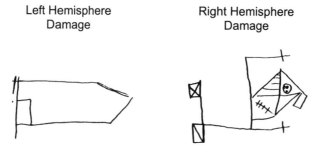

Figure 1.6 The standard Rey-Osterrieth figure used in neuropsychological examinations (top). The patient with left hemisphere damage drew the overall form with little detail (lower left). The patient with right hemisphere damage drew many local details but organized them incorrectly (lower right). (Adapted from Robertson & Lamb, 1991.)

Yet findings such as these suggested that both hemispheres might contribute to processing spatial information. On the basis of the Rey-Osterrieth test only, it is not clear whether the problems exhibited in patients' drawings should be considered perceptual or motoric. Early work in this area indicated a motor problem. The patients were described as having constructional apraxia, a label that emphasized that the drawing problem stemmed from distorted motor representations. According to this theory patients with left hemisphere damage had trouble generating the motor programs required to fill in details, whereas those with right hemisphere damage had trouble generating large-scale motor plans. This view downplayed possible perceptual contributions, but this may have been because techniques to properly address the question had not yet been developed.

The original studies of constructional apraxia for parts and wholes were reported by McFie and his colleagues (McFie, Piercy, & Zangwill, 1950; McFie & Zangwill, 1960). Others soon supported their findings that this constructional apraxia for wholes was linked more to right than to left hemisphere damage (Black & Strub, 1976; Costa & Vaughan, 1962; Gainotti & Tiacci, 1972; Piercy, Hacean, & Ajuriaguerra, 1960; Piercy & Smyth, 1962). It remained for future research to demonstrate that visual input contributed to these effects.

Balint's Syndrome: Further Evidence for Bilateral Representation of Spatial Cognition

One of the most debilitating visual-spatial problems occurs when both parietal lobes are damaged, resulting in Balint's syndrome or what has been called dorsal simultanagnosia in cognitive neuropsychology (Farah, 1990). These patients report seeing only one object or one part of an object at a time. Again, it is hard to imagine what this would be like.

We take it for granted when we awaken each morning that we will see several objects in the room. There is the hateful alarm clock with bright numbers on its digital screen. The dog yawns and stretches where she lies at the foot of the bed. There are bedposts and windows behind her, and a robin outside sings. The leaves on the trees sway in the wind.

Suppose that you awaken one morning and all you can see is the bird outside your bedroom window. You cannot stop gazing at that one bird. Your attention appears to be captured by the object. Your dog is within fixation, but you do not see her nor do you know where she is. You do not see the window or the bedpost, and you have difficulty moving your attention from the bird. You may know there must be other objects in the room, but you have no idea where they are. You are not even sure where the bird you see is located. You have lost the spatial layout of your bedroom entirely, and you do not know where to reach for the alarm clock, nor can you move from your bed to the door. You are not paralyzed. You just do not know where things are, and perhaps because you do not know where they are, you cannot move your attention to them and away from the bird you now see. In time, the bird may vanish as the object of your attention to be replaced by the perception of your dog. One thing abruptly and rather randomly is replaced by another without your control, and this is how it would be all day and perhaps for the rest of your life.

Obviously, this would be a terrifying experience. You would be a prisoner in the space of your own body except for one bizarre link to a single object. You would not be blind, although your problems might be mistaken for blindness. Blindness does not cause people to lose a sense of space or attentional control. Blind people know where to reach for the alarm clock. They can attend to spatial locations. They know where things are even though they cannot see them.

A person with these symptoms would be classified as having Balint's syndrome. Fortunately, the symptoms are rare in this pure form, although they can be observed in conjunction with degenerative diseases such as Alzheimer's dementia. Pure cases began to be reported in the literature in the late nineteenth century. Although only a few cases have been thoroughly studied there is a common thread among their problems that has been discussed as a deficit in spatial awareness (see Friedman-Hill, Robertson, & Treisman, 1995; Robertson, Treisman, Friedman-Hill, & Grabowecky, 1997).

These patients generally exhibit fixation of gaze with no primary motor deficit (oculomotor apraxia). They do not track moving objects well, losing sight of the target as it moves away from fixation. It is as if the patients do not know how to move their eyes to see objects that they want to see. Their spatial deficits can result in a complete inability to correctly report the location of objects or to even crudely locate an object near the upper or lower boundary of a large computer screen. They may have difficulty saying whether an object is moved away or toward them and they exhibit no startle response when a hand moves rapidly toward their face and stops only inches from their eyes. They cannot reach accurately for the one object that they can see and are often at chance when reporting its location (although locations on their own bodies are correctly reported, demonstrating a lack of primary spatial confusion). Not surprisingly, these patients have great difficulty in activities of every-day life and require constant care.

Given the infrequent occurrence of relatively pure cases of bilateral parietal damage resulting in Balint's syndrome, only a few cases have been reported (Balint, 1909; Baylis, Driver, Baylis, & Rafal, 1994; Coslett & Saffran, 1991; Michel & Henaff, 1996; Friedman-Hill et al., 1995; Robertson et al., 1997; Holmes, 1918; Holmes & Horrax, 1919; Humphreys & Riddoch, 1993; Tyler, 1968; also, see reviews by De Renzi, 1996 & Rafal, 1996). To our knowledge, all of these cases have had bilateral damage in occipital-parietal cortex. These deficits may therefore seem irrelevant in a book about functional differences between the hemispheres. It is somewhat surprising, however, that no one emphasized the increased severity of the spatial and attentional deficits in these patients compared to patients with unilateral right hemisphere damage and neglect. If spatial abilities were lateralized to the right hemisphere, then additional damage to the left hemisphere should not increase the visual-spatial problems to the extent that they do when bilateral damage occurs. It is clear, however, that it does.

The representation of space must be a combined effort by the two hemispheres. The computations that contribute to this representation appear to be divided in such a way that right hemisphere damage produces more severe overt visual-spatial problems than does left hemisphere damage. Damage to both parietal regions, however, produces profound loss in visual and spatial abilities accompanied by a loss in spatial awareness.

Data collected with these types of patients play a large role in theoretical development today and will be discussed in detail in subsequent chapters of this book. Our emphasis will be on perception and encoding in areas of the cortex that are assumed to be involved in relatively early stages of analysis. This is not to say that motor planning and performance are not lateralized as well, but theories based on later stages of lateralization should first rule out explanations that can be accounted for by perceptual differences.

Spatial Deficits: Summary

Studies of deficits in spatial cognition have added at least three important aspects to the study of hemispheric specialization. First, such studies pointed to the folly of describing functional hemispheric asymmetries in terms of a "major" and "minor" hemisphere, a nomenclature that suggests the right hemisphere either plays a back-up role to the left hemisphere or is somehow subservient to it. On certain types of tasks, lesions of the right hemisphere are more devastating than lesions of the left hemisphere. Not only are disorders of spatial attention more likely to be observed following right hemisphere lesions, but the long-term problems experienced by these patients in everyday life can be considerably greater than those experienced by patients with left hemisphere lesions.

Second, the detailed study of disorders of spatial cognition emphasized the need for a more sophisticated approach to the study of spatial processing and its link to neural systems. The same criticism that was leveled at Gall and the adherents of phrenology could also be applied to the early work of the neuropsychological diagram makers. Complex cognitive domains such as language and spatial cognition could not be linked simply to brain locations. Rather, these processes involve numerous component operations distributed over a number of different areas. Spatial deficits may occur because of a problem in analyzing the parts of an object or scene or in integrating these parts into a coherent whole or for a myriad of other reasons. Spatial problems may also arise because of an inability to orient to a region of space or an inability to maintain an internal representation of part of the external world (see Rafal & Robertson, 1995). As in the study of language, the early taxonomies were crude, providing only the roughest partitions. More detailed analyses were required to reveal that a complex task such as spatial reasoning requires both the contribution of a large number of component processes associated with many different brain areas and a great deal of computational power.

A third, related conclusion is that it is too simplistic to assume that hemispheric specialization occurs at the level of tasks such as language or spatial cognition. As described throughout this chapter, spatial deficits can arise from lesions of either the right or left hemisphere. As will be discussed in chapter 6, the same holds for language. The right hemisphere has also been linked to certain paralinguistic and linguistic processes. Thus, if we take language and spatial cognition as two representative cases, both hemispheres provide contributions to each task domain. By making this claim (by no means a new one), we do not wish to suggest that each hemisphere contributes equally to all tasks or that they process information identically. But we should not expect that a theory of hemispheric specialization can be articulated in terms of task-defined goals such as speech decoding or the construction of representational space. We will need to consider the computations required to achieve the task-defined goals.

THE HISTORICAL IMPACT OF SPLIT-BRAIN RESEARCH

One of the most important historical events for the investigation of hemispheric specialization in neuropsychology occurred as a by-product of the search for new medical procedures to treat intractable epilepsy. One of the more radical interventions involved a procedure in which surgeons isolated the two halves of the brain from one another by severing the corpus callosum, the massive bundle of fibers that connects the left and right cerebral hemispheres. This procedure renders what is often called the "split brain."

Epilepsy is a common neurological disorder that affects a large segment of the population. The defining feature of epilepsy is recurrent electrographic seizure—the high-frequency bursting of millions of neurons in close synchrony. The causes of these seizures are many. In some cases seizures are preceded by a traumatic event such as a stroke, car accident, or high fever. In others, the seizure activity is idiopathic and occurs in the absence of any detectable anatomical abnormality. Seizures may originate consistently from a given brain region such as the temporal lobes or limbic structures, or they may have a widespread origin. In all cases the seizure activity tends to spread quickly, disrupting consciousness as the brain is sent into a wild oscillation of overactivity.

Many treatments have been developed for controlling epilepsy. The most common are drug treatments that use medication to inhibit excessive neural activity. In a small percentage of cases, however, these medications are insufficient. Patients may have several seizures per day, resulting in severe disruption of function. It is for the treatment of these patients that invasive surgical interventions have been developed. The strategy typically takes one of two forms. In one case the goal is to resect the neural tissue that is the source of seizure activity. In the other case the goal is to eliminate the means by which the seizure activity is propagated over the brain. It is in these latter instances that the split-brain operation, or commissurotomy, is employed. The procedure is often effective. Seizure activity can be greatly retarded, and many patients show relatively mild behavioral changes following recovery from the procedure. This does not mean that there are no persistent neurological deficits. In most cases candidates for this operation are severely impaired prior to the operation.

The fact that postsurgical behavior may appear only slightly abnormal in patients who undergo this operation is puzzling, given that the split-brain procedure essentially disables the transfer of information across the two cerebral hemispheres. It seems unfathomable that the 200 million fibers of the corpus callosum serve such a small functional purpose. Indeed, a closer examination of these patients has provided strong evidence for hemispheric specialization and has yielded important insights into how the two hemispheres may integrate information in normal processing.

Much of the early work was conducted by a research team composed of Joseph Bogen, Roger Sperry, and Michael Gazzaniga. These researchers performed extensive cognitive testing of a group of approximately 25 patients. Their studies have now become classics in the field (Bogen & Gazzaniga, 1965; Gazzaniga, 1970; Gazzaniga, Bogen, & Sperry, 1962, 1965; Sperry, 1968).

The fibers of the corpus callosum have widespread projections. Most common are those projections linking together homologous areas in the right and left cerebral hemispheres. These connections are reciprocal. In general, an area not only is innervated by a comparable area in the opposite hemisphere, but sends fibers back to that same region. When the callosum is split these transcortical connections are lost. The two sides of the brain are disconnected from one another. If the surgical procedure also includes the anterior and posterior commissures as well as the massa intermedia, several subcortical structures are also segregated from their homologous partners.

The cortex of the two hemispheres is anatomically independent after commissurotomy. In normal subjects we can lateralize the presentation of

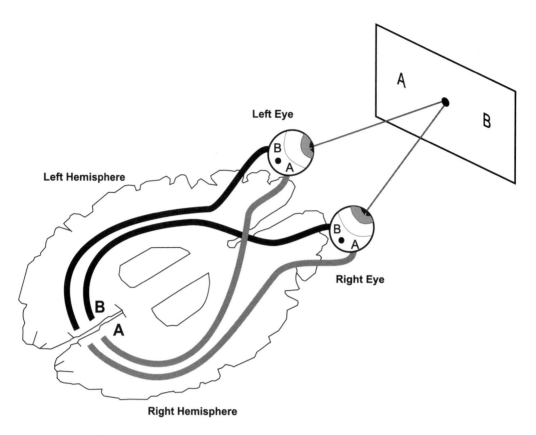

Figure 1.7 Drawing of visual system organization that results in stimuli presented in the left visual field (A) being projected to the right visual cortex and stimuli presented in the right visual field (B) being projected to the left visual cortex. Eyes are fixated on the central dot.

a stimulus to project the input to one hemisphere. For example, if a visual stimulus is flashed on the left side of space from foveal fixation, input will be into the right visual cortex. From the anatomical projections from the eye to the brain we know that the stimulus will first arrive in the right hemisphere, the side contralateral to the stimulus (figure 1.7). But it would be naive to assume that this information is processed solely in that hemisphere. Transcortical transfer occurs very rapidly. For example, responding with the right hand (controlled primarily by the left hemisphere) to a stimulus in the left visual field is slower by a few milliseconds than responding with the left hand to the same stimulus.

Thus, with healthy people there is no way of knowing whether a response to a lateralized stimulus is driven by processing within the contralateral hemisphere or whether the response reflects the joint effects of both hemispheres after transcallosal interaction. In the split-brain patient the possibility for interhemispheric transfer through the corpus callosum is eliminated. Stimuli presented in the right visual field are projected to the left hemisphere and have no cortical-cortical connection over which to engage the right hemisphere (although subcortical pathways exist).

Disconnection of function can be seen in the patient's motor behavior, especially right after the operation. During recovery the two hemispheres often act to achieve different and conflicting goals (Springer & Deutsch, 1981). One side may want to wear a red dress, the other side, a blue dress. The right hand may pull the red dress off a hanger, only to have the left hand hang it back up.

Such dramatic examples are rare in the behavior of these patients after a certain recovery period. The patients develop strategies to make their lives as normal as possible. It would be unusual for information to remain isolated in one hemisphere or the other without being affected by experience. For instance, most people quickly move their eyes around the visual field. For commissurotomy patients, this would allow the stimulus to be projected to both hemispheres (also, the central region of space appears to have a bilateral representation). The patients also develop specialized strategies to cope with their predicament, such as reaching for objects with both hands to ensure that somatosensory information is projected bilaterally (see Gazzaniga and Hillyard, 1971).

Given the presence of these strategies, it has required carefully controlled experiments to explore the segregated processing of the cerebral hemispheres in the split-brain population (Zaidel, 1975). The study of these patients provided powerful converging evidence to the patient studies for the dominant role of the left hemisphere in language. In one early study (Gazzaniga, 1970), the patients' ability to read lateralized words was tested. The subjects were required to fixate a central fixation point, and a stimulus was flashed in either the left or right visual field. Words that were flashed in the right visual field were nearly always reported correctly. In contrast, when words were presented in the left visual field and projected directly to the right hemisphere the patients were rarely able to report the stimulus.

The problem for the right hemisphere does not appear to be related to a general lack of knowledge. Rather it seems to be one of accessing and/or producing verbal labels. To observe this it was necessary to use nonverbal stimuli such as pictures of common objects. Split-brain patients were able to name the objects only when the stimulus was presented to the left hemisphere. If the task was changed so that the response was also nonlinguistic, however, they performed comparably regardless of whether the stimulus was projected to the left or right visual field. For example, when shown a picture of a ball in the left visual field, they could then select this object when allowed to touch several unseen objects with their left hand (Gazzaniga, 1970). Further evidence of the separation of processing came from the fact that they failed on matching tasks if the input and output channels depended on different hemispheres. Objects seen in the left visual field could not be matched with objects felt with the right hand.

A conclusion that emerged from these early studies was that the two hemispheres were of roughly comparable competence in their perceptual capabilities. Perceptual processes were segregated in the split-brain patients but there was no specialization of perceptual function. Either hemisphere could perform the requisite operations so long as the tasks did not require the linguistic functions of the left hemisphere.

It was not clear how this apparent equipotentiality could be reconciled with the data from the study of patients with spatial disorders like unilateral neglect. One argument was that the split-brain patient was abnormal, not only because of the commissurotomy, but also because these patients had suffered countless seizures over an extended period of time. Given their histories, it would be imprudent to expect similar patterns of hemispheric specialization in split-brain patients, as were seen in other types of patients, such as those with stroke. It might also be concluded that compensatory strategies used to deal with impairments were different for patients who underwent commissurotomy and for patients who suffered cortical lesions of either the right or left hemispheres.

Although these caveats are important, subsequent investigations demonstrated striking similarities between the drawings of patients with right hemisphere damage and drawings directed by the left hemisphere of split-brain patients (Gazzaniga et al., 1965). For the commissurotomy patients right-handed drawings (controlled by the left hemisphere) necessarily reflect processes limited to the left hemisphere because no callosal transfer was possible. For the patients with unilateral right hemisphere damage the drawings are assumed to be dominated by the intact left hemisphere. In both cases, the drawings were disorganized and often unrecognizable, despite the fact that many relatively obscure details were included.

Paralleling the findings for patients with unilateral left hemisphere strokes (intact right hemisphere), the results for the split-brain patients showed that they were able to produce properly organized and recognizable drawings with their left hands (right hemispheres). These results were obtained even when the patients were right-handed. Right-handed drawings did include more details than left-handed drawings, but the overall structure was still disorganized. The right-handed split-brain patients were also much more proficient in reproducing complex geometric designs when using their nondominant, left hands (figure 1.8).

It was not clear how these qualitative differences were to be interpreted in these early findings. If the percept was intact in each hemisphere, one might conclude that the drawings reflected differences in response selection. In motor production hand differences have been described in terms of the spatial scale at which movements occur (Guiard, 1987; Previc, 1991). For right-handers the dominant hand is usually required to make

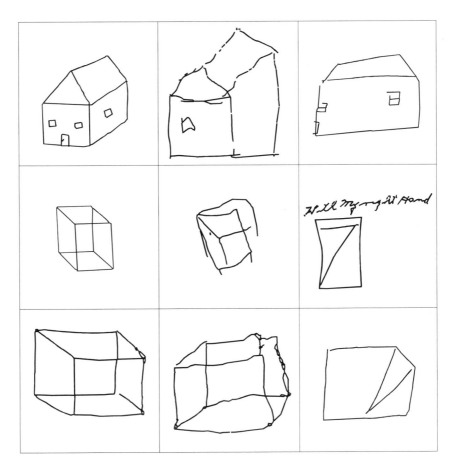

Figure 1.8 Standard (left-most column) and drawings by a commissurotomy patient. The drawings in the middle column were made with his left hand (controlled by his right hemisphere), and those in the right column were made with his right hand (controlled by his left hemisphere). Although the patient was right-handed, drawings with his left hand more closely captured the overall configuration. (From Gazzaniga, 1967.)

fine movements that require precise detail. The left hand is used for maintaining stability. The left hand holds a bowl while the right hand stirs the spoon. The left hand holds the matchbook steady while the right hand is used to strike the match. Perhaps these asymmetries in motor performance produced similar biases in drawings, an argument reminiscent of those made for constructional apraxia.

Over the last two decades, however, a great deal of evidence has begun to accumulate suggesting that similar differences can be found on perceptual tasks, although ascertaining these differences required more sensitive measures. The earlier evidence suggesting perceptual equipotentiality likely resulted from the use of crude measures such as overall error rates or patient drawings. Reaction-time measures indicate that this equivalence is illusory. For example, a recent study (Robertson, Lamb, &

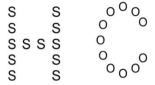

Figure 1.9 Examples of hierarchical letter patterns: a global *H* created from local *S*s and a global *C* created from local *O*s. (Adapted from Navon, 1977.)

Zaidel, 1993) with split-brain patients employed hierarchical letter stimuli (figure 1.9). Because all stimuli were shown in peripheral vision, where acuity is decreased, global targets were responded to more rapidly than local targets. The stimuli were also presented briefly in the right or left visual field. For the split-brain patients the normal reaction-time advantage for global targets was enhanced relative to that of control subjects when the stimuli were presented in the left visual field and reduced when the stimuli were presented in the right visual field.

As had been found in earlier studies, both hemispheres were capable of making discriminations whether the targets were global or local. The differences were only in terms of milliseconds in reaction-time measures. Although the two hemispheres are similar in their overall perceptual functions when using gross measures, there are subtle differences in how they process features of the stimulus.

THE IMPACT OF COGNITIVE PSYCHOLOGY

Developments in cognitive psychology question the assumption of a simple correspondence between complex tasks and brain areas. Cognitive psychologists have sought to develop detailed theories of how we process information in order to accomplish particular tasks. As the theories mature they become more complex. For example, what had been lumped into a single box labeled "reading" became elaborated into a theory that includes letter identification, whole word recognition, and semantic activation (Coltheart, 1985). As time progresses these component operations can be expected to be further fractionalized.

Similar trends can be found in the literature on object recognition. For example, a recent computer model elaborates seven essential stages that are required for recognizing an object (Hummel & Biederman, 1992). The initial processing stages are devoted to decomposing the image into component parts, the latter stages to linking the parts into a coherent whole. Although this decomposition and then reconstitution may seem inefficient it offers a number of computational advantages. For example, by enumerating the parts and their relations recognition can occur even when the object is viewed from novel or unusual positions.

The part/whole distinction, which shows reliable hemispheric differences, has a long history in the study of cognition and perception. A central question has focused on the dynamics of perception: Does perception begin by processing individual parts and then put the parts together to form wholes, or does it begin with an analysis of the whole followed by subsequent parsing into parts? Introspection would seem to favor the latter interpretation. We do not have a sense that we recognize a telephone by carefully examining the stimulus to determine whether there is a receiver, a number pad, and a cord. But this introspection contradicts reason. How could we derive a global representation that was not created out of an assemblage of component parts?

Indeed, when we build an object in the physical world, construction of the whole requires that we produce all of the parts and then put them together. We build a wall by placing a series of boards in a row, one after the other. If the arrangement of the parts is altered, the wall too is altered. If building a house can serve as a metaphor for building a perceptual representation of an object, then we might expect processing to occur in a piecewise, cumulative manner (e.g., from lines and edges to shapes). The associative view of cognition motivated by behaviorism and prevailing during the middle of this century would be an example of an approach that would embrace this view.

Max Wertheimer, the patriarch of the Gestalt school of psychology, was one of the first to disagree with the behavioristic approach. He presented several demonstrations showing that the percept of the whole could not always be predicated on the basis of its perceptual parts (Wertheimer, 1938). The sum of the parts was different from the whole. A melodic sequence of notes will be perceived as the same melody whether played in the vicinity of middle C or in a higher or lower key. The tune can quickly be recognized even though each of the parts has been substantially altered. It is the *relationship* between the parts that is important and not their exact identity. In vision, the percept of a diamond standing on its tip can be changed to the percept of a square when the shape is surrounded by a rectangle (Koffka, 1935) (figure 1.10). The part has not changed in the figure, but its percept is changed by the addition of a more global figure. The identity of one part is affected by the orientation of the other. Again, the key factor is the relationship between the parts.

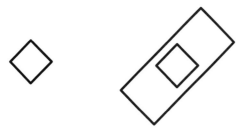

Figure 1.10 The diamond (left) is perceived as a square (right) when the tilted global rectangle defines a tilted "object-centered" orientation. (Adapted from Koffka, 1935.)

The influence of the gestaltists was widespread during the early part of this century, and they continue to have an influence on current cognitive theory (see Robertson, 1986). In the 1930s neurologists like Kurt Goldstein were quick to incorporate Gestalt ideas, including those of perceptual function, into clinical assessments (Goldstein, 1995). Gestalt thinking also played a major role in loosening the hold of behaviorism on experimental psychology. Behaviorism sought to account for complex behavior as the end result of the successive chaining of individual stimulus-response pairs independently formed by appropriate reinforcement. The Gestalt approach offered an alternative. In contrast to the behaviorists' devotion to the parts, early cognitive theorists like Edward Tolman and David Krech redirected psychological investigation to the molar aspects of behavior—the overall goals that constrain an animal's learning processes. When learning a maze, rats first demonstrate knowledge of the general layout of the maze and only later exhibit learning of individual turns and alleys (Krechevsky, 1938). Later studies with humans (Krech & Calvin, 1953) revealed similar effects with perceptual learning tasks. When people were given a series of visual problems and then were tested on what they had learned, they learned the wholes faster than the parts.

With the advent of cognitive psychology in the late 1960s, the focus of study changed. Psychologists felt less compelled to restrict their theories to observable behaviors. Instead, they sought methods to develop theories that emphasized the internal representation and transformation of information that supports observable patterns of behavior. For visual perception the questions about parts and wholes again became central. What defines a set of sensations as a whole versus a part? Do wholes or parts or both direct further processing of the scene? What sorts of interactions occur between these different levels of representation? How does attention affect the perception of wholes and parts?

Investigations into these questions were aided by the development of methodologies and paradigms that allowed fine-grained analysis of the operation of mental behavior. Of key importance was the refinement of chronometric methods (Posner, 1978), or the use of temporal measures and manipulations. Psychologists had long been interested in the speed with which people responded to stimuli, but researchers such as Michael Posner and Saul Sternberg were instrumental in showing how theoretical issues could be addressed by comparing response times in well-controlled experiments.

Implicit in their work was the recognition that neural processing takes time. The human brain cannot keep pace with the speed of a modern computer, at least not in terms of the time it takes to transmit information from one unit (neuron or bit) to another. It takes time for sensory transducers to send their signals through the central nervous system, and each synapse within the brain adds additional processing time before a response can be made. When a given percept results from the interactions between millions and millions of neurons, each firing hundreds of times, measurable differences can be observed as the experimenter manipulates the type of information that is available or the task the subject is required to perform.

Chronometric methods allow us to test theories of how perceptual recognition arises. They serve as a useful tool in identifying functional components of a cognitive task and their interactions in a distributed system. In the area of part/whole perception, a classic example is a study conducted by Navon (1977). This study is especially important because it has had a large impact in neuropsychology. Navon presented his subjects with patterns with a large global form made from several smaller local forms (see figure 1.9). Because the patterns contained information at different levels or at different spatial scales these patterns are referred to as hierarchical stimuli.

Navon used larger letters and forms created from the repetition of smaller letters and forms. Subjects were asked to press a key to identify the larger global form in one block of trials and the smaller local forms in another block of trials. Some experiments measured reaction time to perform this task and others measured the display time needed for a person to accurately perform the task. To avoid large acuity differences between foveal and peripheral vision the stimuli were presented in either the right or left visual field for just a few milliseconds before the subject responded. Navon measured the speed at which subjects were able to identify targets at different levels of stimulus structure. He reasoned that representations that were derived with the most speed would be associated with faster response times.

The results showed that subjects were much faster at identifying the global forms than the local forms, and that the global form interfered with the speed at which local forms could be identified but not vice versa. For example, during a response to a local target *H*, a global *S* (also a possible target) slowed reaction time, but during a response to a global target *H*, a local *S* had no effect. On the basis of these two effects Navon proposed a theory of global precedence. Perception begins with a derivation of the representation of the overall form and then proceeds to an analysis of the local elements.

Together, the faster response times and differences in interference were interpreted as revealing several aspects of part/whole perception. Consistent with the arguments of the Gestalt school, the global shape had precedence in perception. Perception of the whole did not require perceptual identification of the parts. Moreover, part perception was affected by the perception of the whole. Global information interfered with the speed of a local response, whereas local information had no effect on the speed of a global response.

Broadbent (1977) was the first to suggest that global precedence was due to attention being pulled to the global form by the lower spatial frequency content (roughly lower spatial resolution) at the global level (see chapter 2 for descriptions of spatial frequencies and how they relate to these types of patterns). Others proposed parallel processing models in which local features (although not necessarily identity) influenced the perception of a global form and vice versa (Palmer, 1980, 1982). Kimchi and Palmer (1982) demonstrated that global precedence was limited to cases in which the local forms were not perceived as texture, in a study reminiscent of those performed by Eric Goldmeier, an investigator from the early Gestalt school of psychology (Goldmeier, 1972).

More recent research with hierarchical figures has led to a softening of Navon's strong claims. As one might expect, global precedence is limited. If the global shape is too large, subjects will become faster at identifying the local elements (Kinchla & Wolfe, 1979). The patterns of interference have also been found to be more complex and subtle than was first suspected. For instance, Lamb & Robertson (1990) found that the speed required to identify a global or local form was not simply a function of stimulus size on the screen, but was also calibrated to sizes of stimuli presented throughout a block of trials. When the stimulus set contained stimuli between 1.5 and 6 degrees visual angle, global precedence was present at 3 degrees. When the set contained stimuli between 3 and 12 degrees visual angle, however, local precedence was present at 3 degrees. Global precedence then appeared at 6 degrees. In a later study, Robertson, Lamb, & Zaidel (1993) found no relationship between interference from the global form and the speed at which local forms could be identified. Still others found that response speed was affected by the ratio and density of global to local size (Martin, 1979a) as well as by where the stimulus was presented on the fovea (Lamb & Robertson, 1989).

In retrospect, these findings were predictable. When looking out over a landscape, we quickly recognize the trees scattered along a hillside. The ability to identify the species, however, may depend on a number of factors. In some cases the global shape may be sufficient: the overall shape of a fir is seldom confused with that of a drooping willow. In other instances, at least for the naive naturalist, species identification may depend on an analysis of individual leaves. There are many factors that will influence this process. Not only must we be standing at a reasonable distance to resolve the leaves' individual shape, but our perception will further depend on leaf density as well as other properties. Nevertheless, under many circumstances perception can begin with the parts. When we are napping at the base of a tree, its global shape is obscured, but identification is still possible as we examine the leaves in view.

Wertheimer was correct, in that the whole could be different than the sum of its parts. Furthermore, he was correct in maintaining that parts could predict the percept of the whole under some but not all situations. It took developments within cognitive psychology, however, to support the priority of the whole over the part in terms of time; temporal priority is reflected in subtle ways such as reaction-time differences of tens of milliseconds. As cognitive science has developed, computational models of part/whole perception have had to account for these effects, focusing on factors such as global and local symmetry (Palmer, 1982), levels of spatial resolution (Watt, 1988), or grouping processes (Enns & Kingstone, 1995). The chronometric method was critical in opening the door to more sophisticated theories of object recognition and in prompting researchers to acknowledge that perception involves a series of representational states that can extract the hierarchical spatial structure of the world.

STUDIES OF LATERALITY IN HEALTHY INDIVIDUALS

The marriage of hemisphere specialization and cognitive psychology began with split-brain research but evolved most rapidly with studies of young, normal college-aged subjects. One of the seminal studies using auditory stimuli was reported by Doreen Kimura (1961). As did the studies of patients with focal brain injuries and the early split-brain research, Kimura's research tested whether the left hemisphere has a distinct advantage over the right in processing linguistic information. Kimura adopted the dichotic-listening task, which had proven useful in the study of selective attention.

This task was developed to mimic processing demands in the natural world, where sensory overload is common. Consider the cocktail party or, more appropriate for today, the wine-tasting party. We may attempt to speak with one individual, but the speaker's voice is intermixed with a multitude of incoming auditory signals: conversations going on about us, music from the compact disc player, the clatter of plates being filled at the buffet table, the children watching a video in the next room. Despite this cacophony of sound, we are quite proficient at focusing on the relevant signal—the words being spoken by our conversational partner.

To explore this ability, dichotic-listening tasks were used. They involve the presentation of two simultaneous messages, one to each ear. In the early studies of attention, subjects had been instructed to attend to one message while ignoring the other. The goal was to assess the fate of the unattended message (Broadbent, 1954; Treisman, 1969). Kimura modified this task by asking subjects to report the information from both ears. Her objective was to determine whether subjects were more likely to report information presented to one ear at the cost of information presented to the other ear.

In the initial studies the stimuli were digits, presented so that one digit was heard in the left ear at the same time as a second digit was heard in the right ear. Kimura found that people were much more likely to report the stimuli presented to the right ear. This effect was dubbed the right ear advantage. It has been interpreted as reflecting an underlying advantage for the contralateral left hemisphere for processing linguistic stimuli.

Without the observations from neurological patient data, this ear bias would probably not have had much impact. It converged, however, with the neurological observations of language deficits produced by left hemisphere damage.

Kimura (1961b) went on to show that patients with left temporal lobe lesions performed worse at the task than did patients with right temporal lobe lesions. In addition, split-brain patients showed a huge right ear advantage in a study using words as stimuli. They succeeded in recognizing words presented to the right ear, but were at chance for words presented to the left ear (Milner, Taylor, & Sperry, 1968; Sparks & Geschwind, 1968).

Subsequent research showed that the right ear advantage could not be attributed to a generic advantage for the left hemisphere (or the right ear). When the stimuli were melodies, the advantage shifted to the left ear (Kimura, 1964; also, see chapter 5). Thus, the side of the ear advantage was dependent on the type of stimulus material being processed.

At the time, these results were surprising since other work had found no ear advantage with monaural stimuli. It was well known that visual information was lateralized. Information from each visual field was projected initially to the contralateral hemisphere. But this segregation of information does not hold as strictly for audition. In addition to the dominant contralateral projection from each ear, there are ipsilateral projections as well (Rosenzweig, 1951). Yet Kimura's work indicated that functional asymmetries could be revealed when the system was taxed. The dichotic procedure put the two hemispheres into competition with each other. This competition allowed the right ear advantage for linguistic stimuli to surface. A corollary of this interpretation is that each hemisphere is primarily driven by stimuli from the contralateral ear.

Some of Kimura's conclusions have been challenged over the years. Ear differences can be obtained with monaural presentation if precise chronometric measures are used (Catlin & Neville, 1976). In addition, it is now believed that, as with vision, auditory information is lateralized, not in terms of ears, but in terms of the side of space from which the signal originates. Thus, each ear may project to both hemispheres, but auditory inputs from one side of space will be projected to the contralateral hemisphere. Thus, a sound coming from a person's left will be projected to the right hemisphere, following the contralateral pathway from the left ear and the ipsilateral pathway from the right ear (Morais & Bertelson, 1975).

Nonetheless, it would be difficult to overestimate the impact of Kimura's work. Her research introduced a methodology that seemed to make it possible to explore laterality effects in people with intact, fully functioning brains. It was hoped that questions of hemispheric specialization no longer required the researcher to have access to neurological populations. Studies could now be conducted on the experimental psychologist's favorite research subject: the undergraduate college student. Armed with the tools of cognitive psychology and with the belief that lateralized stimuli produce asymmetric activation of the two hemispheres, these researchers generated an explosion of articles on hemispheric specialization that has continued unabated to the present time (unfortunately not always to the benefit of the field).

These studies have explored a wide range of tasks involving the modalities of vision, audition, and somatosensation. Two basic approaches have been employed. Most prevalent has been the use of lateralized stimuli. For vision, this involves the brief presentation of stimuli in either the left or right visual field (see figure 1.7). For audition, stimuli are presented either dichotically, as in the early Kimura studies, or monaurally. A smaller literature has emerged that explores differences in somatosensory perception (e.g., Bradshaw, 1986).

Another approach has been to combine tasks in such a way as to tax one hemisphere more than the other. These studies involve the dual-task methodology. Subjects are asked to perform two concurrent tasks to examine patterns of interference between the tasks. For example, suppose we were to accept that language selectively activates the left hemisphere. One could then compare what happens when a language task is combined with a motor task that involves either the right or left hand. The simplest dual-task prediction is that the language task will produce more interference for right-handed performance since both of these tasks would be expected to require left hemisphere processing resources (Kinsbourne & Cook, 1971).

A basic premise underlying this approach is that the degree of interference will be related to the cerebral distance between the component operations required for the two tasks (see Kinsbourne, 1975). Of course, if the two tasks do not use any common resources, no interference should emerge, regardless of the side of hemispheric involvement. Nonetheless, the dual-task paradigm has added another methodology for exploring functional hemispheric asymmetries in normal individuals.

These methods, of course, have their limitations. A critical assumption has been that differences in performance with lateralized stimuli nearly always reflect functional differences between the cerebral hemispheres. This is an extremely strong assumption. Researchers have tended to ignore or downplay the fact that asymmetries in brain function cannot be directly observed with these methods. It requires a leap of faith to assume that there is a straightforward mapping between lateralizing a stimulus and producing disproportionate activation throughout the contralateral hemisphere. Normal subjects have an intact corpus callosum, which provides for the rapid transfer of information from one hemisphere to the other. Many cells in areas outside early visual cortex respond to stimulation on both sides of the fovea (see Gattass, Sousa, & Covey, 1985).

Recently, investigators have developed elaborate methods to determine when collosal relay or one hemisphere's direct access to information can account for visual field differences in normals. For example, Zaidel, Clarke, and Suyenobu (1990) identified the types of data patterns that would be expected if information entering one hemisphere had to be transferred to another hemisphere to be processed (i.e., collosal relay). One would expect a correlation between performance in one visual field and the other as difficulty of the task varied. One would also expect this correlation, however, if attention were directed to one visual field and then to the other. As Zaidel et al. noted, an absence of correlation could be more informative, suggesting qualitative differences in processing that depend on the hemisphere of input. Their approach is one example of the more sophisticated methods being developed to determine when typically subtle performance differences with items presented directly to one hemisphere or another may implicate functional hemispheric differences in normals and when they may not.

Despite these advances, too many investigators continue to rely almost solely on data from normals and simple visual field differences to address the complex issue of hemispheric specialization: A study is run presenting stimuli in the right or left visual field and it is immediately concluded that any differences must be due to hemispheric differences. There are at least two problems with this approach. First, the visual field differences found in studies with normal subjects tend to be rather small, and replication has often been a problem (Efron, 1990). But it is the positive results, the ones that show differences in performance as a function of the visual field of presentation, that are published in the journals. It is difficult to publish null results or failures to replicate. And considering that laterality studies often operate in a relatively binary world (i.e., obtaining a right or left visual field advantage versus none at all), the possibility of finding a significant effect when one does not actually exist is relatively high.

The first problem leads directly to the second. The best development of theory generally occurs when people consider the evidence that appears to disconfirm a theory or belief. Theories need to be falsifiable. We can generate a large number of studies that are in accord with a particular hypothesis, but much stronger evidence is obtained when we can devise experiments that pit two hypotheses against one another. As with much psychological research, laterality studies rarely compare two divergent theories (but, see Zaidel et al, 1990). More often the experiments seek to provide confirmatory evidence for a hypothesis. If the results do not come out as expected, interpretation is difficult, and the results may sit in a file marked "failed experiments." Was there a problem with the method or the theory? If a small change was made, say, in the visual angle of the stimuli would the results come out differently?

Obviously, caution is in order. Theories of hemispheric specialization based on findings from normal subjects receive support when other sources of data converge with those observed in normals and vice versa.

There are problems with any methodology if it is used in isolation. Data from patients may reflect neural reorganization or the development of strategies. One cannot simply assume that the absence of a function means that the patient has normal cognition minus a part. It is always possible that interactions between remaining functions produce new methods of processing information. Furthermore, damage in one area may affect processing in another, and damage in one hemisphere may affect processing in the intact hemisphere. The latter possibility is especially likely given the large number of collosal connections between analogous areas of the right and left hemispheres.

Other methods such as functional imaging pose a different set of problems. The signal-to-noise ratio of neural activity is relatively low for most of the current measures, meaning that the absence of a signal is difficult if not impossible to interpret. In addition, the temporal resolution of such methods is very low. If a stimulus produced symmetry in a positron emission tomography (PET) or functional MRI (fMRI) study, it is difficult to evaluate differences that may exist in milliseconds of time. Some investigators are currently trying to combine imaging measures with timing measures, such as those that occur from scalp evoked potentials, to address many of these problems (Heinze et al., 1994; Mangun & Heinze, 1995).

Given the inadequacy of one method by itself, it seems that the best theories should predict and be predicted by observations in neurological patients with right or left hemisphere damage. They should be consistent with findings in normals and should use other techniques such as event-related potentials and functional imaging. It is better still if they can be supported by split-brain data and visual field differences in the performance of normal subjects. Under such circumstances the pitfalls associated with the assumptions of any one method are less troublesome. The theory proposed in the following pages meets these criteria.

THE NEED FOR CONVERGING EVIDENCE

General interest in functional differences between the two hemispheres of the human brain originated in the nineteenth century with observations of patients with unilateral brain injuries. As the sciences specialized and matured this interest became relatively isolated within the medical community. Neuropsychology was not part of mainstream psychology, due at least in part to the dominance of behaviorism's emphasis on observable events rather than on internal processes. The split-brain studies, coupled with the emergence of cognitive psychology in the 1950s and '60s, provided a tremendous boost to the study of hemispheric specialization.

Indeed, laterality research can be viewed as one of the first examples of the benefits that occurred as the result of the cross-fertilization of the different disciplines in psychology and neurology. Some of the most prominent researchers in this field moved freely between the study of normal and neurologically impaired function. Today hemispheric specialization is studied by researchers with varied backgrounds that include neurology, anatomy, pharmacology, psychiatry, psychology, computer science, and genetics. The study of the relationship between the brain and cognition has become an active interdisciplinary endeavor, an approach that is epitomized by the emergence of a new field, cognitive neuroscience (Gazzaniga, 1995).

In the following chapters we present a theory of hemispheric specialization in perception. The findings motivating this theory entail all of the methodologies described in this chapter as well as results based on new technologies designed to reveal the function of the active, healthy brain. Much of the work with normal subjects, including our own, is not immune to the criticisms raised in the preceding section. We will argue, however, that these concerns are mitigated by our reliance on converging operations and our attempt to integrate the results obtained with healthy individuals with those discovered in the study of people with neurological disorders. Moreover, a central feature of this work is our attempt to integrate laterality results across a range of tasks. In doing so we will offer novel interpretations of certain findings in the literature that have been difficult to explain within traditional theories of hemispheric specialization. In this way we seek convergence both across methodologies and across task domains.

This theory must be viewed within a historical perspective. Early studies of hemispheric specialization focused on identifying tasks that were associated with one hemisphere or the other. The simplest dichotomy was the attribution of language functions to the left hemisphere and spatial abilities to the right hemisphere. But this dichotomy has run into a number of problems. Each hemisphere contributes to performance of a complex task whether the task is linguistic or spatial. This is not to say that the hemispheres' contributions are identical; the two hemispheres extract information from the sensory input in slightly different ways. They cooperate with one another, rather than simply providing a replication of function.

Over time the emphasis has changed from attempting to catalog the roles of the two hemispheres on particular tasks to asking questions about how the different processing abilities of different areas of each hemisphere contribute to asymmetric function. This is not to deny that certain tasks are closely tied to a particular region of one hemisphere or the other. Areas of the left hemisphere clearly play a dominant role in language, and areas of the right hemisphere are more important for moving about in a three-dimensional world. But the focus has shifted to questions about why these differences occur. What is it about the processing of linguistic information that entails left hemisphere function?

The theory proposed here centers on the idea that there is a subtle yet fundamental difference in how the two hemispheres process early perceptual information. It suggests that the principles that convert raw sensory input into recognizable auditory and visual objects may be similar across the two hemispheres but with a different emphasis. After developing this computational hypothesis we can then ask to what extent these differential capabilities contribute to functional hemispheric asymmetries in tasks like language comprehension, spatial cognition, object recognition, and the control of attention. One of our underlying goals is to integrate historically disparate lines of research into a coherent framework.

2 A Theory of Hemispheric Asymmetries in Perception

Information can be represented at different spatial scales. Consider figure 2.1, one of Mandelbrot's computer art pieces from his book *Fractals*. The individual triangles can be seen, but their organization and repetition create structure at multiple levels.

In the real world large objects are not made out of smaller versions of those same objects. Similarly, the constituent parts of a scene are not miniature replicas of the scene. Mandelbrot used a recursive technique to exaggerate the fact that our perception of a scene and its parts is dependent on the relative sizes of the different sources of information. In this manner his work touches upon a central issue that arises when we think about the perception of complex scenes. How do we recognize both the scene and its parts? Is perception analytic, proceeding from an analysis of simple parts to build a synthetic whole? Or do the early stages of perception involve identifying the basic overall shapes with later processing required for the identification of the smaller details? As described in chapter 1, this has been a question of debate throughout the twentieth century. It is quite possible that the solution involves a compromise of these two extreme positions.

REPRESENTATIONAL ASYMMETRIES IN THE CEREBRAL HEMISPHERES

In this book we argue that the two cerebral hemispheres amplify different sources of information when processing visual objects. A compelling demonstration of why this hypothesis is needed is provided by the study of people who have suffered neurological trauma. Figure 2.2 shows the drawings of two patients, each of whom had suffered a stroke that damaged the cerebral cortex. For one of the patients the lesion produced by the stroke was restricted to the right hemisphere; for the other patient the lesion was in the left hemisphere. Each patient was shown the figures in the left column of figure 2.2 and asked to reproduce them.

The productions by the two patients could hardly be more different. The patient with right hemisphere damage has clearly identified the basic

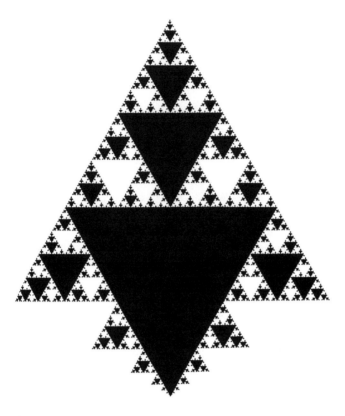

Figure 2.1 A recursive drawing in which each element is a simple triangle. Larger-scale triangles emerge through the configuration of the elements. (From Mandelbrot, 1977.)

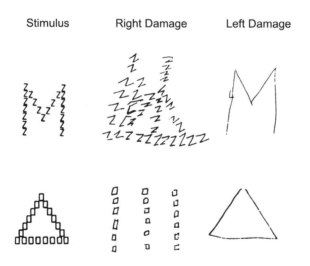

Figure 2.2 Two patients were asked to reproduce the drawings shown on the left. The patient with a right hemisphere lesion drew repetitions of the correct elements, but failed to draw the global configurations. The patient with a left hemisphere lesion drew the correct global shape but either included the incorrect local elements or else missed them entirely. (From Delis et al., 1986.)

elements of the stimuli and appears to understand that these elements must be linked to form the objects. For example, in trying to reproduce the triangle he faithfully draws a series of boxes and even gets as far as organizing these boxes into three collinear segments. This patient fails, however, to organize these segments into the correct global configuration. In striking contrast, the patient with left hemisphere damage is able to reproduce the global outlines of the letter *M* and the triangle. But this patient leaves out the details! Note that this patient can represent the parts of the object: The *M* is made up of four segments and the patient produces each of these. But, with the exception of an erroneous *L* hanging on the left side of the *M*, the drawings fail to show any evidence that this patient has correctly perceived anything other than the global shapes of the letters.

Taken together the two patients show what neuropsychologists have labeled a "double dissociation." The patient with left hemisphere damage reproduces the global shape while either ignoring the local elements or mistaking their identity. The patient with right hemisphere damage reproduces the local elements but is unable to link the local elements together into the appropriate global configuration. The fact that each patient's productions do contain information at the level ignored by the other patient implies that perception at one level is not dependent on perception at the other. It is not necessary to perceive the whole in order to apprehend the parts; similarly, the whole can be seen even when the perceiver fails to apprehend the fine structure of the parts. Double dissociations such as these provide strong evidence of separable processing mechanisms.

The double dissociation evident in the drawings of figure 2.2 are consistent with three important conclusions. First, information is represented at different spatial scales. The boxes of the triangle are at a smaller scale than each of the sides of the triangle and the sides, in turn, are at a smaller scale than the larger shape formed by their configuration. Second, processing leading to one level of shape representation (e.g., the identity of the elements) is not dependent on processing of other levels (e.g., the identity of the overall shape). Third, if we assume that these patients' behavioral deficits represent a breakdown in normal processing we can restate our original hypothesis more precisely. In particular, we hypothesize that the left hemisphere is biased to amplify information contained at smaller spatial scales than is the right hemisphere. The corollary also holds: the right hemisphere is biased to amplify larger scale information than is the left hemisphere.

But how do we define small and large? Are they defined on some sort of absolute scale? Or are small and large defined with respect to one another? Consider figure 2.3 from the Margaret Wise Brown's childhood story, "Two Farmers." On an absolute scale the big farmer, his barn, and even his chickens tower over the world of his minuscule neighbor. But if

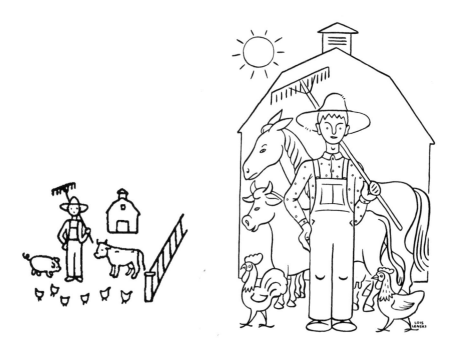

Figure 2.3 Relative size is maintained within the respective worlds of the two farmers. From Brown, 1947.

we restrict our attention to the small farmer, then the objects once again are perceived in terms of their relative sizes. We will argue throughout this book that the difference in how the two hemispheres amplify information is one of relative scale rather than absolute scale. Specifically, the left hemisphere is biased to amplify information at a relatively finer scale than is the right hemisphere. The right hemisphere, in contrast, is biased to amplify information at a larger scale.

FREQUENCY-BASED REPRESENTATIONS

The phrases "small scale" and "large scale" may at first seem clumsy. We could just as well talk about the "small" and "large" objects in a scene. We have chosen to speak of information as existing somewhere on a scale because this terminology nicely maps onto a way to describe a visual scene in a mathematically precise manner. This formalism is based on the analysis of a visual scene in terms of its spatial frequency components. Figure 2.4 depicts a set of gratings in which the brightness varies sinusoidally along the horizontal direction. The cyclic transition from dark to light is least rapid for the grating at the top and becomes more rapid as you move down the page. Given a measure to describe a unit of space, the spatial frequency of each grating can be specified. For example, if we assume the figure spans the page, then the bottom grating has a spatial frequency of 8 cycles/page since the brightest and darkest regions each occur eight times. Similarly, the top grating has a spatial frequency of 2 cycles/page. In vision, the typical unit of space is degrees of visual angle, which provides a way to describe any scene in terms of the image on the retina. Thus, if the lower grating in figure 2.4 is viewed at a distance so the eight cycles span 2 degrees of visual angle, the pattern would be 4 cycles/degree.

Speaking of visual information in terms of spatial frequencies is useful for a number of reasons. We not only have a precise way to describe the information in each grating, but we also have a continuous scale on which to make comparisons between different gratings. Moreover, the ability to describe a visual stimulus in terms of its spatial frequency content is not limited to stimuli such as the pure sinusoids shown in figure 2.4. Consider what happens if we create more complex patterns by superimposing a set of sinusoids of different frequencies or by phase shifting (i.e., horizontally displacing) a set of sinusoids of identical frequency (figure 2.5).

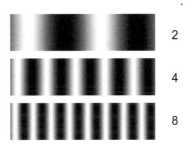

Figure 2.4 Three gratings in which luminance along the horizontal direction is varied according to a sinusoidal function. The rate of variation is manipulated by adjusting the frequency of the sine waves that are used to generate the stimuli.

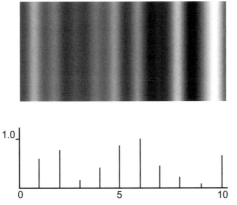

Figure 2.5 The complex image at the top is created by combining a set of sinusoidal functions with a particular phase relationship. The power spectrum of this image is shown at the bottom. Component frequencies are at 2, 3, 5, and 10 Hz.

Although these patterns do not look as regular as the pure sinusoid gratings the spectral content of the stimulus is still known—it contains the component frequencies used in the synthesis. That is, regardless of the phase structure between the components the synthesis process does not introduce novel frequencies.

More importantly, the converse of the synthetic process is also true. Any complex pattern can be described as the sum of a set of sine waves, with each sinusoid at a particular frequency, amplitude, and phase. This extremely powerful concept is referred to as Fourier analysis. Using Fourier analysis we not only can decompose the synthesized waveform of figure 2.5 back into its component parts, but we can do a similar analysis on any visual stimulus, be it a photograph of the Golden Gate Bridge or Mandelbrot's recursive drawing. Indeed, the application of Fourier analysis is not limited to the visual domain. A similar analysis can be performed on complex sounds such as speech. With audition, the signal is analyzed into sound frequency components rather than spatial frequency components.

The appeal of Fourier analysis in the study of perception, however, extends beyond its mathematical properties. It has been proposed that some of our perceptual systems operate as if they perform a Fourier analysis (Campbell & Robson, 1968; De Valois & De Valois, 1990). This idea is most easily grasped in the auditory domain. The primary receptors of sound reside on the basilar membrane of the cochlea, a cavity in the inner ear. By placing electrophysiological recording devices at different places on this membrane, the response properties of the cells can be determined by varying the sound frequency of an auditory stimulus. Experiments such as this have determined that each cell responds to a limited range of frequencies (Kiang, 1965). There is a narrow region of frequencies at which the response of the cell is maximal and there is a bandwidth around this preferred frequency at which responses are elicited, but at submaximal rates. Consequently, auditory receptors operate as band-pass filters. Moreover, the preferred frequencies vary in a systematic manner across the basilar membrane. High-frequency pure tones produce the greatest activity near the base of the membrane; cells near the apex are most highly activated by low-frequency pure tones. Complex sounds will produce activity across the membrane, but the component frequencies are reflected in the distribution of activity across this tonotopic map. It is as if these early receptors are performing a biological Fourier analysis.

Similar ideas have been proposed for visual receptors, although the application is less straightforward for this modality. Two square waves are shown in figure 2.6, straddling two hypothetical visual receptors. Each receptor is modeled to have a center region that is excited by light and inhibited by darkness, as well as a surrounding region that is excited by darkness and inhibited by light. Consider first the activity produced

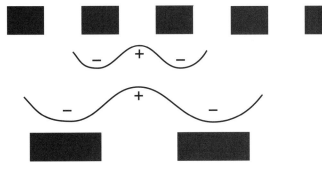

Figure 2.6 The visual receptors specialized for the frequencies shown in the middle will have very different responses to the two square wave stimuli. The smaller receptor will be maximally activated by the higher frequency stimulus (top) because the bright band falls within the excitatory zone (+) and dark bands fall within the inhibitory zones (−). The larger receptor will show little response to the higher frequency stimulus because both dark and light regions of the stimulus fall within its excitatory and inhibitory zones. The larger receptor will be maximally responsive to the lower frequency stimulus (bottom).

in the different receptors by the high-frequency stimulus. If the small receptor is centered over the brightest region then the light regions of the stimulus will only activate the center region. The surround will not provide any inhibition since this area is stimulated by the dark regions. Thus, this cell will respond vigorously. In contrast, the large receptor will be silent (or weakly activated) if it is positioned at the center of the light region of the stimulus. Thus, the input to the center region will also come from the dark regions of the stimulus (and light regions of the stimulus will activate the inhibitory surround). In general, the opposite occurs for the low-frequency stimulus: The large receptor will be maximally activated by the low-frequency stimulus, whereas the small receptor will tend to generate a weak response.

As in audition, visual receptors such as these operate as band-pass filters. Each receptor is most responsive to a particular spatial frequency, and the response level is attenuated for stimuli that contain component frequencies that are distant from the preferred frequency. A large body of behavioral, computational, and electrophysiological evidence has accumulated over the past 30 years demonstrating that cells in the visual pathways can be characterized as spatial frequency filters (see De Valois & De Valois, 1988). Although the response properties of these cells do not always implicate center-surround types of mechanisms, their activity is restricted to a limited range of spatial frequencies. Given that the preferred frequencies span a sufficiently large range, the activity across a set of these receptors would be analogous to a mathematical Fourier analysis.

Before returning to the issue of laterality two final points should be made explicit. First, simple stimuli such as sinusoidal gratings are handy tools for the experimenter; such stimuli, however, are not seen in the real world. There are real objects that may resemble the square wave patterns shown in figure 2.6. For example, the posts of a picket fence, the windows on a skyscraper, or the texture of a woolen blanket provide a repeating pattern. More important, the operation of receptors like those shown in figure 2.6 will be the same regardless of whether the stimulus contains periodic patterns. If the stimulus were to simply contain one black bar and one white bar we would also see a difference in the responsiveness of the two receptors depending on the size of the bars. The ecological validity of a stimulus such as this is not in question; it provides a reasonable approximation of an edge.

Second, we have described the receptors in figure 2.6 as if they were performing a Fourier analysis. We could just as easily argue, however, that the large receptor is useful for detecting large objects (e.g., wide bars) and that the small receptor is useful for detecting small objects (e.g., narrow bars). The debate about whether visual cells represent features such as edges and corners (Hubel & Wiesel, 1977) or whether these cells are biological Fourier analyzers is not central to this book. The important point is that the visual system represents information at different spatial scales. Spatial frequency terminology provides a concise description of visual stimuli without neglecting their complexity. Natural objects contain information at multiple scales.

EVIDENCE FOR LATERALIZATION OF FREQUENCY INFORMATION

The basic premise of this book is that the two hemispheres differ in how they process complex information. Stated in frequency terms, our proposal is that processing in the right hemisphere is biased toward low-frequency information and processing in the left hemisphere is biased toward high-frequency information. Sergent (1982) first proposed that there was a fundamental asymmetry between the two hemispheres in the representation of high and low spatial frequencies in vision, and the hypothesis has been echoed by a number of researchers over the past decade (e.g., Kitterle, Christman, & Hellige, 1990; Kosslyn, Chabris, Marsolek, & Koenig, 1992). An important feature of our proposal is that this frequency distinction applies across different perceptual modalities. We will present evidence showing that a parallel asymmetry holds in audition, although here the stimuli are described in terms of sound frequencies (Ivry & Lebby, 1993). The frequency hypothesis may also extend to the temporal domain. Here the hypothesis would be that the left hemisphere is specialized for processing information changing over high temporal frequencies (Tallal, Miller, & Fitch, 1993). In contrast, the right hemisphere is more adept at representing information that is modulated more slowly over time.

A second central property of our theory is that the processing asymmetry is mediated by attentional mechanisms. The asymmetrical representations introduced by the cerebral hemispheres do not result from differences in the population of receptors feeding into each hemisphere. People are sensitive to a wide range of frequencies and both hemispheres are capable of representing the entire spectrum of information. Depending on the task, however, we may choose to attend to a limited range of this information. The hemispheric asymmetry arises following the selection of the appropriate information and therefore reflects differences in processing beyond early sensory processes. This property leads to a lateralization effect that holds in terms of relative frequency (i.e., the relatively lower and higher frequencies in the selected region) rather than absolute frequency.

In the next section we introduce a framework for a computational model that accounts for how similar laterality effects might be observed across different perceptual modalities. Before introducing the framework we review representative studies involving visual or auditory stimuli that were critical to the development of the current theory.

Asymmetries in Visual Perception

The frequency hypothesis is intended to account for asymmetries that may arise in the perception of complex stimuli. Nonetheless, we begin with a discussion of experiments using simple stimuli since these provide the best direct assessment of the frequency hypothesis.

In exploring hemispheric differences in the processing of visual information the traditional paradigm with normal subjects is to use lateralized stimuli. A fixation point at the center of the display screen is provided so that the experimenter can control the subjects' direction of gaze. The stimulus is then presented to either the left or right of this fixation point. The neural connectivity of the brain is such that information presented to the left visual field is projected to the right hemisphere and information presented to the right visual field is projected to the left hemisphere (see figure 1.7). As noted in chapter 1 this crossed connectivity does not ensure that only one hemisphere will be stimulated. The fibers of the corpus callosum provide rapid interhemispheric communication. Two assumptions, however, motivate the belief that lateralized stimuli preferentially activate the contralateral hemisphere. First, because the ipsilateral hemisphere requires transcortical transmission, there may be some loss in the fidelity of the signal. Second, the ipsilateral hemisphere will only receive its input after the contralateral hemisphere has had a head start in processing. Moreover, as will be discussed later, converging evidence can be obtained in the study of people with neurological disorders in which either processing in one hemisphere is disrupted or else the connections between the hemispheres have been severed.

Fred Kitterle and his colleagues have published a set of papers that consistently show visual field asymmetries in the processing of spatial frequency information. In the most relevant study for our present

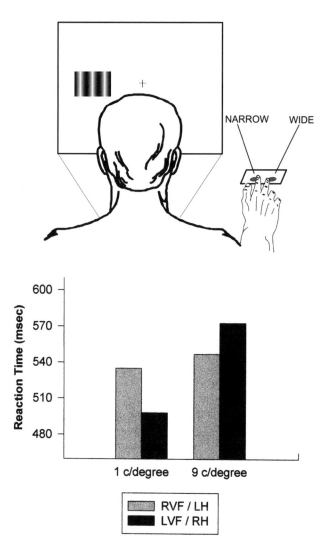

Figure 2.7 Subjects had to judge whether the stripes of a grating were narrow or wide (top). The subjects kept their eyes fixed on the cross at the center of the screen and the gratings were presented in either the left visual field (LVF) as shown or right visual field (RVF). Mean reaction time for the two stimuli as a function of visual field is shown (bottom). Subjects were faster to correctly classify the wide, low-frequency stimulus when it was presented in the left visual field and the narrow, high-frequency stimulus when it was presented in the right visual field. (Adapted from Kitterle et al., 1990.)

purpose (Kitterle et. al, 1990, Experiments 4 and 5) a sinusoidal grating was presented on each trial, either to the left or right visual field. The spatial frequency of the grating was either low, 1 cycle/degree, or high, 9 cycles/degree (figure 2.7). The brightness of the stimuli was also varied, although all were presented at suprathreshold levels of intensity. The subjects' task was to identify whether the stimulus had "wide" stripes (low-frequency stimulus) or "narrow" stripes (high-frequency stimulus), and the primary dependent variable was reaction time.

The laterality hypothesis regarding spatial frequency would predict that the right hemisphere would show an advantage in identifying the lower frequency member of the stimulus set and that the left hemisphere would show an advantage in identifying the higher frequency member. The overall reaction time is the result of a number of processes, however, and it is unlikely that all of these processes would reflect asymmetric processing in the two cerebral hemispheres. For example, subjects might show an overall advantage in identifying the wide-striped stimulus simply because it is easier to detect the larger stripes. Or subjects may identify stimuli presented in the left visual field faster, perhaps because of a general alertness advantage sometimes found for the right hemisphere (Posner, Inhoff, Friedrich, & Cohen, 1987). Thus, the prediction derived from the laterality hypothesis is less constrained: The critical expectation is that there will be an interaction between the variables of stimulus frequency and the side of presentation.

The predicted interaction was obtained (figure 2.7). Subjects were faster in identifying the 1 cycle/degree low-frequency stimulus when it was presented in the left visual field and assumed to be primarily processed within the right hemisphere. In contrast, response latencies to the 9 cycle/degree high-frequency stimulus were faster when this stimulus was presented in the right visual field and, thus, primarily projected to the left hemisphere. Two main effects were also found. Subjects were faster overall in identifying the 1 cycle/degree stimulus, and responses tended to be faster for the brighter stimuli. Nonetheless, the laterality effect was found at all three levels of brightness. These results were replicated in a follow-up experiment in which the brightness was held constant but the exposure duration of the stimuli was manipulated (range: 20–160 ms). Thus, in these identification tasks with simple stimuli a striking laterality effect was obtained. The right hemisphere showed a consistent advantage in identifying the low-frequency member of the stimulus set, whereas the left hemisphere showed a relative advantage in identifying the higher frequency member of the set. Similar results were found by Kitterle and Selig (1991) using a larger range of spatial frequencies.

The importance of spatial frequency information is made clear in another study reported by Kitterle, Hellige, and Christman (1992). In this experiment, there were four stimuli. Two of these were sine waves oscillating at frequencies of either 1 cycle/degree or 3 cycles/degree. The other stimuli were two square waves. While sine waves consist of just a fundamental frequency—the frequency at which the pattern repeats—square waves are composed of a fundamental frequency and all the odd harmonics of that fundamental. Thus, a square wave with a fundamental frequency of 3 cycles/degree contains information at 6 cycles/degree, 12 cycles/degree, 18 cycles/degree, and so on. In one task the subjects had to determine whether the bars were wide or narrow, requirements similar to those of the study described previously. In this task the subjects' judgments could be based on the fundamental frequencies. In the second task the subjects had to decide whether the bars had sharp edges (i.e., square waves) or fuzzy edges (i.e., sine waves). For this task higher frequency information is essential (figure 2.8).

A crossover interaction between task and visual field was obtained. The wide versus narrow task was performed more rapidly when the stimuli were presented in the left visual field. In contrast, the edge determination task showed a significant right visual field advantage. These results underscore our contention that hemispheric asymmetries in perception are critically dependent on the processing demands required for a particular task. The exact set of stimuli led to reversed asymmetries for the

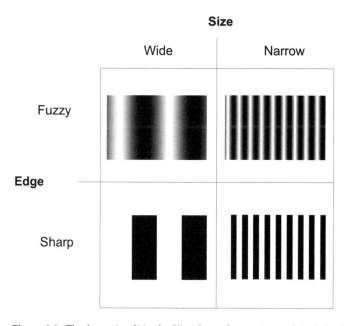

Figure 2.8 The four stimuli in the Kitterle et al. experiment (1992). In the size task subjects had to classify the stimuli along the horizontal dimension, distinguishing between the stimuli on the basis of their fundamental frequencies (1 or 3 cycles/degree). In the edge task subjects had to classify the stimuli along the vertical dimension, distinguishing between the stimuli on the basis of their component structures (sine or square wave). The size task requires analysis of lower frequency information; the edge task requires analysis of higher frequency information.

two tasks. Processing lower frequency information (i.e., the fundamental frequency) was sufficient for the wide versus narrow task, for which there was a right hemisphere advantage. In contrast, the edge determination task required processing of higher frequency information; in accord with the frequency hypothesis, the left hemisphere appears to be more adept at making these judgments.

In the experiments reviewed to this point absolute and relative frequency have been confounded. For example, in Kitterle et al. (1990) the 1 cycle/degree stimulus is both relatively lower than the 9 cycle/degree stimulus and also has the lowest spatial frequency content of any of the stimuli tested. Christman, Kitterle, and Hellige (1991), however, demonstrate that visual field asymmetries emerge as a function of differences in relative frequency. The stimuli in this experiment were compound gratings in which either two or three sinusoids were superimposed at random phases. On each trial one of these stimuli was briefly shown in either the left or right visual field, and subjects were required to identify which stimulus was presented.

Two stimulus sets were tested in separate blocks of trials. In one set, the low-frequency condition, the duplex pattern was composed of 0.5 and 1.0 cycle/degree sinusoids and the triplex pattern was composed of sinusoids at 0.5, 1.0, and 2.0 cycles/degree. In accord with the frequency hypothesis subjects were faster to identify the duplex pattern when it was presented in the left visual field. This follows, since the triplex pattern includes higher spatial frequency information compared to the duplex pattern. In the other set, the high-frequency condition, the duplex pattern was composed of 4 and 8 cycles/degree sinusoids and the triplex pattern was composed of sinusoids at 2, 4, and 8 cycles/degree. Note that for this set the 2 cycle/degree component creates a triplex pattern with lower spatial frequency information than is contained in the duplex pattern. A crossover interaction was observed for this condition. The duplex stimulus was identified more rapidly in the right visual field and the triplex stimulus was identified more rapidly in the left visual field.

Taken together, the results convincingly demonstrate that the laterality effects are based on differences in relative frequency. If the effect were one of absolute frequency then the addition of a 2 cycle/degree sinusoid should have had the same effect, regardless of the other frequency components. The inclusion of the 2 cycle/degree component, however, had the opposite effects for the two conditions. Thus, high and low frequency are determined on a relative basis according to the range of frequencies forming the stimulus sets.

Asymmetries in Auditory Perception

The studies discussed in the previous section provide evidence consistent with the hypothesis that there are asymmetries in how the two cerebral hemispheres utilize spatial frequency information. We have conducted a series of experiments to investigate whether an analogous asymmetry is found in auditory perception (Ivry & Lebby, 1993). In this domain, of course, frequency has a much different meaning. Rather than referring to the repetition of a spatial pattern, frequency in audition refers to periodic changes in sound pressure. The response of peripheral receptors can vary in a phase-locked manner with these changes in sound pressure, at least for lower frequency sounds. For example, a 100 Hz tone will cause some auditory fibers to generate approximately 100 spikes/second. At the cortex, however, frequency is no longer represented in an analog fashion, but has been transformed into a place code. Auditory cortex contains a tonotopic representation in which there is an orderly relationship between the location of cells and the stimulus frequency that produces the optimal response. Thus, the locus of activity within auditory cortex can subserve sound frequency identification and discrimination similar to the manner in which activity within visual cortex may subserve size judgments based on variations in terms of spatial frequency tuning.

Anatomical and behavioral considerations make the study of laterality effects in audition less straightforward than in vision. In vision there is a clear anatomical segregation of input from the two visual fields; the primary visual cortex in the left hemisphere receives input from receptors sensitive to visual events in the right visual field and the reverse holds for the right hemisphere. Such an anatomical segregation does not apply to the auditory pathways. Ascending neurons from an ear project to both contralesional and ipsilesional auditory cortices. The bilateral representation of monaural inputs has been further demonstrated in electrophysiological studies. For example, in both animal (Rosenzweig, 1951) and human studies (Celesia, 1976; Majkowski, Bochenek, Bochenek, Knapik-Fijalkowska, & Kopec, 1971) cortical evoked potentials are observed over both hemispheres following the presentation of a sound on either the right or left side of space. In the human studies the latencies of these potentials are roughly identical, indicating that the ipsilesional activity does not result from transcortical transmission via the corpus callosum.

Nonetheless, laterality studies in auditory perception have been predicated on the assumption that the contralateral hemisphere provides a stronger representation of a lateralized stimulus. Evidence supporting the asymmetric representation hypothesis has come from numerous sources (for a cogent review, see Phillips & Gates, 1982). Anatomical results indicate that, although a significant number of auditory afferents project to the ipsilateral hemisphere, the majority of fibers from each ear ascend to the contralateral hemisphere (Kelly, 1981; Brodal, 1981). Functional evidence for asymmetric processing can be found in a variety of electrophysiological studies. Single-cell recordings in auditory cortex of both monkey (Brugge & Merzenich, 1973) and cats (Phillips & Irvine, 1981) show larger responses following contralateral stimulation, whereas evoked potentials recorded from the contralateral hemisphere tend to be larger in both humans and nonhuman species (Rosenzweig, 1951; Celesia, 1976; Majkowski et al., 1971; Tanguay, Taub, Doubleday, & Clarkson, 1977). More recently, neuroimaging studies of cerebral blood flow (Lauter, Herscovitch, Formby, & Raichle, 1985) and of magnetic evoked responses (Makela et al., 1993) have demonstrated greater activation in the contralateral hemisphere. A third source of electrophysiological evidence comes from the classical neurological studies of Penfield. While developing a surgical treatment for chronic epilepsy Penfield stimulated the exposed cortex of awake patients. When the stimulations occurred in the vicinity of primary auditory cortex the patients would report hearing sounds emanating from the contralateral side of space (Penfield & Perot, 1963). Correspondingly, unilateral lesions of the temporal lobe tend to impair the patient's ability to discriminate auditory information when the stimuli are restricted to the contralesional ear.

Note that in this discussion of hemispheric asymmetries in audition, the question has centered on whether each hemisphere is more strongly activated by stimuli in the contralateral ear. This is a different question, however, than the one that has been asked regarding visual perception. In vision, the contralateral organization is not in terms of the projections from the two eyes but rather in terms of visual fields. An analogous situation may hold in audition. There may be a functional lateralization of auditory processing, but the asymmetry is best described in terms of auditory hemispace (Phillips & Gates, 1982). Sounds emanating from the right side of the head are represented in the left hemisphere and sounds emanating from the left side of the head are represented in the right hemisphere. Indeed, cats with unilateral lesions of the auditory cortex are unable to localize contralesional sounds (Jenkins & Masterson, 1982; Jenkins & Merzenich, 1984). These study results led Jenkins and his colleagues to propose that spatial information derived from audition is represented solely in the hemisphere contralateral to the stimulus location.

Taken together, the evidence strongly supports the assumption that at a functional level the contralateral hemisphere is dominant in processing both dichotic and monaural stimuli. Because we were interested in conducting an experiment that closely paralleled the visual studies of Kitterle et al. (1990), we chose to use monaural stimuli in our studies (Ivry & Lebby, 1993). The design of our initial auditory experiments was slightly more complex than that of the visual studies, however, because we wanted the study to provide a strong test of the relative frequency hypothesis. Each stimulus was composed of a pair of superimposed sinusoidal tones (table 2.1). One of these tones was the target; the other was an irrelevant distractor. There were two sets of six stimuli each. For the low set, the frequency of the distractor tone was always 1900 Hz. The

Table 2.1 Frequency components of the stimuli and assigned response categories in Experiment 1 of Ivry and Lebby (1993)

Low Set of Sounds

Irrelevant Frequency	Target Frequency	Response Category
1900	192	low
1900	195	low
1900	198	low
1900	202	high
1900	205	high
1900	208	high

High Set of Sounds

Irrelevant Frequency	Target Frequency	Response Category
200	1860	low
200	1876	low
200	1892	low
200	1908	high
200	1924	high
200	1940	high

On each trial, a single stimulus composed of an irrelevant frequency and a target frequency, was presented to either the left or right ear. Subjects classified the sound as "low" or "high," and were provided feedback. In separate blocks of trials, the target frequency was either the lower component or the higher component.

frequency of the lower component was varied, ranging from a low of 192 Hz to a high of 208 Hz. Thus, for the low set the stimuli differed in terms of the frequency of the lower frequency component. For the high set the frequency of the higher component of the duplex varied from a low of 1860 Hz to a high of 1940 Hz, and the distractor tone was held constant at 200 Hz. The duration of each duplex stimulus was 150 ms.

The low and high sets were presented in separate blocks of trials. During each trial, a duplex stimulus was presented to either the left or right ear. The subjects' task was to determine whether the stimulus was one of the relatively low or relatively high members of the set. Given that there were six stimuli in each set and that the range of target frequencies was fairly small, the task was much more difficult than that used by Kitterle et al. (1990) in their initial visual studies. For that reason, the dependent variable was accuracy and the subjects were given feedback throughout the experiment whenever they made incorrect judgments.

Of primary interest was whether the frequency asymmetry observed in visual perception would generalize to audition. If the asymmetry did generalize, then we expected that subjects would be better at discriminating low-frequency targets when those stimuli were presented to the left ear and that discrimination would be better for high-frequency targets when those stimuli were presented to the right ear. But how should low and high be defined? The design of our experiment provided a means to evaluate the contribution of absolute and relative frequency to any observed laterality effect. If the effect were one of absolute frequency, then there would be an ear by stimulus set interaction. In other words, subjects would be better at judging the frequency of the low set of tones when they were presented in the left ear in comparison to when those tones were presented to the right ear. Similarly, a right ear advantage would be found for the high set of tones. Thus, an absolute frequency difference would be evident in comparisons between blocks of trials. In contrast, if the laterality effect were one of relative frequency, then there would be an ear by stimulus interaction within a block of trials. Specifically, judgments would be more accurate for the lower frequency members of a set when they were presented to the left ear and more accurate for the higher frequency members of a set when they were presented to the right ear.

As can be seen in figure 2.9, the results clearly supported the relative frequency hypothesis. The top two panels of figure 2.9 show the percentage of errors for each stimulus in the low and high sets, respectively. Subjects were more accurate in assigning the lower frequency members of both sets to the low category when those stimuli were presented to the left ear. The opposite was found for the higher frequency members of each set, which were accurately assigned to the high category when presented to the right ear. The results can also be presented in terms of bias: subjects were more likely to label each tone "high" when that tone was presented to the right ear than when the same stimulus was presented to the left ear. That bias was roughly equivalent for all the members of each set, although, of course, the overall number of "high" responses increased with frequency.

There was no evidence to support the absolute frequency hypothesis (figure 2.9, bottom panel). Although subjects were better at labeling the high set of stimuli, that effect was similar for the two ears. In agreement with the results of the visual experiments using sinusoidal gratings, the laterality effect in audition was observed to be in terms of relative frequency. Follow-up studies replicated these findings and demonstrated that the laterality effects can be found with both reaction-time and accuracy measures.

MOTIVATING A UNIFIED THEORY OF HEMISPHERIC SPECIALIZATION IN AUDITORY AND VISUAL PERCEPTION

An important question that needs to be addressed is why hemispheric asymmetries are similar in vision and audition. Consider what is required when we attend an art gallery opening. The visual array is replete with

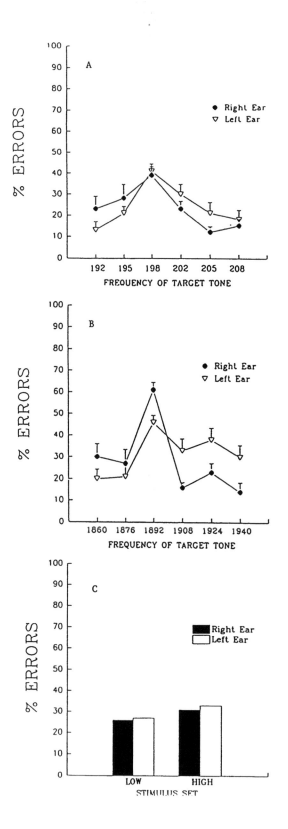

complex information: the moving throng of people, the table of appetizers, the art on the wall. Moreover, the auditory system is flooded with different sounds: the music played over the sound system and the buzz of numerous conversations. From this vast array of sensory input, our attention restricts what we look at and hear. Each painting may cover a subsection of the wall and depict an overall scene, but we can choose to examine the details, the fine gradations in shading or the use of broad strokes to define edges. In audition, we may attend to the interpretations offered by a friend while ignoring the music. Moreover, in certain situations, it is essential that we are able to attribute these sounds to their appropriate objects. For example, we may engage a friend in a conversation. Attentional capabilities allow us to focus on this person—monitoring the speaker's gestures and actions while listening intently to his or her speech.

Common Goals in Processing Visual and Auditory Information

The need to represent information at multiple scales and select a subset of that information is common to both modalities. These problems of multiple scales arise at what Marr (1980) has called the computational level of theorizing, and any theory of perception must address them. While a wide range of mechanisms may suffice for perception, a theory of perception must be able to account for how we select task-relevant information and represent the selected information. There are similar constraints in both vision and audition, and they can be expected to exert pressures on how perceptual and attentional systems evolve to solve these problems of selection.

A central tenet of cognitive psychology is that complex tasks such as perception and attention are performed via the coordinated activities of separable component parts. For example, there does not exist a single visual processor, but rather a set of specialized processors, each adept at representing certain aspects of the stimulus (Zeki, 1993). One processor might be specialized for representing shape information; another for representing color information. By distributing processing across a set of specialized modules, the demands on any single processor are reduced and the final percept can be achieved more efficiently. Distributed processing has proven to be an essential component of many theories of visual and auditory perception.

Figure 2.9 Subjects learned to classify tones composed of two nonharmonic frequencies. Top and middle panels: When the sounds were presented to the left ear classifications were more accurate for stimuli assigned to the "low" category, regardless of whether the target frequency was the low- or high-frequency component of the stimulus. When the sounds were presented to the right ear classifications were more accurate for the stimuli assigned to the "high" category. Bottom panel: There were no laterality effects in terms of absolute target frequency. (From Ivry & Lebby, 1993.)

Our approach to understanding hemispheric specialization builds on this notion of distributed processing. As discussed in chapter 1, early theories of laterality tended to focus on task-based distinctions such as verbal versus spatial. More recent theorists have taken a more computational approach, arguing that it is not the task but the type of representation that distinguishes the functions of the two hemispheres. For example, Kosslyn (1987) has proposed that the left hemisphere is specialized for representing categorical information (e.g., is X above Y?) whereas the right hemisphere is specialized for representing coordinate information (e.g., is X far from Y?).

Our hypothesis—that frequency information is asymmetrically represented in the two hemispheres—offers a different computational tack. It provides a mechanism for how we may efficiently represent information at multiple scales by asymmetrically distributing the chore across the two hemispheres. Given a complex visual input, each hemisphere need not be equally efficient in its representation of the entire spectrum of information. Instead, the right hemisphere is biased to amplify lower spatial frequency information while the left hemisphere is biased to amplify the higher spatial frequency information. Functional asymmetries in the performance of different tasks will result from such distributed processing. For example, the right hemisphere will prove more adept at tasks requiring the identification of the global shape of an object since low-frequency information is required for this task. Or, in audition, tasks that require analysis of the harmonic structure of music—information carried in the higher frequencies—can be expected to be performed better by the left hemisphere. In our theory, the appropriate level for describing hemispheric specializations is not in terms of tasks such as music or language. Rather, task-based differences emerge as a function of whether the critical information is contained in the relatively higher or lower frequencies. Further discussion of how performance of different tasks depends on the analysis of either lower or higher regions of the frequency spectrum is provided in chapters 3–6. For now we simply wish to make the point that the asymmetric representation of frequency information offers another example of how the brain favors a distributed form of representation.

Evolutionary Perspectives

The preceding discussion presents an argument for why the two hemispheres might emphasize different regions of the frequency spectrum. But that hypothesis does not offer an explanation for the similarities between vision and audition in how the asymmetry is organized. Again, it is important to keep in mind that in vision we are dealing with spatial frequencies, whereas in audition the variation is of sound frequencies. Just because the same mathematics can be used for both modalities does not mean there is a functional similarity.

It is possible that the apparent similarities in hemispheric specialization for vision and audition are coincident. A basic evolutionary pressure may have led to the differential representation of frequency information, resulting in a left hemisphere that favors higher spatial frequencies and a right hemisphere that favors lower spatial frequencies. An independent adaptive process may have been operating in audition, and simply by chance, the partitioning of higher and lower sound frequencies may have paralleled the asymmetry observed in vision. Indeed, given that processing in one modality is asymmetric, by chance alone the probability is .50 that an asymmetry in the other modality would result in a similar organization.

A common causal mechanism may also have led to the development of parallel asymmetries in vision and audition, even though these asymmetries are unrelated. It has been proposed that the developmental time course for the two hemispheres is asynchronous. The anatomical record indicates that regions within the right hemisphere mature earlier than do homologous areas in the left hemisphere (reviewed by Geschwind & Galaburda, 1987). Cortical landmarks in the superior temporal lobe of the right hemisphere appear at an earlier point during fetal development (Chi, Dooling, & Gilles, 1977), which suggests that regions in the right hemisphere associated with auditory processing may become functional at an earlier point in time. The uterine environment is not silent. The fetus is exposed to the internal sounds of the mother, including the steady beats of her heart and the rumbling of food as it passes through the digestive system. In addition, external sounds penetrate the embryonic sac. Such sounds are not identical to those reaching the mother's ear. Like the walls that separate two offices, the mother's skin, bones, and organs attenuate high frequencies. Low frequencies, on the other hand, are minimally filtered, and the evidence suggests that a newborn baby is already sensitized to information carried in this region of the spectrum. For example, two-day-old infants show a preference for their native language (Moon, Cooper, & Fifer, 1993). It is likely that such an ability depends on the languages' different prosodic structures—information that is primarily conveyed by the fundamental frequency of the speech signal.

Given developmental asynchrony, prenatal processing may be primarily dependent on the right hemisphere, and thus the right hemisphere would develop a specialization for prosody perception at an early age. Such development would be consistent with the evidence showing that in adults deficits in prosody perception are associated with lesions of posterior areas of the right hemisphere (see chapter 6). Assuming that the right hemisphere of an infant remains biased toward the lower region of the spectrum, the later-developing left hemisphere would be in a position to dominate in the processing of high-frequency sounds, which provide the primary cues for discriminating the phonetic sounds of speech (Turkewitz, 1988). In this view, hemispheric asymmetries in audition may persist across the life span, due to the combination of genetic triggers that guide the development of the two hemispheres and the types of information that become available during maturation.

Analogous arguments have been offered to account for the hemispheric asymmetries in vision (Hellige, 1993). For this modality, experiential factors can only come into play after birth, given the dark void of the uterine environment. Although the newborn is exposed to the same complex visual world as the adult, her brain is not able to process the information in the same manner. At birth, the visual system is most responsive to coarse information, which is carried at the lowest spatial frequencies (reviewed in de Schonen & Mathivet, 1989). Sensitivity to higher frequencies emerges during the first 6 months of life. If we assume that the right hemisphere is more mature in the neonate, then we can propose the development of a visual processing asymmetry parallel to the asymmetry proposed in audition. The right hemisphere may become biased to process global information carried by lower frequencies; given the brain's propensity for a division of labor, the left hemisphere may then become specialized to emphasize information carried by relatively higher frequencies. In summary, a single causal factor—the differential maturation rates for the two hemispheres—could independently lay the foundation for the emergence of parallel asymmetries in the brain's processing of sound and spatial frequencies.

However, there exist certain correlations that may favor a processing system organized to link corresponding spectral regions in vision and audition. First, larger objects tend to produce lower sounds than smaller objects. This correlation exists between different types of objects and within a single class of objects. An example of the former situation is evident in comparisons of the vocalizations of different animals. The spectrum of the bellowing cries of an elephant contain much more power at lower frequencies than does the song of a canary (figure 2.10). That correlation is also found in inanimate objects. Compare the sounds produced when a large tree is toppled with those produced by dropping a pencil. In those examples, the differences can occur over a couple of orders of magnitude. The same correlation is also found within a single class of stimuli, but over a smaller range. For example, the pitch of human speech is correlated with size. The pitch of male speakers is typically an octave lower than that of female speakers, a difference that is generally correlated with the size of the speakers (or at least with the length of their vocal tracts). Moreover, the most painful high-frequency human sounds are produced by the smallest members of our species, newborn babies.

Second, correlations between spatial and sound frequencies can also be found within a single object. Consider how frequency information changes as a function of distance. If we are directly in front of the stage at a rock concert, we can hear all the sounds of the different instruments,

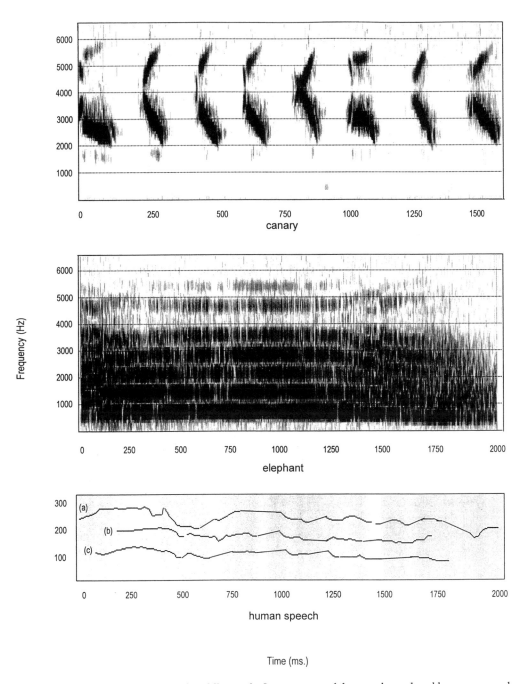

Figure 2.10 Top and middle panels: Spectrograms of the sounds produced by a canary and an elephant. There is a correlation between the size of the animal and the distribution of energy in the spectra. Larger animals tend to have more power at lower frequencies than smaller animals. Bottom panel: The correlation between size and pitch also characterizes differences within a species. The three contours are the fundamental frequency for three speakers saying the sentence, "I am using both sides of my brain." Speaker *a* is a six-year-old boy, Speaker *b* is an adult female, and Speaker *c* is an adult male.

A Theory of Hemispheric Asymmetries in Perception

ranging from the low-pitched rhythm of the bass guitar to the high-pitched clang of the cymbals. At that distance, we are also able to observe the entire scene in exquisite detail. Our perception changes drastically if we are seated at the back of the concert hall. Here, both the high spatial and high sound frequency information is lost or severely attenuated. Our auditory percept is dominated by low-frequency sounds such as those produced by the bass guitar. Similarly, we can no longer see the intricate finger movements of the guitarist or the steady motions of the drummer. Only the general outlines of the band members remain visible.

At this point, there is no clear way to decide whether the parallel hemispheric asymmetries in vision and audition are fortuitous, whether they emerge independently from a common causal agent, or whether they result from common evolutionary pressures. Ideas on the evolution of cognition offered by Jerrison (1980) and Rozin (1976) lead us to favor the latter interpretation as a working hypothesis. These theorists acknowledge that cognitive processes have evolved to solve specific problems. For example, representing spatial frequencies may have been an efficient mechanism for analyzing complex visual scenes. Over the course of time, however, a mechanism that is useful in one domain may come to be exploited by processing systems in other task domains. That is, a computational process originally derived for one purpose may become accessible for other purposes. It seems reasonable to assume that a later-evolving system would adopt an organizational structure that had been derived for earlier evolving systems.

Ivry (1993) has used the accessibility idea to argue for the emergence of generalized timing properties of the cerebellum. Timing capability may have originally been restricted to the regulation of the timing of movements. Over time, other processing systems that required precise timing may have come to utilize the timing capability of the cerebellum, extending the task domain of the cerebellum to perception and sensorimotor learning. Exploitation of a unique computational capability in multiple task domains, however, does not mandate that the same, or even overlapping, neural elements are used in all situations. For instance, the cerebellum may be composed of an infinite number of timing mechanisms rather than a single clock (Ivry, 1996).

In a related fashion, parallel asymmetries in hemispheric specialization may have arisen in vision and audition, even though neural structures within each hemisphere may remain linked to one modality or the other. The similarities in the asymmetries exist at a more general level. Whether they also reflect shared neural mechanism remains to be seen.

THE DOUBLE FILTERING BY FREQUENCY THEORY

The theory presented here is intended to capture the general similarities in hemispheric specialization in perception. Three basic ideas are emphasized. First, there is the notion of frequency-based representations as a way to capture information at multiple scales in both vision and audition. Second, as a form of distributed processing, frequency information is assumed to be asymmetrically represented in the two hemispheres. Third, in both visual and auditory perception a selective attention process results in laterality effects that are based on differences in relative frequency rather than absolute frequency. We begin with a descriptive overview of the theory. In chapter 7 we describe an implemented computer model that incorporates these ideas.

We have reviewed evidence supporting our contention that in both vision and audition the cerebral hemispheres show a consistent asymmetry in the representation of relative frequency information. To repeat, in vision this asymmetry holds for the processing of spatial frequency information (Kitterle et al., 1990; Christman et al., 1991). The left hemisphere is more adept at identifying relatively high spatial frequency patterns. In contrast, the right hemisphere is more adept at identifying relatively low spatial frequency patterns. As shown by Ivry and Lebby (1993), an analogous effect can be found in audition, but here the stimulus dimension is sound frequency. In subsequent chapters we argue that the basic dichotomy between processing of high and low frequencies provides a parsimonious way to account for a wide range of laterality effects obtained in a range of tasks using more complex visual and auditory stimuli.

Before turning to this review, we provide a framework for a computational theory that captures the essential characteristics of our laterality hypothesis. We will refer to this theory as the double filtering by frequency theory (DFF). The DFF theory is intended to identify the basic components of our theory of hemispheric specialization. Figure 2.11 provides a sketch of the critical processing stages that lead to asymmetries

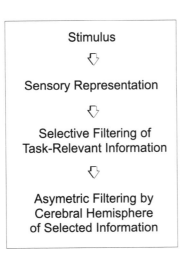

Figure 2.11 An overview of the processing stages in the DFF theory.

A Theory of Hemispheric Asymmetries in Perception

in the representation of frequency information. Our sketch is not intended to capture all aspects of processing from peripheral receptors to conscious percepts. Instead, it is limited to three stages that are necessary for producing laterality effects: an initial sensory representation, followed by two filtering stages that operate on frequency-based representations. We outline the properties and assumptions associated with each processing stage in the following sections.

Sensory Representation of Frequency Information

The first processing stage concerns the sensory representation of the stimulus. Building on our earlier arguments, we assume that this sensory representation is in terms of spatial and sound frequency information for vision and audition, respectively. Although the extraction of a frequency-based representation is performed at many levels of processing, we are concerned here with the input to the cerebral hemispheres. Specifically, we assume that at the initial cortical stage of processing the input is similar for the left and right hemispheres. Asymmetries between the hemispheres will result from postsensory stages of processing.

A detection paradigm is typically used to investigate the question of sensory acuity. In the standard form of experiments in visual perception subjects must determine whether or not a particular spatial frequency grating was presented. The critical manipulation involves the contrast between the light and dark portions of the grating. For a high contrast grating there is a large difference in luminance between the brightest and darkest regions of the grating; for a low contrast grating the difference is smaller Contrast sensitivity is operationalized by determining the contrast at which subjects accurately detect the stimulus at some defined criterion level (e.g., 70%). With foveal viewing under daylight conditions, humans show an inverted U-shaped function in contrast sensitivity over frequency. Sensitivity peaks around 5–6 cycles/degree and drops steadily as frequency is decreased or increased. The upper limit under these viewing conditions is around 50 cycles/degree (see De Valois & De Valois, 1990). However, as the viewing conditions are altered, either by decreasing the luminance of the background (De Valois, Morgan, & Snodderly, 1974) or by increasing the eccentricity of the grating (Rovamo, Virsu, & Nasanen, 1978), the range is considerably narrowed and peak sensitivity shifts to a lower frequency.

This paradigm has been modified to test for laterality effects in contrast sensitivity. In these experiments the subjects are required to fixate on a center point on a display and the gratings are presented in either the left or right visual field. Kitterle and Kay (1985) presented stimuli in a 2 degree aperture, centered 2 degrees to either the right or left of fixation. Across a range of frequencies the contrast sensitivity functions were identical for the two visual fields, regardless of the orientation of the gratings or the eye used to view the stimuli.

Using a variety of alternative paradigms, other researchers have similarly failed to find any laterality effects in contrast sensitivity (Peterzell, Harvey, & Hardyck, 1989; Rose, 1983; Szelag, Budohoska, & Koltuska, 1987). Of note here is Experiment 2 of Kitterle et. al (1990), which used reaction time as the dependent variable. In this experiment subjects were faster to detect suprathreshold gratings when the stimuli were presented in the left visual field. However, the left visual field advantage held steady across variations in frequency, contrast, and stimulus exposure. Thus, the series of experiments reported by Kitterle et al. (1990) show a striking difference between detection and identification. Whereas there is no laterality effect for the former task, a robust effect of visual field is found for identification. That dissociation bolsters our assumption that hemispheric asymmetries arise at postsensory stages of processing.

The situation is less clear for auditory perception. A number of studies have found ear differences in detection sensitivity (e.g., Chung, Mason, Gannon, & Wilson, 1983; Kannan & Lipscomb, 1974; Ward, 1957). Chung et al. (1983) performed a meta-analysis on pure-tone audiograms obtained from 50,000 industrial workers who worked in noisy environments. For males the right ear was more sensitive than the left ear at all frequencies tested; the difference in sensitivity was greatest between 2000 and 6000 Hz. With females the laterality effect was considerably reduced and only achieved conventional levels of statistical significance for the lowest frequency tested, which was 500 Hz. Ward (1957) reported a similar laterality effect in males in his tests of a group of military men who had been exposed to jet engine noise and extensive gunfire.

Those results suggest that there may be hemispheric differences in the sensory representation of sound frequencies. Previc (1991) has argued that the greater sensitivity for mid-range frequencies in the left hemisphere arises from differences in the peripheral apparatus required for sound transmission and that the asymmetry underlies the dominance of this hemisphere in speech perception. Although the merits of that argument are debatable, we must keep in mind that, unlike with vision, there is evidence suggesting an auditory laterality effect in terms of the sensory representation of frequency information.

Nonetheless, the laterality effects found in auditory detection tasks cannot provide a complete account of the results of Ivry and Lebby (1993). Remember that the ear asymmetries in those studies were in terms of relative frequency rather than absolute frequency. That is, the right ear bias for identifying the relatively high-frequency stimuli was found for targets varying around either 200 Hz or 1900 Hz. A similar left ear bias was found for identifying the lower frequency stimuli, regardless of whether the variation was in the lower or higher component tone. Thus, independent of any asymmetries in the representation of sensory information, additional mechanisms are required to account for laterality effects in identification or discrimination tasks. The discrepancy between detection and identification or discrimination is similar in both vision and audition.

The First frequency Filtering Stage: Attentional Selection of Task-Relevant Information

Whether or not there are small hemispheric differences in the representation of the sensory signal, we assume that each hemisphere is capable of representing the full range of frequency information present in the perceiver's current environment. At any point in time there are several stimuli contributing to this input; the world is filled with a host of objects and sounds. As our experience suggests, however, we are able to focus our attention on those aspects of the scene that are most relevant to our current goals. We are able to selectively attend to task-relevant information. When standing on the sidewalk waiting to cross the street, we can rapidly scan in both directions to determine the distance of approaching cars. But, if we notice a ladybug on the sidewalk and choose to study the pattern of black dots on her back, we may not notice the cars whizzing past. Attention, of course, is not completely volitional. If a car honks at us as we wander into the street, we automatically orient toward the sound.

Selective attention has always been at the center of interest in psychology. Indeed, it can be easily argued that the emergence of cognitive psychology as a discipline was inspired by the problems that arose when it was recognized that animals had limited information processing systems (Broadbent, 1958). One important issue has been how to characterize selective attention (see Egly, Driver, & Rafal, 1994). Do we select to focus on particular regions of space, biasing processing to objects and sounds that occupy that space? Or is attention allocated to objects, entities within the world that are demarcated by rapid, scene-parsing processes?

Within a spatial focus or within an object the frequency content can be quite widely distributed. The first filtering stage in the DFF theory is intended to capture the fact that selective attention, whether it operates on restricted spatial regions or on objects, determines which region of the sensory spectrum will be elaborated for further processing. That mechanism determines which frequencies will be amplified in subsequent representations and, correspondingly, which frequencies will be attenuated. The constraining forces for this selection process are twofold. First, properties of the stimulus dictate the range of frequency information. When presented with a large object, we view a range of frequency information that extends to relatively lower frequencies than we see when we view a smaller object. Second, within the range of frequency information the demands of the current processing task may dictate that some information is more useful. That is, attention is construed as involving both automatic (e.g., range adjustment) and flexible processes. The peripheral apparatus may be capable of transforming the entire visual and auditory scene into a frequency-based representation, but the processing goals of the perceiver require that attention be allocated to a restricted region of the input. It is that selection process that leads to the laterality effects that occur in terms of relative frequency.

Consider the auditory experiments of Ivry and Lebby (1993). Each stimulus is a duplex tone containing one target frequency and one irrelevant frequency. The subject knows in advance whether the critical information will be carried by the lower or higher frequency component of the stimulus. Thus, performance would be optimized if the subjects were able to selectively attend to the target region of the auditory spectrum.

A depiction of the proposed attention process is given in figure 2.12, which shows a condition in which the target frequency is the lower component of the duplex stimulus. Note that while the stimulus contains power at only two frequencies (i.e., 196 Hz and 1900 Hz), the sensory representation is assumed to blur that fact. Detectors optimally tuned to frequencies in the neighborhood of the two component sinusoids will be activated. The initial filtering mechanism is assumed to select for further processing that stimulus information which is relevant for current processing goals. Thus, in frequency space that attentional mechanism can be described as a narrow band-pass filter. Information in the neighborhood of the target frequency is selected for further processing; distant frequencies are attenuated. If the target frequency is from the low set of sounds (e.g., between 192 and 208 Hz), then information from detectors tuned to that region of the frequency spectrum will be selected for subsequent processing. Information in the vicinity of the 1900 Hz irrelevant tone will be ignored. When the target is determined by variation in the high-frequency component, the reverse occurs. The initial filtering mechanism amplifies information from detectors tuned to the high-frequency region of the spectrum while attenuating output from low-frequency detectors.

Experiments in both visual and auditory perception clearly demonstrate that subjects are able to selectively attend to a restricted region of spatial or sound frequencies. Consider an experiment reported by Scharf, Quigley, Aoki, Peachey, and Reeves (1987; see, also, Schlauch & Hafter, 1991). Subjects were tested on an auditory detection task in which they had to decide which of two intervals contained a pure-tone stimulus. Each trial began with the presentation of a suprathreshold cue. After a silent interval, two sequential noise-filled intervals were presented, separated by a 350 ms silent period. For one of the intervals, a pure tone was superimposed on the noise; the subjects' task was to decide which of the two intervals contained this stimulus.

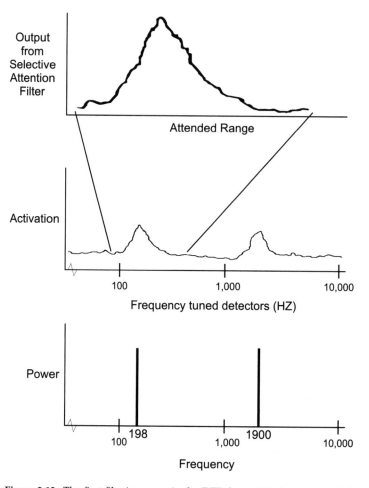

Figure 2.12 The first filtering stage in the DFF theory. The bottom panel shows the power spectrum of one of the stimuli in the Ivry and Lebby experiments (1993). The middle panel shows hypothetical activation across a band of frequency-tuned detectors. Subjects know that the critical information is carried by the lower frequency component, and attention is therefore directed to this region of the spectrum (top panel).

There were two main conditions. In the Perfect Cue condition the frequency of the target stimulus was always the same as the cue. A range of frequencies were tested, each in separate blocks of trials. In the Probable Cue condition the frequency of the cue was always 1000 Hz. The frequency of the target was also 1000 Hz on 75% of the trials. Thus, on these trials, the cue was "valid." On the remaining 25%, the cue was "invalid," since the target frequency was different from 1000 Hz. On half of the invalid trials the target frequency was lower than 1000 Hz and on the other half it was higher than 1000 Hz. The frequency difference on invalid trials varied between subjects, ranging from a difference of 400 Hz for some subjects to a difference of just 25 Hz for other subjects.

Figure 2.13 shows the results (Scharf et al., 1987). Regardless of the frequency of the cue, subjects identified the correct interval in over 90%

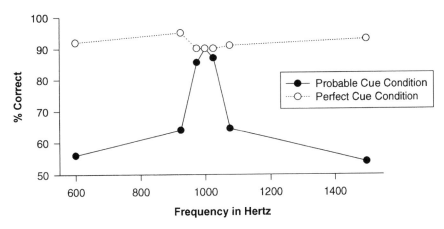

Figure 2.13 Attention can be directed to a particular frequency. The filled circles show how well subjects were able to detect a sound when they were expecting a 1000 Hz sound. Performance is quite accurate around the expected frequency and falls off dramatically for more distant frequencies. The results cannot be attributed to poorer sensitivity for the noncued frequencies. If subjects are directed to expect the target at the other frequencies on separate trials (open circles), performance was almost perfect. (Adapted from Scharf et al., 1987.)

of the trials in the Perfect Cue conditions. Thus, attention could readily be directed to any of the test frequencies. Now consider the results for the Probable Cue condition, in which the cue led subjects to expect a 1000 Hz target. When the cue was valid performance was quite accurate. Indeed, there was no difference in performance in valid trials compared to performance in the Perfect Cue condition with a 1000 Hz target. As the frequency of the target in the invalid trials became more different from the cue, however, performance deteriorated rapidly. Indeed, if the frequency of the target was just 75 Hz off the cued frequency (925 Hz or 1075 Hz), subjects were barely better than chance at determining which of the two intervals contains the target. For the most distant invalid target frequencies, performance was at chance.

Those results indicate a number of important characteristics of the selective attention process in audition. First, as shown by the uniform results in the Perfect Cue conditions, subjects demonstrate excellent flexibility in focusing on the task-relevant frequency. Scharf et al. did not include a control condition in which no cue was given and the target could appear at any one of the stimulus frequencies. However, Johnson and Hafter (1980) performed a similar experiment and found that there are benefits associated with pure-tone cues. Without a cue a target had to be louder in order to be detected than when the same target was preceded by a cue.

Second, there is a cost associated with selective attention. Detection of targets at non-cued frequencies is reduced. Moreover, the band-pass characteristics of the selective attention mechanism for this task appears to be extremely narrow. It is also important to note that the deployment of attention in this task need not be driven by the cue. Scharf et al. (1987) obtained similar results when experienced subjects were simply informed of the target frequency probabilities and the cue was eliminated.

Similar results have been obtained in tasks relating to visual perception. Davis (1981; Davis & Graham, 1981) used a similar procedure with low contrast sinusoidal gratings. The subjects' task was to indicate which of two intervals contained a stimulus. In Fixed Frequency conditions the stimulus frequency was invariant within a block of trials and ranged between blocks from 1–16 cycles/degree. In Mixed Frequency conditions the subjects were informed that in 95% of the trials the spatial frequency of the stimulus would be 4.0 cycles/degree. In the remaining trials the spatial frequency of the stimulus was either lower or higher. Rates of detection of the 4 cycles/degree stimulus was essentially unchanged between the two conditions. In contrast, detection of the low-probability stimuli was markedly reduced. For example, detection of a 1 cycle/degree stimulus was at chance in the Mixed Frequency condition, presumably because the observers restricted their attention to information in the vicinity of the expected 4 cycle/degree stimulus. The fall-off in performance for probe frequencies that were higher than the expected frequency was not as dramatic, but was still considerable.

In both modalities, the evidence indicates that attention can facilitate processing of frequency information, which can be selected to reflect current processing demands. Thus, this attentional mechanism serves as the first filtering process on a frequency representation. The tasks used by Ivry and Lebby (1993) favored the selection of a narrow region of the auditory spectrum. In contrast, many situations would require attention to be broadly tuned. The subject may not know which region of the spectrum will contain the relevant information, or identification of the stimulus may require processing of a wide range of frequencies. For example, as is discussed in chapter 6, speech perception entails analysis of information across a broad spectrum. We assume that, as a default, the full range of spectral information is selected by the first filtering operation. This filter can, however, focus on a restricted region of information as a function of task demands. (For simplicity, we have lumped those two attentional processes—range assessment and range adjustment—into the first filtering stage. It remains possible that these operations are performed by separable mechanisms.)

The Second Frequency Filtering Stage: Asymmetric Processing of Selected Information by the Two Hemispheres

The process model developed to this point does not postulate any differences in the representations derived by the two hemispheres. The sensory representation is assumed to be (approximately) symmetric, and the first filtering stage provides an attentional mechanism for amplifying the task-relevant region of the sound and/or spatial frequency spectrum.

To account for hemispheric asymmetries it is necessary to add another processing stage, a stage at which additional filtering is performed on the selected information. Specifically, it is proposed that information undergoes differential filtering in the two cerebral hemispheres when higher-order analyses are required, as in identification or discrimination tasks. Processing in the right hemisphere is characterized as a low-pass filtering operation. In contrast, left hemisphere processing is characterized as a high-pass filtering operation. The central hypothesis of the DFF theory is that the output of those filtering operations underlies many of the laterality effects reported in visual and auditory perception.

Figure 2.14 shows a simple depiction of what is meant by low-pass and high-pass filtering of a selected region of frequency information. The bottom part of the figure shows the initial sensory representation and the operation of the attentional filtering mechanism, which is identical to that shown in figure 2.12. As shown in the top part of the figure, the selected information is then filtered for a second time, and it is here that the two hemispheres perform different computations. The shapes of the hemispheric filters convey how different regions of the selected information are amplified and attenuated. The low-pass property of the right hemisphere filter is due to the fact that it amplifies information in the lower frequency range of the selected information while attenuating the relatively higher frequencies. Correspondingly, the high-pass property of the left hemisphere filter amplifies the higher frequency information of the selected range while attenuating the lower frequencies. Hemispheric asymmetries based on relative frequency information thus arise through the transformation of sensory information through two, frequency-based, filtering processes.

Examples of how asymmetric filtering could produce the laterality effects observed by Ivry and Lebby (1993) are given in figure 2.15. The left column depicts sensory representations that might arise to the same stimulus in two separate trials. The actual frequency is indicated by the arrow, and for this stimulus the correct response would be "low." The stimulus is assumed to activate a set of frequency-tuned detectors. The activation is highest in those detectors whose optimal tuning is set to the stimulus frequencies. Detectors tuned to neighboring frequencies are also activated, but to a lesser degree. Differences in sensory representation occur due to variation in vigilance or neural noise. Thus, although the stimulus is the same in both examples, the representation in the top row is of higher fidelity than is the representation in the bottom row.

The second column in figure 2.15 shows the asymmetric filtering operations performed by the two hemispheres, and the third column shows the resulting hemispheric representations. If the sounds had been presented in the right ear, then the high-pass filtering operation of the left hemisphere would result in the representations shown at the right end of the first and third rows. If the sounds had been presented in the left

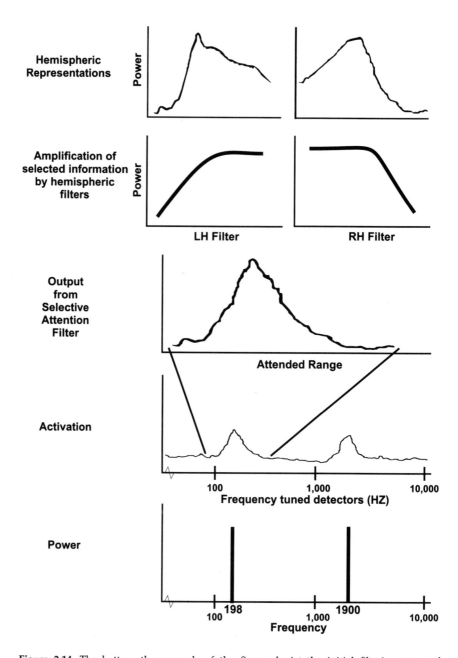

Figure 2.14 The bottom three panels of the figure depict the initial filtering stage of task-relevant information and are identical to figure 2.12. The top part of the figure shows the second filtering stage. The left hemisphere is assumed to operate as a high-pass filter; the right hemisphere is assumed to operate as a low-pass filter. Nonidentical representations emerge when those secondary hemispheric filters are applied to the information selected by the first filtering stage.

ear, then the low-pass filtering operation of the right hemisphere would result in the representations shown in the second and fourth rows.

In these examples, the hemispheric representations were obtained by simply multiplying the activation and amplification levels for each frequency. This transformation is quite rudimentary, and the actual process most likely involves more complicated computations such as convolutions operators, nonlinear activation functions, and competitive processes (De Valois & De Valois, 1990; Marr, 1982). However, the goal here is simply to demonstrate how errors can occur, given asymmetric filters.

Perceptual judgments are based on the activation function that results from the asymmetric filtering process. A simple decision rule would be to base the judgment on the point of greatest activation. In the auditory experiments of Ivry and Lebby, the subjects' decisions were categorical: a stimulus was identified as being either lower or higher in frequency than the average frequency for that set. To reflect this binary decision, the region below the midpoint is shaded in figure 2.15. If the point of greatest activation falls in the shaded region, the subject will respond, "low"; otherwise the subject will respond, "high." In rows 1–3, the peak activation is from an output unit that falls within the shaded region. Thus, the response is correct for these trials. In row 4, the output unit that is most strongly activated falls outside the shaded region. The response on this trial would thus be "high" and would be incorrect. The shift into the incorrect "high" region is the result of high-pass filtering of a stimulus, which produced a noisy sensory representation. The high-pass filter amplifies the high frequency "noise."

To summarize, figure 2.15 shows the critical processing stages of the DFF theory that lead to laterality effects from frequency-based representations. Although these examples were derived to account for asymmetric representations of sound frequencies, the same mechanisms could be applied to spatial frequency representations. The essential feature of the theory is that laterality effects in perception may result from an asymmetric postsensory filtering stage, with the left hemisphere filter characterized as a high-pass filter and the right hemisphere as a low-pass filter. In other words, the asymmetric filters impose a bias in terms of which frequencies receive the greatest amplification. The initial filtering, used to select a range of frequency information, allows the asymmetries to be based on relative frequency rather than on absolute frequency. If information across the entire sensory spectrum was passed on to the hemispheric filters, laterality effects would be expected in terms of absolute frequency.

Before concluding this chapter, we want to make a few final points concerning the DFF theory. First, the low- and high-pass filters depicted in figure 2.15 are extreme: there is little fall-off in amplification for frequencies on one side of the midpoint, and there is a sharp cutoff for frequencies on the other side. Those choices were made to make clear the

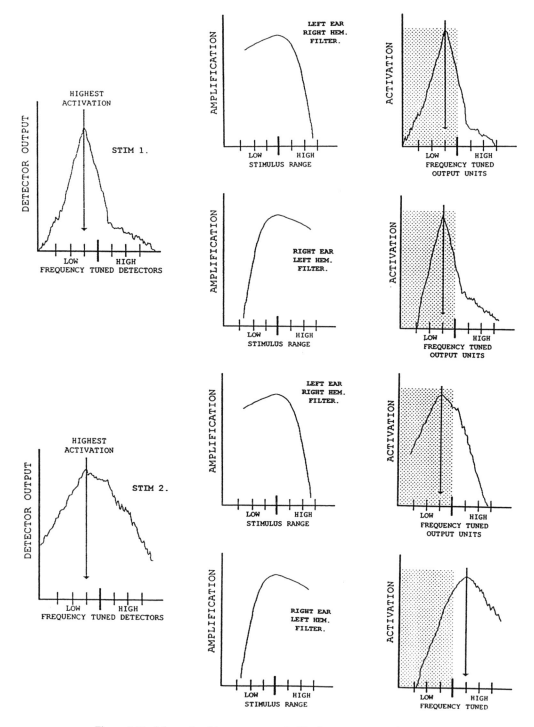

Figure 2.15 Schematic of how asymmetric filtering can account for the biases reported by Ivry and Lebby (1993). The hemispheric representations (right column) follow two filtering stages and serve as the basis for the perpetual classifications. Subjects will respond "low" when the peak activation falls to the left of the criterion point (thick hash mark on the

basic assumptions of the theory. We do not know of any biological or psychophysical data that favor such radically shaped filters, and we believe it is a fertile area for future research to explore.

A more important question centers on whether the selection and asymmetric filtering mechanisms constitute two distinct processing stages. In the following two chapters on visual perception and attention, we review neuropsychological evidence that suggests that those two filtering processes are independent. Specifically, we will review data that indicate the two mechanisms can be disrupted independently and that the critical neural areas associated with each mechanism are distinct.

At a computational level, however, there is an alternative way to conceptualize how a filtering mechanism might yield an asymmetry in the representation of frequency information. In that alternative the hemispheric filters are assumed to be symmetric, but the spectral positioning of the filters is asymmetric. Within the selected region the left hemisphere filter is centered at a higher frequency than the right hemisphere filter (figure 2.16). Asymmetric representations would be created by offsetting the position of symmetric filters.

Note that, over trials, it would appear as if the left hemisphere was operating as a high-pass filter and that the right hemisphere was operating as a low-pass filter. Moreover, even within the alternative model, there are really two different aspects to the filtering process. One aspect concerns selecting the range of the filtering process; that is, the extent of frequency information that is critical for achieving current processing goals. The second aspect concerns the positioning of the filters. It continues to be the second component that would produce different representations for the two cerebral hemispheres. As in the basic version of the DFF theory, two filtering operations are required to account for asymmetries in terms of relative frequency.

SUMMARY

This chapter provides the motivation for and a description of the double filtering by frequency theory of hemispheric specialization in perception. We began by pointing out that information in the world is contained at multiple scales. Frequency-sensitive detectors provide the nervous system with one means for representing this multiplicity, using common computational mechanisms in both vision and audition. Moreover, experimental results suggest that, across the two modalities, there are similarities in how the two hemispheres asymmetrically represent frequency

horizontal axis) and "high" when the peak activation falls to the right of that point. In all four examples, the correct response is "low." However, the combination of a noisy sensory representation and the left hemisphere's high-pass filtering operation leads to an error in the bottom row.

A Theory of Hemispheric Asymmetries in Perception

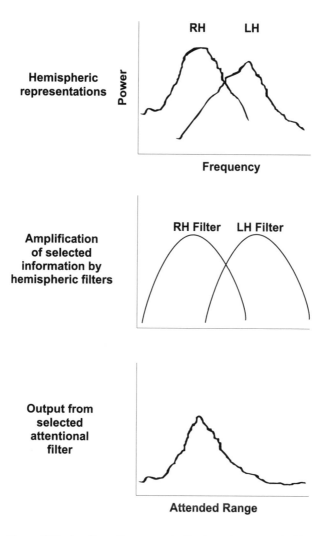

Figure 2.16 An alternative conceptualization of asymmetric filtering by frequency in the two hemispheres. In this scheme both hemispheric filters are symmetric. However, the right hemisphere filter is centered over a lower frequency than is the left hemisphere filter. This offset will create asymmetric representations. Note that this model also contains two filtering stages, one associated with selection of task-relevant information and the second associated with the nonidentical placement of the left and right hemisphere filters.

information. At the heart of the DFF theory is the idea that symmetric sensory representations undergo two filtering stages. First, an initial filtering process selects task-relevant frequency information. Second, the two hemispheres impose asymmetric filters on the selected information. The asymmetric filtering operation yields nonidentical representations, which may differ in how well they provide the information required to perform particular tasks.

In the following chapters we turn to the behavioral and neural evidence that has motivated the DFF theory. The theory offers a parsimonious framework for integrating laterality results across a wide range of task domains. In addition, we identify predictions generated by the theory and places where our theorizing is at odds with other accounts of hemispheric specialization. At present, evaluation of the DFF theory is still in its infancy, and the theory is best seen as one post hoc interpretation of disparate empirical findings. How well the DFF theory meets the challenge of accounting for the existing laterality literature is an important prerequisite for determining its value as a generator of novel tests of hemispheric specialization.

3 Visual Perception: Lateralization in Simple and Complex Patterns

Objects are seldom viewed in isolation. Pillows are typically seen in the context of bed sets, couches, or chairs; doors appear in the context of buildings; an eye is accompanied by a nose and a mouth. The visual system has evolved in a world where objects are spatially related to other objects both metrically (as with one object being located at some distance from another) and hierarchically (as with one object being a part of another). Studies of functional hemispheric differences have consistently shown that hierarchical patterns are processed differently by the two hemispheres. In this chapter we focus on experiments that have demonstrated these differences, and we discuss the relevance of the DFF theory, introduced in chapter 2, in accounting for these findings. We begin with discussions of experiments using simple stimuli and progress to studies using more complex stimuli. Issues of anatomical areas involved in the differences are also included, as are alternative accounts that have been proposed.

COMPUTATIONAL PROBLEM

Spatial relationships between objects vary in complexity. For instance, one object may be separated from another object by a distance (the pillow may be tossed across the room), or one object may be embedded in another to produce a part/whole relationship. An eye is a local part of a more global face, and a face is a local part of a more global head. Several aspects of this type of part/whole relationship are important. First, an object's status as a part or a whole is relative: a face is a local part of a head but it is also the global whole containing eyes. Second, the more global an object is, the larger it is. Third, this type of part/whole relationship is perceptually different from a logically similar relationship between angles and lines that can be arranged to form a shape. For instance, the horizontal line that defines the front edge of a desk is embedded in the rectangular figure that is the desk as a whole. Yet what we perceive is not a hierarchical stimulus with one object (the edge) embedded in another object (the desk). Instead, we see a desk, and if anything, the drawers as its local parts.

It is likely that a different computational process takes place in the perception of the part/whole relationship of the drawer to the desk than takes place in the perception of the relationship of the front edge to the desk, since our perception of the two are so vastly different. The differences in computational processes are also evident in the patient drawings shown in figure 2.2, which were introduced in the previous chapter. What computations are necessary to perceive the part/whole relationship itself? How does the brain determine where an object is in a hierarchical structure, and in turn, how does that influence what the object is perceived to be?

These questions are reminiscent of a different dichotomy that has been central in recent theories of visual perception; namely, the two processing pathways through the visual cortex that are proposed to be involved in the analysis of "what" versus "where" (Ungerleider & Mishkin, 1982). The dorsal "where" pathway runs through the parietal lobe and has been implicated in certain types of spatial analysis, such as locating an object in one location versus another. The ventral "what" pathway runs through the temporal lobe and is implicated in object recognition. It turns out that the ventral system is also involved in global/local shape identification, whereas the dorsal system seems to be more involved in selective attention to a given level or relative size. That is, the principles governing part/whole perception of objects may have some similarity to those governing perception of objects separated in space and defined by discrete locations.

The ubiquity of hierarchical structures in the natural environment, and our seemingly effortless ability to perceive these structures, brings up a pressing problem that applies across types of spatial structure. How does individuation of potential objects occur? One answer for simple spatial structure is that objects are separated in coordinate space. An object on the left side of space could be perceived as separate from one on the right simply because they are spatially separated on the retina. They may also be separated in body space or in environmental space, since these are spaces that still have a metric structure.

The problem is larger than this. Even if we perceive a certain distance between parts and know the coordinate space in which the distance occurs, that knowledge provides little information about whether the two separated parts are parts of a larger object. So, the problem of perceiving hierarchical spatial structure cannot be solved simply by noting where a global object falls versus a local object in metric space. Something more is needed.

Thus, it would seem that different processes must be involved in determining where an object is in hierarchical space than are involved in determining where it is in coordinate space, even if some underlying principles might be the same, such as the need to parse a stimulus into "blobs" that can act as candidate objects. One feature that consistently differentiates global from local objects is size, or more precisely, relative size or relative resolution. Relative size may be used at least as a beginning step to meet the computational goal of perceiving what potential objects are present and how they might be spatially related to one another.

There are other features that may help solve this problem of parsing into candidate objects but they are not sufficient to account for the data that will be discussed in this chapter. Familiarity surely plays a role in object identification, even when other cues that may be used to discriminate objects are not evident (figure 3.1 shows an example). Although shape familiarity can speed the perception of objects, it does not appear to be necessary for the perception of part/whole perceptual organization. In figure 3.2 the smaller shapes are perceived to be parts of a larger shape even though they are not particularly familiar.

The spatial arrangement of local elements may also be important. This can be seen in the examples in figure 3.3. The *A* is perceived to be an integral part of the *H* when it is aligned with the other local elements, but much less so when it is offset. But note that the relative resolution or size of items within a defined area would also seem to be useful in

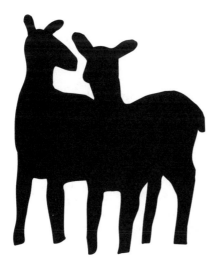

Figure 3.1 An example of top-down control of perception. We perceive two deer, not one with two heads and six legs.

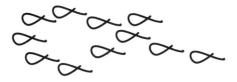

Figure 3.2 Although both the global and local forms are unfamiliar objects, the hierarchical structure of the form can be readily seen.

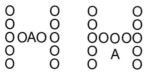

Figure 3.3 The *A* in the figure on the left appears to be more integrated with the global form than the *A* in the figure on the right.

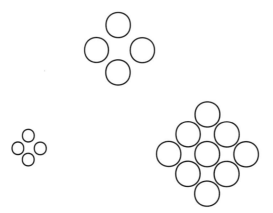

Figure 3.4 The two patterns on the bottom are both similar to the standard on top but in different ways. The lower left-hand pattern differs in overall size but maintains the relative size of the global and local levels of the standard. The lower right-hand pattern differs in overall size and number of local objects but maintains the absolute size of the local elements. Most people judge the pattern on the left as more like the standard than the pattern on the right.

determining the part/whole relationships (figure 3.4). For instance, the *A* in the right pattern would more likely be seen as a part of the global form in figure 3.3 if we moved away from the page. The relative sizes of global form and of all its local elements would covary. That information could then signal that the global and local items are linked as a unit, which could overcome the initial perception of an *A* unattached to the global *H*. Although motion is an important cue for object integration and segregation, it is not necessary for perceiving part/whole relationships per se. This exercise points to important properties of part/whole determination. First, it demonstrates that in static displays there is a continuum of the likelihood that an element will be perceived as part of a global form. Second, an extra feature such as motion can bind the parts together more firmly because, especially with motion, the relative size is maintained. It would seem, then, that part of the computational solution for perceiving objects that are composed of individual parts could be to make use of relative size or spatial frequency information. Regardless of how we view a face, from a few inches away or from a great distance, the eyes, nose, and mouth will retain the same relative size, surrounded by the contours that define the shape of the face.

One theory that has been proposed in cognitive psychology to solve the part/whole problem (discussed in chapter 1) posits that perceptual analysis begins with the most global object (Navon, 1977). However, a computational model that conforms to that aspect of global precedence theory does not capture the complexity of the problem to be solved. A system in which the global form of a scene or object always had to be perceived before the local form would quickly become inefficient and cumbersome. Each time the scene changed, we would have to first identify the larger objects in the visual field, then the next largest object, and so forth until the object of importance was attended. Under those conditions, it could take a lifetime to read this book. Every time the page changed or a new line began, perception would be compelled to begin again at the most global level. For those reasons, global precedence theory—with its claim that global information cannot be ignored—seems incomplete. Although global attention must play some role (see chapter 4), early visual segregation of a visual scene need not be a slave to global information. A more efficient system would be one of divide and conquer, which is what the DFF theory proposes.

In this chapter we discuss the evidence from normal and brain-damaged populations that initially motivated and provided support for the DFF theory. In addition, we begin to make finer distinctions within the hemispheres that are important in visual processing differences between the two hemispheres. Sensory factors are also considered, and alternative theories to account for global/local by hemisphere interactions are evaluated. In chapter 4 we examine the proposed contributions of spatial attentional processes to hemispheric differences and discuss their interaction with bottom-up perceptual effects that are the topic of the present chapter.

LATERALITY EFFECTS IN VISUAL PERCEPTION: EVIDENCE FROM STUDIES WITH HEALTHY YOUNG SUBJECTS

Normally, people do not see parts floating in a haphazard space, but rather see those parts as forming a coherent whole. Yet people with brain damage can experience such segregated percepts. The essential premise of the DFF theory acknowledges both of these perceptual facts. We postulate that the two hemispheres are each capable of representing the full complexity of the visual scene. But, we also argue that the two hemispheres do not represent that information with identical fidelity. Rather, the visual system in humans and other animals appears to have evolved to use a different strategy. The right hemisphere is biased toward global features of a scene, whereas the left hemisphere is biased toward details or local features.

As pointed out in chapter 1, the first hints of the functional asymmetry in organization emerged from the study of patients with neurological disorders. It was the study of abnormal perception that helped to reveal the differences in function of the two hemispheres in spatial cognition. It is important that these data be complemented by the study of normal perception. It is always possible that people who study the visual experience of neurological patients are studying a qualitatively different form of perception. Compensatory strategies or new neural interactions may produced unique forms of perception. Moreover, brain injury does not just produce negative symptoms or the loss of certain capabilities. It can also introduce positive symptoms or the manifestation of new forms of behavior. With this in mind, we begin our discussion of visual perception by reviewing some of the critical studies that have assessed visual laterality effects in healthy subjects. Discussions in later sections will demonstrate that the evidence from various populations converge to support similar conclusions that are consistent with the DFF theory.

Experiments with Simple Gratings

Whereas the natural world provides a dazzling array of visual complexities, the scientific investigation of vision has benefited from the development of simple experimental paradigms. As discussed in chapter 2, the use of sinusoidal gratings has proven to be a powerful tool in the study of vision. The information content of those stimuli can be easily described and manipulated. One-dimensional sinusoidal gratings provide perhaps the simplest stimulus. A single parameter, brightness, is varied as a function of position. The rate of variation determines the spatial frequency of the stimulus.

As pointed out in the preceding chapter, any complex stimulus can be formally described as the sum of a set of sinusoids. Moreover, it has been shown that the responses of visual cells vary as a function of the spatial frequency components of visual input. We propose that different representations arise because of the ways in which the two hemispheres perform postsensory processing on spectral information. With this in mind, the most direct tests of the DFF theory come from studies in which the stimuli are sinusoidal gratings.

Chapter 2 provided a brief review of a few such studies. The key finding is that people are faster in identifying a stimulus composed of "thin" stripes or gratings (i.e., high spatial frequency) when the gratings are presented in the right visual field compared to the left visual field; conversely, a stimulus composed of "thick" stripes or gratings (i.e., low spatial frequency) is more quickly identified when presented in the left visual field. This interaction between visual field and "thickness" of the stripes provides support for the hypothesis of hemispheric specialization based on the analysis of spatial frequency information.

While such an interaction is impressive, it is also important to note the presence of a consistent null effect when the task is changed. Visual field differences have not been reported when subjects are merely asked to detect a grating, regardless of whether the stimulus is composed of "thin" or "thick" lines (Kitterle & Kay, 1985; Kitterle & Christman, 1991; Rao, Rourke, & Whitman, 1981). Those null effects can be found when stimuli are shown above threshold and are clearly perceived, as well as when the stimuli are presented near threshold. "Near threshold" in this case simply means that the brightness level of the stimuli is at a level where people are just above chance in detecting the stimulus. "Above threshold" in this case refers to a luminance level at which the stimuli are clearly visible. Measures other than reaction time (e.g., accuracy) are required under near threshold conditions. Varying the luminance, and therefore the perceived brightness, produces large differences in response times and detection. As would be expected, performance is better for brighter stimuli than for dimmer ones. Nonetheless, laterality effects have not been found in detection tasks with sinusoidal gratings.

Taken together, the results from visual field studies comparing identification and detection tasks suggest that hemispheric differences emerge at later stages of processing, after the initial representation of spatial frequency information. The visual field effects arise when subjects have to discriminate or identify which stimulus appeared. They arise when subjects have to make a judgment based on relative spatial frequency: "these bars are wider than the other bars"; "there is a thin as opposed to a wide bar in the stimulus." In simple detection tasks relative analyses are not necessary. It is not necessary to determine whether the stimulus is "wide" or "thin," but only that a stimulus is present.

Our conclusion that the hemispheres do not differ in initial registration is based on a null effect in detection studies, which is not a strong result on which to base any conclusion. It is possible that there are small hemispheric differences in the representation of absolute frequency (Zani & Proverbio, 1995; but also see Rebai, Mecacci, Bagot, & Bonnet, 1989). Whether or not such small differences exist, however, we must still account for the hemispheric differences in terms of relative frequency as well.

If future evidence does support an absolute frequency difference, a later stage that responds to relative frequency would still be necessary in order to account for the evidence we have discussed in this section and in chapter 2. Under conditions in which the absolute frequency remained the same but the task required comparisons of the relatively lower or relatively higher frequency, relative frequency predicted the direction of visual field differences.

Whatever the case turns out to be concerning lateralization of absolute frequency, the evidence is very strong that hemispheric differences appear rather early in visual processing and can be attributed to the higher and lower spatial frequency information in the stimulus.

Implications and Importance of Relative Frequency

The data as a whole suggest that if subjects do not need to attend to the spectral content of a stimulus, laterality effects may not be found (Sergent, 1983). That hypothesis helps account for some of the null results that have been reported when spatial frequency content has been manipulated but has not been very useful in performing the task (such as with detection). This may also be the basis of the difference in the data discussed at the end of the last section.

When there was no need for the subjects to utilize the spectral content of the stimuli in performing the task, laterality effects were not evident. Simple detection does not yield visual field differences. Laterality effects emerge when there is a need to select certain frequency information for use in further processing. The behavioral data have shown that differences in relative frequency analysis arise because of differences that result as a function of that selection process. When a subject must identify a shape at one level or the other, the absolute size of the overall pattern cannot account for the visual field differences. Thus, it becomes critical to examine the relationship between the spatial frequency content of the stimuli and how a particular task exploits that information. The DFF theory does not predict that simply reducing the energy in the higher or lower frequencies of a stimulus will reveal hemispheric differences. Laterality effects should emerge when those manipulations change the specific frequency content that is useful for performing a particular task. If the frequency spectrum is reduced to the extent that it is no longer easily available for use in further processing or to the extent that there is only one frequency present and relevant (as in a sinusoidal grating and a simple detection task), then visual field differences may not emerge.

Consider one of the simplest manipulations of frequency information: changing the viewing distance between an observer and a stimulus. For example, if the stimulus is moved away from the viewer, then in absolute terms the spectrum will shift to higher frequencies. Indeed, information that had been carried at the lowest absolute frequencies for the close viewing distance will no longer be present at the farther distance, and information carried at the highest frequencies for the close viewing distance will also be lost when it exceeds the limit of human resolution. This example provides a mechanistic account of how the ability to perceive fine details is lost when things become distant (figure 3.5).

If a car is viewed from a distance of 5 feet, it may cover most of the visual field; as a whole stimulus it produces a very low fundamental frequency, and objects as parts (e.g. the windows of the car, the side mirror, the keyhole on the handle used to unlock the door) are defined by higher frequencies. As the car drives away, the keyhole may be the first to exceed the limits of higher frequency resolution, and it will no longer be visible. The car will continue to be perceived as a whole object,

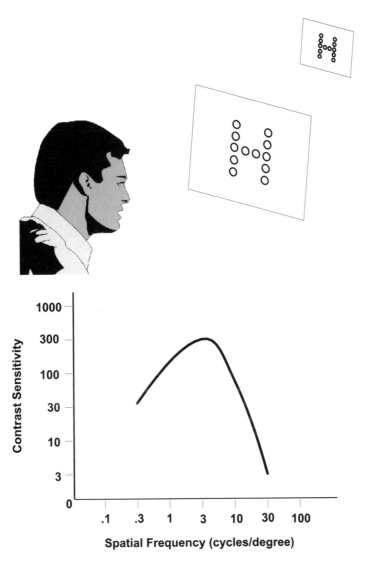

Figure 3.5 Stylized mean contrast-sensitivity function for different spatial frequencies. oving a figure away from an observer decreases the absolute lower spatial frequencies in the pattern. However, the spatial frequency of global to local elements remains constant.

but as it moves, its fundamental frequency will be represented in vision with higher and higher absolute frequencies. Nevertheless, whatever this higher frequency may be, it will continue to be the lowest frequency that defines the car relative to the frequencies that define the windows.

In figure 3.5 the close, large *H* could have a fundamental frequency somewhere in the range of 3 cycles per degree, but the *H*'s frequency would be much higher in the distant, smaller *H*. Yet the lowest frequency in the hierarchical letter pattern would be defined by the global *H*. A change in viewing distance would not by itself be expected to produce changes in laterality effects. That is, if an observer were asked to identify an object at the two distances, we would not expect there to be a left visual field advantage for the close distance and a right visual field advantage for the far distance. The manipulation of distance changes the absolute spatial frequency values. It does not affect relative frequency information, except when the stimulus surpasses the frequencies that can be resolved by the visual system.

On the other hand, suppose that an identification task requires an analysis of a particular part of an object. For example, we might be trying to find a friend who wears framed glasses in a crowd of people. The glasses would be carried in the relatively high-frequency portion of the signal, while the outline of the friend's face (along with the outlines of other faces in the crowd) would be carried in a relatively lower frequency portion. Therefore, the left hemisphere should provide a slight advantage, due to the relatively higher fidelity needed to identify the friend based on the glasses. If we could measure a laterality effect in such an instance, we would expect it to exist in this case. The advantage should occur regardless of viewing distance (within acuity limits), as the glasses will continue to be carried in the relatively high-frequency range across changes in absolute frequency. Of course, if the person were at a distance at which the glasses were no longer perceivable, then the laterality effect would be lost, but so would the perception of the glasses themselves.

Experiments with Complex Stimuli

Studies of laterality with normal subjects have been conducted using more complex patterns than sinusoidal gratings, such as the hierarchical letter pattern used by Navon (figure 3.5). Recall that the overall shape of those stimuli may be a letter such as an *H* or *S* created from the repetition of local-level letters, which may also be the letters *H* or *S*. Of course, other forms can be used, such as a *C* created from *O*s or a triangle created from rectangles, and so on. Navon instructed subjects to identify the global form in one block of trials and the local form in another block of trials in his initial studies.

As described in chapter 1, Navon observed two primary findings. First, global identification occurred faster than local identification. Second, global information interfered with local identification, but local information did not interfere with global identification. That is, identification of the local letter occurred even more slowly when the global shape was inconsistent with the local elements, as opposed to when it was consistent. This result, effecting only the local form, has been termed *global interference.*

Navon was interested in normal visual function and in issues surrounding global or local precedence. Although he presented stimuli in the right or left visual field, he collapsed over visual fields when analyzing his data. It was only later that others showed visual field differences for the speed of global and local identification. Martin (1979b) was the first to demonstrate a visual field difference in responses to global and local forms using Navon's patterns and methods. In each trial a hierarchical letter pattern was presented in either the right or left visual field; subjects were directed to report the local letter in one block of trials and the global letter in another. Local letters were responded to more rapidly in the right visual field than in the left. Global letters were responded to more rapidly in the left visual field than in the right, but that effect did not reach significant levels. As in Navon's studies, responses were faster overall in global trials, and in local trials global interference was evident.

A few years later Sergent (1982) also reported a visual field difference in identification of global and local letters in hierarchical letter patterns. She changed the procedure to a divided attention task, and made the task somewhat more difficult by adding a memory set. Subjects were told to report whether or not a letter from the memory set occurred in each stimulus. The target letter could appear at either the global or local level. The subjects were not directed to attend to one level or the other. They were simply told to report a target if it was present, regardless of the level at which it appeared. Like Martin, Sergent found a right visual field advantage for local responses. In addition, the left visual field advantage for global targets reached significant levels in her studies.

Other studies have linked analysis of forms in hierarchical letter patterns directly to the spatial frequency content of global and local information. The global advantage in speed of identification is reduced or eliminated when low spatial frequency energy is reduced, as in figure 3.6 (Hughes, Fendrich, & Reuter-Lorenz, 1990; Lamb & Yund, 1996: Robertson, 1996). Under such conditions the hierarchical structure of the pattern remains, but the lower frequencies are all but eliminated. Both the global and the local shapes can be resolved only through the remaining higher frequency information. When low spatial frequency energy is reduced, global forms are identified at about the same speed as are local forms. Note that this procedure eliminates the relative frequency information that normally defines global and local shapes. Both global and local forms are defined in terms of absolute frequencies.

Other studies using quite different procedures have also linked global and local identification to the spatial frequency content of the pattern. Shulman, Sullivan, Gish, and Sakoda (1986) used an adaptation procedure. They had subjects stare at a sinusoidal grating and then they presented subjects with a hierarchical letter pattern. In one block of trials subjects were required to report the letter at the local level, and in another block they were required to report the letter at the global level. The gratings the subjects stared at were either high or low frequency. As predicted, adaptation to higher frequencies slowed local responses, and adaptation to lower frequencies slowed global responses.

Figure 3.6 Examples of a hierarchical letter pattern made from contrast-balanced dots that reduces the energy in low spatial frequencies.

Shulman and Wilson (1987) went on to show that attention to a global or a local target affected detection of higher or lower frequency gratings. They directed subjects to identify the global or local letter in a Navon pattern, and then presented subjects with a grating with either lower or higher frequencies. When attention was directed to the global level, detection of lower frequency gratings improved; when attention was directed to the local level, detection of higher frequency gratings improved. There were both perceptual and attentional links between identification of a global pattern and lower frequencies and between identification of a local pattern and higher frequencies. Those results demonstrate that spatial frequencies are used in the identification of global and local forms. The results of Shulman and colleagues were collected using only central presentation, so visual field differences could not be evaluated.

Other investigators attempted to test the spatial frequency hypothesis by indirect manipulation of spatial frequencies. Those manipulations included blurring the patterns, an effect that reduces high-frequency information; presenting the stimuli at different retinal eccentricities; manipulating presentation duration; and varying the size of the stimulus patterns (see Hellige, 1993). As noted previously, it is not sufficient to assume that altering the spatial frequency content will produce predictable changes in laterality effects. It is also necessary to consider how such changes alter the percept of relative frequency that can be used to complete the task.

For example, at some point, blurring can reduce the perception of a two-level pattern to a single-level pattern. This can be accomplished simply by looking at one of the patterns in figure 3.3 with squinted eyes. Although there would continue to be a relatively high and relatively low frequency in the smaller frequency range created by squinting the eyes, the ability to use these different spatial frequencies to perform the task would be more difficult.

This issue becomes important in the consideration of studies in which blurring was used to alter the spatial frequency content and to test the spatial frequency hypothesis. It may also explain why the evidence is mixed from studies using blurring. Jonsson and Hellige (1986) found that moderate blurring of letters in a same versus different task affected right visual field but not left visual field performance. Because blurring affects higher frequency information in a pattern, they concluded that their results supported the hypothesis that higher spatial frequencies are favored by the left hemisphere. Similar results were reported by Michimata and Hellige (1987) using nonsense figures. It should be noted that no independent measures were obtained to assess whether subjects were using the higher or lower spatial frequencies in those tasks. Since the forms were presented in pairs, subjects could have used the overall configuration carried by the lower frequencies, or they may have used detailed, high-frequency information. The frequency that subjects used may have varied depending on the particular stimulus form.

This point is especially important because several other investigators who varied absolute frequency did not find predicted differences even with a great deal of effort and stated sympathy for the idea (Chiarello, Senehi, & Soulier, 1986; Fendrich & Gazzaniga, 1990; Hardyck, 1991; Peterzell, 1991; Peterzell et al., 1989). Nevertheless, it is abundantly clear that visual field differences are affected by clarity of input, presentation duration, retinal eccentricity, and range of frequency components (Hellige, 1980, 1983; O'Boyle & Hellige, 1982; Tayler & Hellige, 1987). These differences were found with different types of patterns than those used by Navon. Until there is direct verification that subjects utilize the relatively high or relatively low frequencies in making their judgments (as opposed to the absolute high or low frequencies), these findings remain ambiguous in terms of their support for or refutation of the DFF theory. If the absolute frequencies are not sufficiently salient, their usefulness will be diminished, and if their usefulness is diminished, they may no longer produce hemispheric effects. An alternative account would hold that there are hemispheric differences that respond to both relative and absolute frequency; this account cannot be completely ruled out at this time. That alternative is at odds with the DFF theory's assumption that sensory representation in the primary cortex is symmetric. However, the remaining stages of processing do not rely on that assumption, and visual field differences in absolute frequency would simply increase the complexity of the theory. We would still need to explain how relative frequency effects arise, and this is one important contribution of the DFF theory to the understanding of functional hemispheric differences.

EVIDENCE FROM NEUROLOGICAL PATIENTS

As discussed at length in chapter 1, evidence from neurological patients first suggested hemispheric differences in visual-spatial abilities. Somewhat surprisingly, the initial support was not from the dramatic and obvious symptoms of unilateral neglect. In moderate to severe forms, unilateral neglect can be observed without sophisticated instruments and with no prompting by the observer. No equipment, tasks, or questions are necessary to notice a person turning away from his or her left side with the head and eyes turned away from the left side as well. Instead, it was the less dramatic differences in patients' drawings and ability to reach upon command that suggested the hypothesis that the two hemispheres may differ in how well they represent spatial information.

McFie and Zangwill (1960) were the first to report a qualitative difference in the drawings of patients with right versus left hemisphere damage (figure 3.7). Several other neuropsychologists and neurologists examined the drawings of their patients and concluded that motor plans were disrupted differently with right or left hemisphere damage (Piercy et al., 1960; Benton & Foegel, 1962; Arrigoni & De Renzi, 1964). Specifically, right hemisphere damage weakened manual output signals for configural or global properties such as overall orientation and location. Left hemisphere damage weakened motor persistence, which is required to draw several local parts or to fill in the details of patterns. In both cases accurate integration of parts and wholes did not appear in the drawings.

Benton (see De Renzi, 1982) was the first to suggest that, in order to draw both the configuration of a scene and its local parts, one had to have both parts and wholes available or explicitly represented. No amount of motor persistence would help if a patient did not perceive the

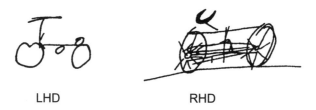

LHD   RHD

Figure 3.7 A patient with left hemisphere damage (LHD) left out the details or local parts of the drawing. A patient with right hemisphere damage (RHD) overemphasized the details by drawing them several times. (From McFie & Zangwill, 1960.)

local parts. Similarly, a patient could not be expected to arrange the parts into a coherent whole if he or she lacked a representation of the global configuration.

Studies conducted during that period also found a correlation between defective drawings and the arrangements of blocks in a Block Design task (Arrigoni & De Renzi, 1964), which is a standard test used in neuropsychological testing. The test begins by showing subjects a standard pattern on a sheet of paper, which remains in front of them for the duration of the trial (figure 3.8). Subjects are then given four or nine cubes with different designs on each side. The task is to arrange the cubes to form the standard pattern. As with drawing tasks, patients with right hemisphere damage are more likely to miss the overall pattern, whereas patients with left hemisphere damage are more likely to miss the details. Figure 3.8 shows an example of the finished product and the stages used to complete the task by a healthy normal subject, by a patient with right hemisphere damage, and by a patient with left hemisphere damage.

More recently, Kramer, Blusewicz, Robertson, and Preston (1989) showed that the different types of errors correlated positively with per-

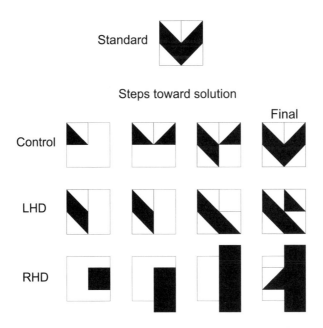

Figure 3.8 Block-design task used in neuropsychological testing. Subjects are presented with a standard pattern (top) and four blocks with darker, lighter, and two-toned sides. Subjects are told to create the standard from the blocks. Examples of the steps a normal control subject and patients may use to perform the task are given below the standard. The patient with left hemisphere damage (LHD) produced the overall configuration of the square but two of the inner blocks were rotated to disrupt the standard's form. The patient with right hemisphere damage (RHD) did not produce the overall square format of the pattern and ended with a vertical line and a protrusion. (Adapted from Kaplan, 1983.)

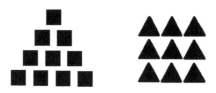

Figure 3.9 The pattern on the lower left has local forms in common with the standard (top), whereas the pattern on the lower right has the global configuration in common with the standard. Judgment of which pattern is more like the standard depends on the size ratio of the global to local forms. (From Kimchi & Palmer, 1982.)

formance on a similarity judgment task that used hierarchically structured visual stimuli. Each subject was given the traditional Block Design task and a series of triads of patterns with global and local levels (Goldmeier, 1972; Kimchi & Palmer, 1982). Each figure in each triad was constructed of geometric forms in which several local forms were arranged to create a global form (figure 3.9). There was a standard pattern at the top of the page, and two test patterns below it. One test pattern was globally similar to the standard (on the right in figure 3.9); the other was locally similar (on the left in figure 3.9). Subjects were asked to judge which test pattern was most similar to the standard. Individuals who were more likely to miss configural properties on the Block Design task were more likely to judge the similarity of the standard and test patterns based on local properties (i.e., they were more likely to choose the left pattern in figure 3.9). Individuals who were more likely to miss details on the Block Design task were more likely to judge the similarity of the standard and test patterns based on global properties (i.e., they were more likely to choose the right pattern in figure 3.9).

The analysis of stages performed while subjects solved the Block Design test further documented that the abstraction of global and local information was related to right or left hemisphere damage. Subjects worked toward a solution in different ways (figure 3.8). It is not just the final product of a spatial reproduction task that is important to consider, but also how the reproduction unfolds. For instance, in the Block Design task, two different patients may each work to an accurate solution, but the way in which they arrive at the same solution may be quite different. Patients with left hemisphere damage tend to make local errors, such as rotating individual elements (Kaplan, 1976). Patients with right hemisphere damage may reach the goal in a piecemeal manner; for example, they may place a block outside the overall configuration and only later notice its displacement.

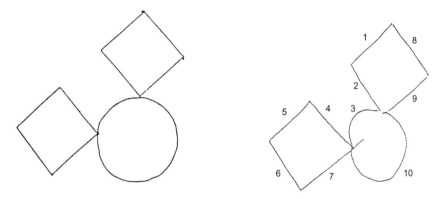

Figure 3.10 The pattern on the right is a patient's drawing of the standard on the left. Although the final product is similar to the standard, the numbers show the order and piecemeal fashion in which it was drawn. The patient started at the apex of the upper diamond, progressed downward to outline the boundaries on the left side, returned to the apex again, and progressed downward to outline the boundaries on the right side. (From Behrmann et al., 1994.)

A particularly good example of such procedural errors was reported by Behrmann, Moscovitch, and Winocur (1994). Their findings are reproduced in figure 3.10. The patient's final drawing closely approximates the target pattern, but the order in which the parts were drawn is quite bizarre. Rather than draw each figure one at a time, the patient began by drawing the left half of the diamond, then proceeded to draw one quarter of the circle, before moving on to the second diamond! Although this patient had strong neurological symptoms of right hemisphere damage (left-sided weakness and a left visual field problem), the patient had suffered a severe head trauma and the CT scans suggested some bilateral involvement.

Hemisphere Damage and Asymmetries on Global/Local Tasks

The drawings of patients clearly suggest hemispheric differences. However, there is still a question of whether local and global deficits reflect general problems in perception or a disconnection between perception and motor output. Is the phenomenon only observed when construction is required, as in drawing or manually assembling block parts to form wholes? This question was debated in neuropsychology for years. Part of the debate was driven by the methods of behavioral testing being used and by the strong emphasis placed on standardized neuropsychological tests. Those tests included several subtests that required manipulation or drawing. The ability to experimentally separate input deficits from output deficits was left for an era in which more sensitive measures were available.

Recent progress in that area was made by combining patient studies in neuropsychology with the methodologies of cognitive psychology. Delis, Robertson, and Efron (1986; also, see Robertson & Delis, 1986) compared groups of patients with unilateral lesions using a variety of tasks involving drawing and perception judgment. The results from the drawing studies, in accord with previous findings, showed a dissociation between right and left hemisphere damage and deficits on global and local features, respectively. (Examples of these drawings were presented in chapter 2). The dissociation pattern was also found in results from a memory-recognition task that required a choice between four alternative patterns. The subjects' task was to indicate by pointing which of the four test patterns was identical to a target pattern that they had seen 15 seconds previously. Only one of the alternative patterns matched the target at both the global and local levels. The other patterns differed from the target at either both levels or at one of the levels. That is, the "global only" alternative contained the correct global form but the incorrect local form. The "local only" alternative contained the correct local form but the incorrect global form. The "neither" alternative contained neither the correct global nor local form.

The patients rarely chose the pattern that was different from the target at both levels (the "neither" alternative). Rather, the two groups diverged in their performance from normal age-matched controls. The group with left hemisphere damage was more likely to choose a globally correct but locally incorrect form ("global only" alternative). The group with right hemisphere damage was more likely to choose a locally correct but globally incorrect form ("local only" alternative).

To test the generality of those effects, both linguistic and nonlinguistic geometric stimuli were included. There were some differences between the two stimulus sets. For example, a group of patients with left hemisphere damage had more trouble (and made more local errors) with the linguistic stimuli, whereas a group of patients with right hemisphere damage had more trouble (and made more global errors) with nonlinguistic stimuli. However, the dissociation between level and the side of the lesion was found for both types of stimuli.

It is difficult to reconcile these results with the hypothesis that laterality effects in part/whole perception are restricted to manual or response-decision rules. However, neither do the results provide direct support for a perceptual interpretation, given the memory demands of the matching-to-sample task that was used. To address this problem, Robertson and Delis (1986) used a task designed to examine global alignment effects in normal subjects (Palmer, 1980). Three equilateral triangles were presented, with each triangle constituting the local elements of the stimulus as shown in figure 3.11. Upon first viewing the figure, subjects were told to report the direction in which the middle triangle appeared to point. Palmer showed that the global alignment influenced the perceived orien-

Figure 3.11 Despite the fact that all the triangles are equilateral, we see them "point" in only one direction at any given moment. The triangles are typically perceived to be pointing in the direction of global alignment (downward and to the left in A; upward and to the left in B). (From Palmer, 1980.)

tation of the central, local element. For example, in figure 3.11A, subjects usually reported the central triangle as pointing downward and to the left toward seven o'clock on an imaginary clock face, but upward and to the left toward eleven o'clock in figure 3.11B.

Robertson and Delis (1986) presented stimuli such as these to healthy control subjects and to patients with left or right hemisphere damage. As in Palmer's study with college sophomores, the subjects' task was to report the direction in which the central triangle appeared to point. A group of patients with left hemisphere damage was more influenced by the global alignment than was the group of matched controls (figure 3.12). The patient group was more likely to say that the triangle pointed in the direction of alignment. A group of patients with right hemisphere damage was less influenced by the global alignment than was the group of matched controls (figure 3.12). This patient group was less likely to say that the triangle pointed in the direction of alignment. Each group diverged from normal performance, and the results were consistent with the global/local differences observed in patients with left or right hemisphere damage during other tasks (such as drawing or discriminating hierarchical letter patterns). When a single triangle was presented alone, no differences between groups were found.

Robertson, Lamb, and Knight (1988) went on to show that the divergence in performance for right and left hemisphere groups could be found in reaction-time measures when the response demands were limited to a button press and when the same button was to be pressed for decisions about either the global or local forms. In a study using hierarchical letter patterns, subjects were told that one of two letters would be present in every trial. In each trial a pattern was presented in the center of the screen for 100 ms. The subjects were required to press one button if the target was an *H* (whether global or local) and a different button if the target was an *S*. The expected results appeared. Right hemisphere damage slowed response time for global targets relative to local, and left hemisphere damage slowed response time for local targets relative to global. Finally, these differences were found in groups of patients with lesions in the region of the left or right temporal-parietal junction but not in patients with damage that did not impinge on these areas.

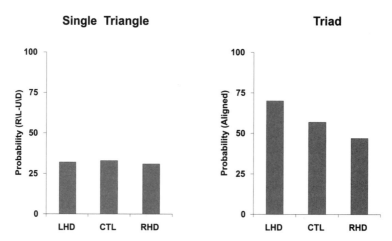

Figure 3.12 Patients with left hemisphere damage (LHD), right hemisphere damage (RHD), and normal age-matched control subjects (CTL) are influenced differently by global alignment of equilateral triangles. When a triangle was presented alone (Single Triangle), there were no differences between groups in the probability of the reported direction of pointing. When triangle triads were placed in alignment (Triad) as shown in Figure 3.11, the probability of reporting the triangle pointing in the aligned direction diverged from controls: probability was higher for the left hemisphere group than for the controls; probability was lower for right hemisphere patients than for the controls. (Adapted from Robertson and Delis, 1986.)

These patient studies are important for several reasons. First, they challenged the idea that spatial deficits in patients were restricted to manual problems. Second, the laterality effects did not appear to be related to different deficits in language abilities. The differences were present in both linguistic and nonlinguistic stimulus sets. Third, the global/local by group interactions were found across a wide range of tasks involving motor, perceptual, and memory skills. The results implicated a central processing difference for visual-spatial cognition. That conclusion is further supported by the converging evidence from reaction-time data using visual field presentation with young healthy college students, which was discussed earlier (e.g., Martin, 1979b; Sergent, 1982).

The 1988 study by Robertson, Lamb, and Knight was especially important because it went beyond the issue of right or left hemisphere damage to address questions about which areas within a hemisphere must be damaged to reveal the hemispheric differences. There were obvious limitations in the original studies by Delis et al. (1986) and by Roberton and Delis. Patient selection was rather crude (based solely on evidence of right or left lesions), and many of the patients had a host of problems beyond those associated with spatial cognition. The data supported years of clinical observations of a basic functional hemispheric asymmetry in spatial cognition and showed that such asymmetry could be studied with more stimulus control than was previously done. There was a consistent relationship between left hemisphere damage and problems in representing local elements and, in a complementary fashion, between right hemisphere damage and problems in representing global elements. The results of their studies began to reveal the areas within each hemisphere that were responsible for those effects, moving beyond a simple left/right dichotomy. Although other types of measures, such as imaging or evoked potential studies, are critical, the studies with patients have begun to reveal the areas that are necessary to support normal functions.

STUDIES IN PATIENTS IN ACUTE AND CHRONIC STAGES: ANATOMICAL AND BEHAVIORAL CONSIDERATIONS

The importance of the right hemisphere in spatial behavior can become obvious after a traumatic event such as a stroke. Such patients may fail to recognize objects or to attend to any source of stimulation coming from the left side of space. With left hemisphere lesions, however, such behavior may not be manifest. With left hemisphere damage there is often the additional problem of major language deficits. Besides the obvious consequences for communication, there are social and emotional consequences as well, and the language problems are often the primary focus of the clinical staff and the family. Patients with left hemisphere damage may find themselves in the frightening position of neither understanding what is being said to them nor being able to speak coherently, and they understandably may show great distress over this condition. Testing for other cognitive deficits during the acute period is often not performed due to the overwhelming salience of language deficits. Language problems also make it difficult to know whether or not a patient understands the instructions for the task at hand.

In contrast, a perceptual deficit is often a profoundly personal problem. Whereas aphasia creates a social interaction deficit that is hard to ignore, perceptual problems can go undetected for quite some time unless they produce an obvious behavioral change, such as continuously turning away from one side. Nevertheless, perceptual problems can be revealed under proper testing conditions.

For example, a patient with left posterior damage and moderate aphasia was examined by one of us soon after his stroke (figure 3.13). When he was shown hierarchical letter patterns, he was very slow to report any shape. When he did, he would always report the identity of the global form and never that of the local form. He did not show signs of having even a general sense of the shape of the local elements. When forced to guess, he was nearly always wrong. His performance was at chance levels even when the experimenter provided a set of alternatives from which he could choose (e.g., was that an *A*, *Z*, or *Y*?).

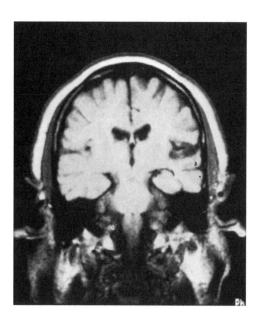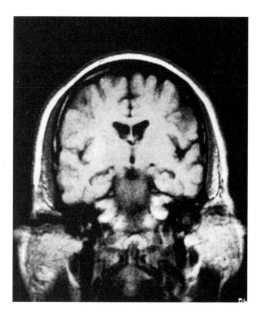

Figure 3.13 MRI scan of patient with left posterior damage and moderate aphasia. Note the lesion on right side of the photograph (left hemisphere) in the superior temporal gyrus.

An obvious question is whether his deficit was due to a problem with visual acuity. When given Snellen's eye test (the chart of letters that graces the walls of optometrists), the patient showed normal acuity. He also was able to identify single elements that were the same size as the local elements used in the hierarchical patterns. He knew that the global letters of the hierarchical stimuli were made from small "things," but he could not identify those things.

As fortunately happens with many stroke victims, this patient made an excellent recovery. A year later, his language problems were rated as mild. At that time he was brought back to the laboratory for follow-up tests. He walked into the office, carried on a conversation with the experimenter, read and signed the consent forms, joked and laughed, and then responded to patterns on a computer monitor for well over an hour without showing any abnormal signs of fatigue. He could easily identify both the local and global shapes of the hierarchical patterns.

But, as with many left-sided patients who are tested well after the acute stage of neurological trauma, this patient continued to show a bias to respond to the global pattern of the stimuli (i.e., he had faster response times to global as opposed to local targets). During the acute stage, that same bias had been so pronounced that it was difficult to find evidence for any representation of the local elements of the patterns. A year later, the deficit was subtle and required a corresponding increase in the sensitivity of the measurement tools. Reaction-time experiments were required to elicit evidence of any lingering global processing deficit, and the deficit was defined in terms of no more than a few hundredths of a second.

Most of the studies discussed below used reaction-time measures to test stable patients with relatively focal lesions. For the most part, the patients had recovered from many of the initial behavioral deficits caused by neurological insult. Although such recovery means that their deficits are more subtle, there are two major benefits in working with such patients to address questions in cognitive neuropsychology. First, they are able to perform relatively complicated tasks. Second, and perhaps more important, the secondary effects of physical insult, such as those due to swelling, have subsided. At this stage of recovery it becomes much more meaningful to relate behavior to anatomy.

Our ability to make claims about which cortical regions are necessary for visual and attentional processing require a rigorous method of patient selection. Patient selection will be described in some detail, since it can serve as a reference for one approach in neuropsychological research to the study of relationships between the brain and behavior. With careful patient selection, group studies are possible, which helps avoid the problems inherent in research involving individual case studies (see Robertson, Knight, Rafal, & Shimamura, 1993).

Patients in the studies described below were chosen on the basis of the location of their lesions and their ability to function at a relatively high level. They were not chosen because they had interesting clinical deficits or because they were part of a series of inpatients with right or left hemisphere damage. They were recruited by neurological staff from a general outpatient population, and most were unknown to us before recruitment.

Subject selection was performed in several stages by a team of neurologists and neuroscience investigators. The first stage required radiological evidence of a unilateral lesion. Every CT or MRI listing in the radiological records of several participating hospitals was scanned. Selected CTs and MRIs were then examined visually. If there was evidence of a focal unilateral cortical lesion that was either anterior or posterior to the fissure of Rolando but outside the primary auditory and visual cortex, the patient's charts were ordered. Evidence of accompanying cortical atrophy, degenerative disease, or other abnormalities that would interfere with lesion articulation were grounds for exclusion. The second stage of selection relied on medical charts to eliminate individuals who had a recorded psychiatric history or history of other medical complications that could interfere with testing and interpretation of data. The third stage included a complete neurological examination performed by a neurologist, as well as structured interviews and tests of visual and auditory function.

The selection procedure effectively eliminated about 95% of the patients who might have been included under less restrictive criteria. From the remaining 5%, patients were recruited who were willing to participate in an extensive neuropsychological testing program. At least six months had elapsed between the time of the acute neurological event and the beginning of testing. This duration extended up to 19 years post-trauma. The subjects tended to be older and retired, but most were still functioning on their own and active in their families and communities.

An important point worth reemphasizing is that these subjects were not selected to be representative of neurological populations as a whole or of a particular neuropsychological syndrome or disease. A priori, we did not know whether they presented any evidence of particular perceptual syndromes such as simultaneous agnosia, neglect, or extinction. Rather, they were selected because of their stable neurological condition, their ability to function well in their everyday lives, and the nature and location of their lesions.

ANATOMICAL REGIONS ASSOCIATED WITH GLOBAL LOCAL DIFFERENCES

Patients in the Robertson et al. study (1988) discussed previously were selected from this group. Groups were formed of patients with lesions centered in either the left or right temporal, the parietal (Lamb, Robertson, & Knight, 1990; Robertson et al., 1988), or frontal lobe (Robertson et al., 1991). Lesion reconstruction software allowed the identification of areas of maximal overlap (hence the term "centered in").

In one set of studies patients were tested on a divided attention task with hierarchical letter stimuli similar to those used in previous studies. Each stimulus contained one of two target letters, an *H* or an *S*, that could appear at either the local or global level. If the target was global, the local elements were composed of one of two distractor letters, either an *E* or an *A*. Likewise, if the target was local, the global configuration formed one of those distractor shapes. Subjects responded by pressing one of two keys to indicate which target was present.

The stimuli were presented briefly at the center of the display. The central presentation contrasts with the approach used in behavioral studies of functional hemisphere asymmetries in young healthy subjects. With those subjects lateralized stimuli are used, the assumption being that such procedures facilitate processing in the contralateral hemisphere. With neurological patients, it is assumed that the damaged area disrupts the critical and necessary computations that affect performance. Undamaged areas must dominate processing if successful performance is to occur. In order to determine what these areas might be, a double dissociation is required. That is, we must be able to show that one aspect of processing is disrupted by damage to one area, while another process is disrupted by damage to another area. Hypotheses of hemispheric differences are supported when this dissociation is found, with damage to homologous areas in each hemisphere. The performance of patients with right hemisphere lesions will be dominated by processing within the intact left hemisphere, whereas the reverse will be true for patients with left hemisphere lesions.

The studies using these high-functioning individuals with known areas of damage showed that the critical area linked to hemispheric differences in global/local processing was the temporal-parietal junction, with some extension into the parietal lobe. Patients with left hemisphere lesions in that area were slow to respond when the target was at the local level (figure 3.14). Patients with right hemisphere lesions in that area were slow to respond when the target was at the global level (figure 3.15).

Note that the lesions represented in figure 3.15 were not isolated to the temporal-parietal junction in every patient. There was a great deal of

LTP

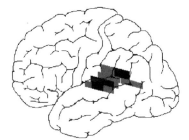 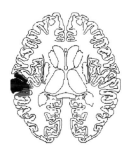 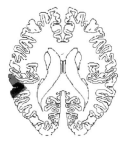

Figure 3.14 Lesion average for a group of patients with left temporal-parietal damage (LTP) who showed a deficit in identifying local shapes. The dark areas are the region of maximal lesion overlap for the group. (Adapted from Robertson et al., 1988.)

RTP

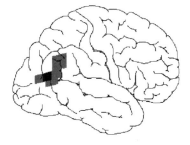 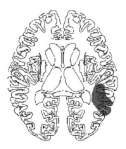 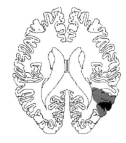

Figure 3.15 Lesion average for a group of patients with right temporal-parietal damage (RTP) who showed a deficit in identifying global shapes. The dark areas are the region of maximal lesion overlap for the group. Heterogeneity was larger for the RTP group than LTP group. (Adapted from Robertson et al., 1988.)

interpatient variability in terms of the foci and extent of the lesions. Nonetheless, by an inclusion criterion, for both group of patients there was maximal overlap in the vicinity of the temporal-parietal junction. By an exclusionary criterion, patients with cortical lesions that did not include temporal regions did not show such performance differences. These other patients had lesions restricted to more superior portions of the parietal lobe or lesions in the dorsolateral frontal lobe of either hemisphere. The data support the conclusion that lesions in association cortex in the temporal-parietal junction are not only sufficient but are also necessary to disrupt normal spatial analysis of hierarchical patterns.

Those findings have been supported by other studies. Doyon and Milner (1991) also reported a global processing deficit in patients who had portions of their right temporal lobes removed as an intervention for intractable epilepsy. They did not find the corresponding local processing deficit in a group of patients who had portions of their left temporal lobe removed. However, the surgical procedures used in lobectomy operations were not developed with the goal in mind of making equal-sized resections. Neurosurgeons often remove as much of the temporal lobe as possible in such cases in order to increase the chance of successfully eliminating seizures. Given the well-known role of left posterior temporal areas in language functions, neurosurgeons can be more aggressive with right hemisphere reactions than with left hemisphere resections. As a result, lesions tend to extend more posteriorly on the right than on the left in patients who have undergone temporal lobectomies. As a group, therefore, right hemisphere lobectomies create lesions that are more likely to encroach on the temporal-parietal junction than do left hemisphere lobectomies. That difference between types of lobectomy patients may account for the fact that the left hemisphere patients in the Doyan and Milner study did not show a local processing deficit; it is also consistent with the critical anatomical area being more posterior in the temporal-parietal region.

Studies with normal subjects using electrophysiological measures have provided converging evidence implicating the posterior temporal lobe in the discrimination of forms in hierarchical stimuli. Heinze and Munte (1993) found a dissociation between global/local performance and left-right event-related potential (ERP) waves over temporal lobe scalp electrodes. The dissociation was found in a part of the waveform referred to as N2, which is a negative shift that occurs between 200 and 400 ms after stimulus onset (figure 3.16). The amplitude of the N2 was greatest over the left temporal lobe when the subject was responding to local patterns, and the amplitude was much reduced over the right temporal lobe when the subject was responding to global patterns (see also Heinze, Johannes, Munte, & Mangun, 1994). Interestingly, early sensory components of the

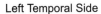Left Temporal Side   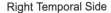Right Temporal Side

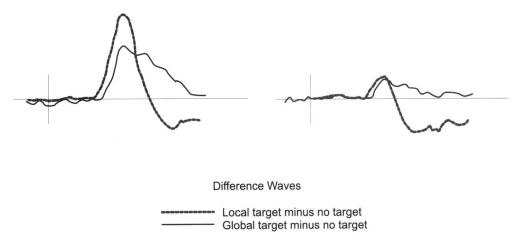

Difference Waves

-------------- Local target minus no target
──────────── Global target minus no target

Figure 3.16 Difference waves in the N2 component of the evoked potential over posterior inferior leads. Note the increased amplitude over the left temporal side for local-target compared to no-target conditions and the elimination of that local dominance over the right temporal side. Standard parameters were selected; negative values are plotted above the line and positive values are plotted below the line. (Adapted from Heinze & Munte, 1993.)

ERP wave that corresponds to early visual processing did not differ between hemispheres and no differences were found over occipital leads. These data are consistent with our hypothesis of symmetrical representation of global and local features in the primary visual cortex, with differences arising at a later stage of analysis.

More recent data—from studies using PET, fMRI, and hierarchical letter patterns similar to those used in studies of patients and normals to measure evoked potential responses—have supported the hypothesis of hemispheric differences. A group of investigators in London (Fink et al. 1996) varied the visual angle of hierarchical patterns and found increased PET activation in the left prestriate cortex during identification of local patterns and in the right lingual gyrus during identification of global patterns. They also found evidence of increased PET activation in the temporal-parietal region when attention was divided. fMRI data show a somewhat different pattern of activation for hierarchical shape patterns (Martinez et al. 1996) Martinez et al. presented stimuli in the right or left visual field and directed subjects to identify the global shape in one block of trials and the local shape in another block of trials. The predicted interaction of visual field and task was obtained in the behavioral data. During a later activation study the stimuli were presented centrally, but the task remained the same. As with the behavioral data, a significant interaction of hemisphere and task resulted. Using as a measurement increased activation in a region of interest, Martinez et al. found the lateralized effect to be associated with posterior inferior temporal lobes. The data tend to support an even earlier visual hemispheric difference than patient data suggest. The data also pose the question of how temporal-parietal damage may affect processing in ventral extrastriate regions.

Hypotheses of interactions between the temporal-parietal junction and extrastriate areas have been supported by visual evoked potential data (Knight, 1997). It is generally believed that the N1 component of the visual evoked potential reflects electrical activity in extrastriate cortex. Patients with lesions in the temporal-parietal junction show decreased amplitude in N1, which presumably reflects feedback to the extrastriate from this area.

Together, the anatomical, electrophysiological, and imaging findings are consistent with the DFF theory. The electrophysiological, imaging, and patient data suggest that visual-spatial information produces symmetrical activation in the relatively early visual stages of analysis. As information is projected to secondary visual centers, differences in activation appear. The electrophysiological and imaging data are consistent with the lesion data in implicating posterior visual areas in the differences. However, they place the difference in an even more posterior and ventral location, suggesting strong interactions between areas within the temporal-parietal junction and extrastriate visual areas. Such interactions have been supported by evoked potential data in patients with lesions in this junction.

It should be emphasized that we are not arguing for a strict segregation of function. That is, we are neither arguing that the right hemisphere is solely responsible for identifying global targets, nor that the left hemisphere is solely responsible for identifying local targets. Rather, our central premise is that each hemisphere is sufficient for abstracting information from both levels but with differential efficiency or speed. We argue that the right hemisphere amplifies relatively low spatial frequency information, which is most associated with the global spatial structure of a pattern. The left hemisphere amplifies relatively high spatial frequency information, which is most associated with local spatial structure of a pattern. Objects at one of the two levels will be perceived more rapidly than objects at the other level, depending on which hemisphere is most involved in the task.

The data are also consistent with two parallel processing pathways that are lateralized in the human brain. One is biased toward the relatively global information in a visual pattern and the other toward the relatively local information. These pathways are not exclusively dedicated to processing information at one level or the other, as is predicted by dichotomous theories of hemisphere specialization. Rather, they contribute to identification of forms at both levels. They simply emphasize different aspects of the visual input. In the language of the DFF theory, they act as high- or low-pass filters of a selected range of spatial frequencies. Such filtering is enough to set into motion a processing advantage in perceiving local or global objects.

GLOBAL/LOCAL ASYMMETRY IS SUPERIMPOSED ON THE SENSORY SIGNAL

One of the main tenets of the DFF theory is that functional hemispheric asymmetries in perception arise from postsensory filtering mechanisms. If that tenet is true, we should be able to change the sensory input within reasonable limits and still observe the typical laterality effect. The evidence from studies using global/local patterns is consistent with this prediction. The data discussed in the previous section from studies with patient groups all used central presentation. However, differences have also been obtained in studies in which lateralized stimuli were presented to patients with focal lesions. In such cases the stimuli can be presented directly to the "good" or "bad" hemisphere. One might expect that under such circumstances, only presentations to the damaged hemisphere would reveal deficits. This has not been the case. Whether patterns were presented centrally (i.e., foveally) or in the left or right visual field (peripherally), the laterality effects were observed.

The use of left versus right visual field presentation is important. When patterns were presented in the periphery the stimuli were directly projected to either the intact or damaged hemisphere. Consider the predictions of the DFF theory for lateralized presentation. First, we assume that the initial sensory representation in primary visual areas contains the entire spectrum of spatial frequencies. That initial representation of frequency information in the right and left primary visual cortex should be intact for all groups of patients and controls. With central presentation, the primary visual cortex of both hemispheres would register the spectrum; with left visual field presentation, the primary cortex of the right hemisphere would register it; with right visual field presentation, the primary cortex of the left hemisphere would register it.

The DFF theory asserts that the visual system performs a second filtering operation after the initial sensory representation of spatial frequencies. If this filtering is associated with the right and left temporal-parietal junctions (and adjoining extrastriate regions), then lateralized input might be expected to have little effect on the direction of performance differences. The reasoning behind this claim is represented in the schematic in figure 3.17.

If the mechanism that performs secondary filtering is eliminated in the left hemisphere, as shown at the bottom of the figure, then visual input may be transferred to the right hemisphere, which is where global biasing takes place. Of course, the right hemisphere would not receive any signals from the damaged site in the left hemisphere, but it could still receive

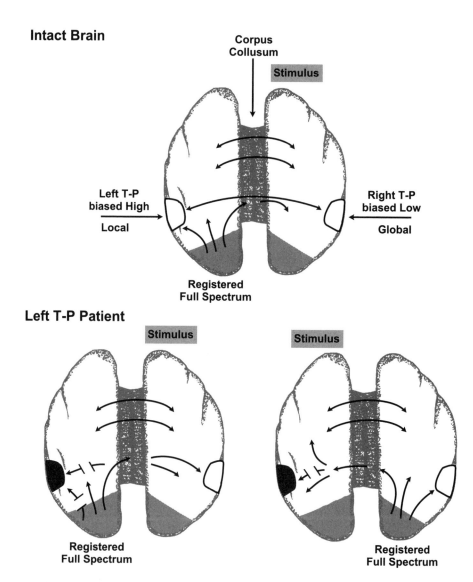

Figure 3.17 The upper drawing represents intact flow between the hemispheres over the corpus callosum under conditions in which the stimulus is directly projected to the left hemisphere (presented in the right visual field). The outlined white areas represent left and right temporal-parietal (T-P) regions. Both the left T-P and the right T-P can receive signals from either visual cortex. The examples in the lower drawings represent the case of a patient with left T-P damage. Signals from stimuli projected directly to the damaged left hemisphere can be transferred to the intact right T-P through the corpus callosum. However, the left T-P cannot receive the signal and is cut off from visual information projected to the damaged hemisphere as well as from normal input signals from the intact hemisphere. For this patient, information presented in the left visual field and thus projected directly to the right hemisphere will also be degraded. In both cases the intact right T-P receives signals representing the full spectrum of information, but the signals are simply delayed when the stimulus is directly projected to the damaged left hemisphere.

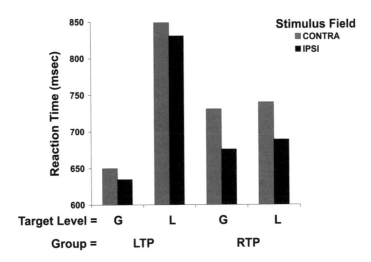

Figure 3.18 Mean reaction time for a group of patients with left temporal-parietal damage (LTP) and right temporal-parietal damage (RTP). The stimuli were presented 5 degrees to the right or left of fixation. The magnitude of the difference in responses to global (G) or local (L) targets was similar whether the stimuli were presented in the contralesional or ipsilesional visual field. Both groups were faster to respond when patterns were presented in the ipsilesional, rather than contralesional, field whether the target level was global or local. There was a global advantage of 118 ms for normal age-matched control subjects (not shown). That advantage increased to 197 ms for LTP and decreased to 11 ms for RTP. The data are consistent with the diagram of the model outlined in figure 3.17.

visual information from striate cortex through extrastriate cortex and the posterior corpus callosum. By that means the local form of a stimulus presented in the right visual field could be identified, although it should take more time. The mean data shown in figure 3.18 support this prediction, although the effects were small. Whether the stimuli were shown in the ipsilesional or contralesional visual field, a global advantage was found for left temporal-parietal patients compared to matched controls, but response times were faster when patterns were presented in the ipsilesional field (i.e., to the intact hemisphere) than when they were presented in the contralesional field (i.e., to the damaged hemisphere). For the right temporal-parietal patients the pattern was the same except that local identification was favored relative to normal controls regardless of the visual field in which the stimuli appeared.

If the damaged temporal-parietal region simply degraded the information from the receiving hemisphere, then one would expect performance to simply be worse overall. There would be a local-over-global advantage for left temporal-parietal groups, but either response time would be slowed or the magnitude of the difference between global and local responses would increase. Instead, there was a global advantage compared to controls whether the patterns appeared in the ipsilesional or contralesional field, with response time being overall faster for ipsilesional presentation. (Note that the transfer of signals shown in figure 3.17 may only hold true for patients with brain damage in which inhibitory connections between homologous regions may be disrupted.)

Lamb et al. (1989) presented subjects with hierarchical letter patterns; the inner edge of the stimulus was presented 2.7 degrees to the right or left of a central fixation point. Presentation durations were brief at 100 ms so that subjects would not have time to move their eyes to the stimulus location. The groups included patients with left or right temporal-parietal damage and a group of matched healthy controls. Subjects were instructed to identify the letter at the local level in one block of trials and at the global level in another block. Figure 3.18 shows the data for each group for their ipsilesional and contralesional fields, collapsed over other factors. Figure 3.19 shows the data from central and peripheral presentation and the degree of global or local bias for each group.

These data also demonstrate an important point: any laterality effect used to evaluate the DFF theory must be evaluated relative to baseline conditions. Crossover interactions should only be expected when stimuli are specifically designed so that control subjects perform equally in the identification of local and global targets. Otherwise, the effects of global and local response time will be either an increase or reduction in the overall advantage for identifying one level over the other.

Failure to consider that point has created much confusion in the laterality literature on spatial cognition. Frequently, hypotheses about differences in global and local processing have been assessed by varying the absolute size or frequency of the stimuli. It is not the absolute frequencies that are critical, however. Global performance need not be better than

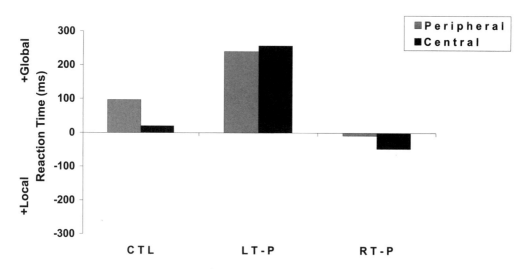

Figure 3.19 Mean reaction-time differences for central and peripheral stimulus presentation (across studies) for groups of patients with left temporal-parietal damage (LT-P), groups with right temporal-parietal damage (RT-P), and age-matched control subjects (CTL).

local performance with left hemisphere damage nor must global performance be better than local performance with right hemisphere damage. If the sensory signal overwhelmingly favors global identification (as it does when placed in the periphery), then global response times will be faster than local response times for both left and right visual field presentation. The laterality effect will take the form of a larger global-over-local advantage with left hemisphere damage and a smaller global-over-local advantage with right hemisphere damage. In studies using normal subjects or patients with resection of the corpus callosum and left or right visual field presentation, the differences occur as larger global advantages when stimuli are placed in the left visual field and as a smaller one when they are placed in the right visual field, (see figure 3.19).

Establishing the appropriate baseline conditions will depend on a number of factors. Local elements may be easy to identify when projected in the fovea, but they are more difficult to identify when the stimuli are presented at more eccentric locations. At more peripheral positions on the retina, the ratio of high to low shifts to favor lower frequencies. That is why sensory representation is quite different for the same stimulus when it is presented at a peripheral location compared to when it is presented to a central location.

For those reasons, one should not expect central and peripheral presentations to produce similar baseline effects on performance during responses to global and local information. Global reaction-time advantages change with visual eccentricity (Amirkhiabani & Lovegrove, 1996). Reaction times are longer and detection is more difficult as eccentricity increases, especially true for local elements (Sergent, 1982; Lamb & Robertson, 1988). The main prediction of the DFF theory is that laterality effects result from higher-order filtering processes superimposed on sensory representations. The absolute global or local advantage is expected to change with changes in retinal acuity, but the interaction between hemisphere or visual field and hierarchical level remains.

These findings demonstrate the importance of examining laterality effects in terms of relative frequency or relative size. This conclusion has been supported by data from a wide range of studies with both healthy normals (Christman et al., 1991; Fink et al., 1996) and patients, and it is found across manipulations of attentional focus (e.g., Robertson et al., 1988) or stimulus size. Independent of this main effect, however, the temporal-parietal groups diverged from normal controls in the same direction as in previous studies.

ASYMMETRIC DIFFERENCES IN SPLIT-BRAIN PATIENTS

Subjects with callosal disconnection can provide converging evidence that visual field differences reflect differences in hemispheric function. Unless the split brain has undergone some form of dramatic reorganization, the direction of laterality effects with split-brain subjects should be similar to those with normal subjects. If local information produces a right visual field advantage in normals, then it should also produce a right visual field advantage in normal subjects. Indeed, we might even expect the differences to be amplified with split-brain subjects, given that communication between the two hemispheres is severely disrupted.

Moreover, data from split-brain subjects can help determine whether or not performance of patients with lesions in a particular area reflects the function of mechanisms associated with the intact hemisphere. For example, subjects with left temporal-parietal damage respond faster to global than to local properties of visual patterns. In the DFF theory, that reflects the operation of intact right hemisphere mechanisms that are biased toward global properties. If that interpretation is correct, then split-brain patients should show similar effects with lateralized stimuli. Under such conditions, only one hemisphere will receive the information, creating a strong version of the situation in which processing is biased toward a single hemisphere.

An alternative conceptualization of hemispheric specialization would be that the two hemispheres function dichotomously. In this view global processing would be the exclusive province of the right hemisphere, and local processing would be the exclusive province of the left hemisphere. Such models dominated the early laterality literature, in which the emphasis was on identifying qualitative differences between the two cerebral hemispheres. Dichotomous models can explain reaction-time differences between visual field presentation in normals by postulating the need for interhemispheric transfer when the information is projected to the "wrong" hemisphere. For example, identification of local patterns would reflect the output of the left hemisphere and would be slower following left visual field presentation, due to the additional time necessary to transfer signals from the right hemisphere to the necessary "place" or "location" in the left hemisphere.

The DFF theory does not assume such a dichotomy. Yet studies using lateralized presentation with normal or brain-damaged subjects have not completely ruled out this dichotomous model. Although it may seem intuitively unlikely, it can be argued that unilateral lesions simply degrade information that is normally processed by one hemisphere. By this logic, a patient with a left temporal-parietal lesion would be slow to identify local targets because the processes needed to extract the information had become less efficient in that hemisphere. Global information would be unaffected because it is the province of the right hemisphere.

Split-brain patients offer an opportunity to resolve these issues because their cortical halves are not connected. Direct cross talk to and from these areas is eliminated. By presenting a stimulus in one visual field, the experimenter can be relatively sure that the information will be processed by the receiving hemisphere (although eye movements and cross-cuing are always considerations that must be controlled). Indirect transfer between cortical areas could occur, but the signal would have to take a highly unusual and circuitous route through subcortical structures. Dichotomous models of part/whole perception lead to the expectation that performance would also be dichotomous. The strong version predicts that performance will drop to chance when the receiving hemisphere is asked to make a judgment usually reserved for its "better half." The left hemisphere should be unable to make global judgments and the right hemisphere should be similarly unable to make local judgments.

The evidence discussed in the following section demonstrates that split-brain patients are able to identify both global and local forms when they are presented in the left or right visual field. Split-brain patients produce a pattern of results similar to lateralized studies of normal subjects using half visual field presentation methods.

Output Measures from Split-Brain Subjects

Are we simply setting up a straw man (or woman) here? Are there really situations in which an isolated hemisphere completely fails to perform a task? Although they are relatively rare, there are examples of such extreme laterality effects. For example, in the language domain, evidence from the study of split-brain patients and from other patients during sodium amytal injections (WADA testing) suggests that there can be complete lateralization of speech functions to one hemisphere (Rasmussen & Milner, 1977). Another indication of extreme lateralization could be the severe problems in part/whole perception experienced by patients in the acute stages after a stroke, who often respond in an all-or-none manner. Even given unlimited time to view an object, acute stroke patients may not produce any evidence of a residual representation at the impaired level (e.g., Delis et al., 1986). Such behavior may be better accounted for by a dichotomous view.

A dissociation consistent with an all-or-none dichotomy was reported in at least one split-brain patient by Delis, Kramer, and Kiefner (1988). First, the patient was asked to draw hierarchical stimuli with his right hand. He drew the local forms. When asked to draw the same pattern with his left hand, he drew the global forms without providing any local details (see figure 3.20). Based on his drawings, Delis et al. concluded that the right hemisphere serves as a global processor and the left hemisphere as a local processor. Each hemisphere, he further concluded, has its own restricted domain that operates in isolation of the of the other.

Note that the evidence that is amenable to a dichotomous point of view involves measures of production, or output. Gazzaniga et al. (1965) also found severe deficits in the ability of split-brain patients to draw local parts of a scene when they used their left hand but not when they used

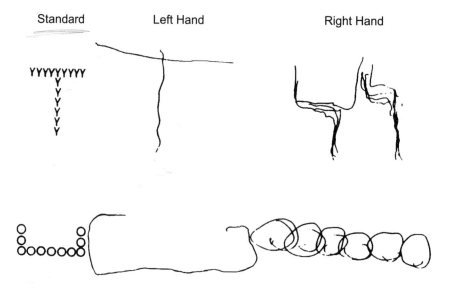

Figure 3.20 The drawing of a commissurotomy patient shortly after surgery. He drew the global form when asked to draw the pattern with his left hand (controlled by his right hemisphere) and the local forms when asked to draw it with his right hand (controlled by his left hemisphere). (From Delis et al., 1988.)

their right hand. It may be that output functions involve a greater degree of lateralization, perhaps as a means of coordinating action. But the question for present purposes is whether or not input is segregated in the same way.

Input Measures and Split-Brain Patients

Input measures do not typically show such drastic distinctions. Studies using reaction-time measures with split-brain patients revealed hemifield differences on the order of only milliseconds for the identification of local and global targets. Robertson, Lamb, and Zaidel (1993) tested three split-brain patients in a study similar to the one used with patients with unilateral, cortical lesions (Robertson et al., 1988). The split-brain patients were long-standing veterans of neuropsychological research. Indeed, they had been part of the original study group of commissurotomy patients tested by Sperry, Bogan, Gazzaniga, and colleagues during the 1960s.

Furthermore, they had participated in studies by Nebes (1972, 1973) in which they were shown pieces of a geometric form and asked to select by touch alone the correct synthesis of the form from three alternatives hidden from view. In one condition they used their left hand to explore the alternatives, and in another condition they used their right hand. Selecting the correct form was far more difficult with their right hand than with their left hand. Nebes concluded that motor selection was affected by the perceptual representations of parts and wholes in the two hemispheres. He suggested that such an effect occurred because parts are better synthesized into global wholes by the right hemisphere; thus, the left hand would perform more accurately.

To explore the role of input processes on global and local identification, Robertson, Lamb & Zaidel (1993) presented hierarchical letter stimuli to either the left visual field, the right visual field, or in both visual fields simultaneously for 100 ms. A focused-attention task was used. On some blocks the subjects were instructed to the identify the global shape. On others they were instructed to identify the local shape.

Contrary to the predictions of a strong dichotomy hypothesis, the split-brain subjects were able to identify global and local patterns in both single field conditions. That is, each hemisphere was able to perceive the shape at either level. Once again, however, there were differences in their performance in the direction predicted by the DFF theory. As discussed earlier, peripheral presentation typically results in an overall global advantage; that advantage was present for the split-brain patients whether the stimuli were presented in the right or left visual field. Yet, the evidence for functional hemispheric asymmetries was still present as well.

The split-brain data converge with data obtained with normal subjects and patients with focal unilateral lesions. Consistent with the DFF theory, each hemisphere can represent the full range of information, but each hemisphere amplifies different portions of that signal. The input differences are quantitative, not qualitative.

Spatial Frequency Differences in Split-Brain Subjects

Do the hemispheric asymmetries in split-brain subjects reflect differential efficiency in responding to higher and lower relative spatial frequencies? To study this question Fendrich and Gazzaniga (1990) presented two sine wave gratings, in either the left or right visual field of two patients. Within a trial, the two gratings had the same frequency, and across trials the frequency varied from 1–8 cycles/degree. The subjects' task was to judge if the two gratings were in the same or different orientation. Such a test required subjects to attend to the orientation of the patterns to perform the task.

Neither patient showed a visual-field-by-frequency interaction, as is found in normal subjects. A left visual field advantage for all frequency pairs was observed for one patient. The other patient actually performed better when high frequency gratings were presented in the left visual field.

However, that testing method does not provide a critical test of the DFF theory. The task did not require the subjects to identify or label the stimuli based on the spectral content of the stimuli. Unlike the studies in which subjects have to decide whether a grating is composed of wide or narrow stripes, the spatial frequency of the stimulus pair used on any particular trial was essentially irrelevant. The information to be extracted in the

Fendrich and Gazzaniga study was orientation. Neither the relative nor absolute frequencies in the stimuli were important for the task.

Of course, it is reasonable to assume that frequency-sensitive cells in the visual pathways were nonetheless activated by those stimuli. That is, the frequency content of the stimuli was represented at various stages of processing. But, the output at any stage of processing would be sufficient to perform the task. Responses could simply be based on consideration of whether the cells responding to the gratings had similar orientation tuning. The output from cells in the earliest visual processing areas—primary visual cortex—could provide sufficient information to perform the task. For that reason, no visual-field-by-frequency interaction would be predicted by the DFF theory.

COORDINATE VERSUS CATEGORICAL DIFFERENCES IN VISUAL FIELD ASYMMETRIES

The DFF theory emphasizes that the two hemispheres produce different representations of a stimulus in a task that requires the use of relative frequency information. Each representation is useful for a different purpose. Amplification of the low-frequency content is useful for making judgments about the global shape of an object. Amplification of the high-frequency content is useful for making judgments about the component parts of an object.

Steve Kosslyn and his associates have provided an alternative explanation of the functional asymmetries in performance that are observed with hierarchical patterns. In Kosslyn's theory, different forms of representation can be useful for solving different computational problems essential to many spatial cognition tasks. In particular, he suggests that the left hemisphere is efficient at deriving categorical spatial information about spatial features, whereas the right hemisphere is efficient at deriving coordinate spatial information from the same stimulus information. Although that idea may initially sound orthogonal to the premises of the DDF theory, it turns out that the differences between the two approaches are not that substantial.

What does it mean to perform categorical versus coordinate analyses of spatial information? Both categorical and coordinate judgments require evaluation of the relationship between two or more stimuli, but in different ways. A categorical judgment requires ordinal information about two objects. Is the picture located to the left of the clock? Did the baseball land inside the foul line? A coordinate judgment requires metric information. How far to the left of the clock should the picture be hung? How close was the baseball to the foul line?

Either type of relation can be considered sufficient for visual recognition. We can recognize a house by detecting certain prototypical features and seeing that they maintain proper categorical relations. The room should exist above the floor. The wall containing the front door usually faces the street, and the windows should be more or less aligned with one another. A coordinate representation would also suffice. We could code the scene as a 40×20-foot wall 3 feet back from the street with an 8×5-foot opening 10 feet from the left vertical wall. The representations may differ, however, in terms of how efficiently they solve certain types of problems. For instance, classifying an object as a chair or table may require little more than a categorical distinction: chairs have backrests above their legs; tables do not. Classifying an object as a particular chair may require other types of spatial distinctions: the chair at the end of the table is 6 inches wider than the one at the side.

Part/Whole as a Categorical/Coordinate Distinction

The categorical/coordinate distinction had its beginning in studies of visual imagery. Kosslyn (1986) hypothesized that parts and wholes in a visual image would show similar hemispheric effects as would parts and wholes in vision. Evidence with a split-brain patient (Kosslyn, Holtzman, Farah, & Gazzaniga, 1985) and with normal healthy subjects supported that idea (Kosslyn, 1987; 1988). Questions or tasks that emphasized the parts of visual images produced better performance by the left hemisphere, and questions or tasks that emphasized wholes produced better performance by the right hemisphere.

At the time, Kosslyn was most interested in the relationship between vision and visual imagery and whether or not similar mechanisms could account for part/whole processes in both (see Kosslyn, 1986). As he collected more data to test his hypotheses, however, he began to ask about computations that could be responsible for the lateralization of processes involved in part/whole representation. In chapter 7 we discuss Kosslyn's computational model at length. For our purposes here we focus on the central tenet of Kosslyn's theory.

Evidence for a Categorical/Coordinate Distinction in Vision

The categorical/coordinate distinction received initial support from studies with normal subjects using lateralized presentation methods. In one study (Kosslyn et al., 1989) subjects were shown a stimulus in either the left or right visual field. The stimulus contained two forms: a fuzzy blob and a dot. The dot was either located on the blob or was placed away from the blob at distances of 1 mm (near) or 10 mm (far).

Different groups of subjects were required to make either categorical or coordinate judgments. In the categorical task subjects indicated whether the dot was located on or off the blob. In the coordinate task they judged whether the dot was far from or near to the blob. As predicted, the categorical judgments (on versus off) were faster when the

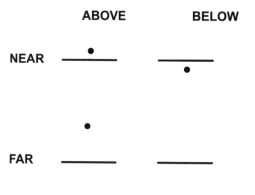

Figure 3.21 Examples of the bar-dot stimuli used in a categorical/coordinate study. (Adapted from Hellige & Michimata, 1989.)

stimulus was in the right visual field, and the coordinate judgments (near versus far) were faster when the stimulus was in the left visual field. An appealing aspect of these experiments is that the stimuli were the same for both tasks.

A similar type of study was reported at about the same time by Kosslyn et al. (1989) and by Hellige and Michimata (1989). In this task, the stimulus consisted of a horizontal bar and a single dot (figure 3.21). The dot was located either above or below the bar. In addition, the dot's distance from the bar was varied. For the categorical judgment subjects had to decide whether the dot was above or below the bar, regardless of its distance from the bar. For the coordinate judgment the subjects had to decide whether the dot was near or far from the bar, independent of whether it was above or below the bar. As in the preceding study, the stimuli were the same in both conditions; only the type of judgment varied.

The critical prediction in those studies was that there would be a task-by-visual-field interaction. That is, the categorical judgments of above versus below would be made more quickly (and accurately) when the stimulus appeared in the right visual field than when the stimulus appeared in the left visual field. In contrast, the coordinate judgments of near versus far would be made more quickly when the stimulus appeared in the left visual field. In both studies a small yet reliable interaction was obtained (Kosslyn et al., 1989; Hellige & Michimata, 1989). There was a reliable left visual field advantage for the near versus far task and a trend toward a right visual field advantage for the above versus below task.

Obtaining similar results with healthy normals has proven somewhat elusive. Rybash and Hoyer (1992) reported a failure to replicate, at least in one of their experiments, although they did find some evidence to support the distinction in another. Sergent (1991) also failed to find the predicted interaction, except when the stimuli were presented at low contrast. Even in the initial studies of Kosslyn et al. (1989), the effects were transient. For example, in their first study the subjects were run on blocks of 24 trials, a method that was necessitated by the fact that the effects ceased to be reliable with longer sessions. Nevertheless, evidence does exist from a few different laboratories implicating a role for the left hemisphere in judging categorical spatial relations and for the right hemisphere in judging coordinate spatial relations. The reverse pattern has not been reported, which is important. If the visual field differences were just a matter of chance, then the opposite pattern should appear as often as the ones that appeared in support of the categorical/coordinate distinction.

There has been at least one study with a large cohort of patients that has supported this distinction. Laeng (1994) tested 60 patients with either right or left hemisphere lesions in a delayed matching-to-sample test. In the sample, two pictures were shown for 5 seconds followed by a delay of 5 seconds. A test figure then appeared with two alternatives. The task was to point to the picture that was the same as the sample.

The test stimulus included the reappearance of the sample and an alternative that was transformed in either a categorical or in a coordinate fashion. For instance, a sample in which a cat appeared to the right of a dog could be paired in the test display with the cat appearing to the left of the dog. This would be a categorical change. The cat changed from "to the right of" to "to the left of" the dog. In other examples, the alternative in the test pattern changed in coordinate space. In our example, the cat would be to the right of the dog in both test alternatives, but the incorrect alternative would have either a larger or smaller separation between the two.

Although the overall number of errors was small (2–3/20), the group of subjects with right hemisphere damage made more errors when the incorrect choice involved a change in coordinate relations than when it involved a change in categorical relations. The reverse was true for the group with left hemisphere damage. They made more errors when the incorrect choice was a change in categorical relations.

The DFF Theory's Alternative Account

The DFF theory's alternative account of the results discussed in the preceding sections returns the emphasis to the spatial frequency information that would be useful in performing the different tasks. Consider Experiment 1 of Kosslyn et al. (1989), in which a dot was placed on, near to, or far from a fuzzy blob. The spacing between the dot and blob was either 0, 1, or 10 mm. For both the categorical and coordinate tasks the 0 mm and 10 mm stimuli were assigned to separate response categories. The assignment of the 1 mm stimulus changed across tasks. In the categorical task, in which subjects had to report whether the dot was on or off the blob, the 1 mm dot was assigned to the same category (off) as the 10 mm dot. In other words, the most difficult discrimination required of the subject in the categorical task was to distinguish between the 0 mm (on) and 1 mm (off) stimuli. In contrast, in the coordinate task, in which the 0 mm and 1 mm stimuli were linked together, the most difficult decision required of the subject was to discriminate between the 1 mm (near) and 10 mm (far) stimulus.

It is easy to see that the relevant spatial frequency information was different for the two tasks. The critical judgment about the 1 mm dot was much finer in the categorical task than in the coordinate task. If we assume that finer discriminations (a 1 mm difference versus a 9 mm difference) depend on higher spatial frequencies, then it can easily be argued that the DFF theory would predict the same interaction as was derived from the categorical/coordinate distinction. Specifically, the right visual field would be favored for making the on versus off (categorical) judgments, and the left visual field would be favored for making the near versus far (coordinate) judgments. Kosslyn et al. (1992) have come to a somewhat similar conclusion.

The usefulness of different regions of the frequency spectrum in performing such tasks can also be seen when comparing the above versus below and near versus far tasks in the studies of Hellige and Michimata (1989). Figure 3.22 shows low-pass filter versions of two of the bar and dot stimuli used in their studies. At the viewing distance reported by Hellige and Michimata, the cutoff is approximately 1 cycle/degree. As can be seen, the near versus far judgments can be readily made with this filtered representation. In fact, the judgment might be facilitated since there are two distinct parts to the far stimulus (the dot and bar), whereas the two parts become blurred for the near stimulus. However, it would be difficult to judge whether the dot was above or below the bar for the

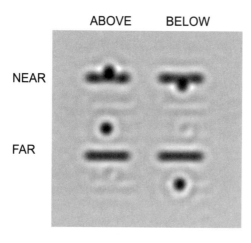

Figure 3.22 Low-pass filtered versions of the bar-dot stimuli shown in figure 3.21.

near stimulus. That is, low-frequency information makes it more difficult to make the categorical judgment of above or below. When the high-frequency information is present, as in figure 3.21, the above versus below judgment would be easier.

In sum, there are at least two ways to account for the laterality effects in these tasks. Kosslyn's account emphasizes the nature of the spatial representation required for the task. The DFF theory focuses on the spatial frequency information that is required to make the judgments.

Another relevant study has been conducted by Cowin and Hellige (1994). They tested two groups of subjects with the bar and dot stimuli using briefly presented lateralized displays. One group made above versus below judgments, and the other group made near versus far judgments. Within each group, two conditions were compared. In one condition the stimuli were high contrast and clear. In the second condition the subjects wore lenses that slightly blurred the stimuli. Such a manipulation primarily affects higher spatial frequencies and leaves low spatial frequency information relatively intact. The results showed that response times on the above versus below task were slowed by nearly 50 ms, but there was little change in response times for the near versus far task. The results suggest that high-frequency information was more important for the above versus below task, a result that is consistent with the analysis offered by the DFF theory. It is not obvious, however, how a theory based on categorical/coordinate spatial relations would account for the selective effects of blurring.

The foregoing discussion is consistent with our contention that the categorical/coordinate distinction can be accounted for by the DFF theory. Higher frequency information appears to be useful for tasks associated with a left hemisphere advantage. Accounting for right hemisphere advantages is less straightforward, since near versus far judgments can usually be made with either high- or low-frequency information. Low-frequency detectors respond faster than high-frequency detectors (De Valois, Albrecht, & Thorell, 1982), but those sorts of differences would hold for absolute frequency and not necessarily for relative frequency. An alternative account might be that low-frequency information is more robust.

A further puzzling aspect of the interaction between visual field and the categorical/coordinate task in normal subjects is that the effect disappears relatively quickly during the course of an experiment. The effects are present only during the first one or two blocks of trials. The DFF theory cannot account for that transiency, but neither is there a straightforward explanation based on the categorical/coordinate account. Some quality of such simple stimuli may make the decision relatively easy as the subject becomes practiced, which may circumvent the need for a divide-and-conquer type of strategy. In other words, the task may become more like a detection task than a localization task.

It is interesting that Kosslyn and his colleagues (Kosslyn et al., 1992) have concluded, on the basis of simulation studies, that there may be differences in how the two hemispheres represent spatial frequency information (see chapter 7). The simulations indicate that coordinate information is better represented by large receptive fields, which would be tuned to low spatial frequencies. In contrast, categorical information is better represented by small receptive fields, which would be better tuned for high-frequency information.

It is rather interesting that in implementing his theory, Kosslyn showed that spatial frequency information must be included to account for the effects he has observed. Although his implementation was based on absolute spatial frequency, there is more convergence than before between the two seemingly different theories to account for hemispheric differences in processing parts and wholes.

Nevertheless, it is important to keep in mind the many differences between Kosslyn's and our theory. It must be emphasized that the frequency distinction modeled by Kosslyn et al. (1989) is one of absolute frequency differences rather than relative frequency differences. A basic tenet of the DFF theory is that differences in the performance of those tasks emerge from the asymmetrically skewed filters after an initial selection stage of a range of frequencies. The selected range may be the same as the absolute frequency spectra, but it does not need to be. Also, the DFF theory is more general, introducing a computational principle that extends across tasks, stimuli, and sensory modalities.

FACE PERCEPTION AND SPATIAL FREQUENCY

Can the DFF theory account for at least some of the hemisphere differences found in more complex perceptual tasks that use objects seen every day in the natural world? One obvious and frequently viewed example of a hierarchical stimulus is a face. A face contains local objects (i.e., eyes, nose, mouth) that are the parts of a more global object. It is not enough just to chronicle the parts to perceive a face. The parts must be spatially arranged in a particular configuration (compare the upper- and lower-left patterns in figure 3.23). There should be two eyes, and they should be horizontally parallel. The two eyes should be located below the hairline but above the nose. The nose should be above the mouth and centered below the eyes. At this level at least, a face is similar to a stimulus such as a global form created from the spatial arrangements of local forms. The local elements in the patterns on the right in figure 3.23 must be placed in specific locations to form the particular global object of an *E* (compare upper and lower patterns).

Faces are also fascinating because they are so important in our everyday lives. We recognize our friends and families by their faces. We look at faces when we talk to people. We note subtle changes in facial expres-

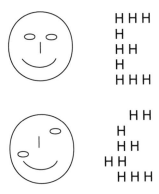

Figure 3.23 Perturbation in the spatial location of one local element changes the overall configuration.

sion that predict an individual's mood or state of mind. Faces can tell us whether a person is friend or foe.

It is clearly important for brains to be able to discriminate between hundreds of faces. We virtually never mistake a stranger's face for our mother's or spouse's. We categorize the thousands of individuals we pass on a busy street as strangers, but we feel a comforting warmth when we recognize a friend among the sea of faces. Yet when brain damage occurs, such abilities can vanish, but they may do so in different ways. For example, familiar faces may no longer be distinguishable from unfamiliar faces (a condition known as prosopagnosia). A neurological patient may not be able to recognize his wife even if he has been married to her for 50 years. Less frequently, patients may lose the ability to perceive whether or not a face is a face; this condition is especially relevant for our thesis.

A large amount of research has been reported on how we perceive and recognize faces (see Bruce & Humphreys, 1994). Our concern here, however, is with possible hemispheric differences in facial perception and whether the DFF theory can account for some of the facial recognition problems that have been reported in the literature.

In neuropsychology it was long believed that the right hemisphere was critical for facial recognition. Individuals with right hemisphere damage had more difficulty on facial recognition tasks than did those with left hemisphere damage (Benton & Van Allen, 1968; De Renzi & Spinnler, 1966; Hecaen & Angelergues, 1962; Levy, Trevarthen, & Sperry, 1972; Milner, 1968; Newcombe, 1969; Warrington & James, 1967). More recent evidence has shown that perception of different aspects of faces can be disrupted by damage to different brain areas (Ellis & Young, 1988). Whether the left or right hemisphere is more involved depends on the task and on the stimulus features (Sergent, 1986). Consistently, prosopagnosia generally requires the presence of bilateral lesions (Damasio & Damasio, 1986).

It is important to keep a critical distinction in mind when evaluating the relevance of the DFF theory to face perception. There is a difference between knowing when a stimulus pattern is or is not a face and recognizing a perceived face as a familiar one. It is a logical necessity that the ability to recognize a face as familiar or not relies on the ability to first perceive the stimulus as a face. The majority of experimental reports of patients with prosopagnosia have focused on recognition of individual faces or on discrimination of one face from another under various transformations, rather than on the recognition of a face as a face per se. Reports of prosopagnosia due to perceptual distortions or primary visual deficits are rare, although not unrecorded (see Ellis, 1986). In those instances the anatomical correlates were uncertain but could possibly be related to temporal-occipital areas, where global/local differences appear.

The first step, then, in relating the DFF theory to face perception is to ask whether perceiving a face as a face relies on spatial frequency analysis. The evidence suggests that low-frequency information is sufficient to perceive a face as a face but that both low- and high-frequency information are necessary to perceive the face as a particular face. Low-frequency information is sufficient for face perception (Ginsberg, 1978; Harmon, 1973). A common example is shown in figure 3.24, in which the blocks of shading represent the average luminance in a particular region. The abrupt contours in shading between blocks introduce higher frequencies. To filter out the high frequencies all you have to do is squint your eyes. This is like performing a low-pass filter: the visual system registers the lower frequencies of the stimulus and filters out the higher frequencies. When this is done, the face as a face is much easier to perceive. However, it may be difficult to say to whom the face belongs without effort.

There is some evidence that the higher and lower frequency information in a face contributes to hemispheric differences in recognition performance. Sergent (1985) asked normal healthy subjects to identify or categorize faces that were presented briefly in the right or left visual field. In one condition the faces were low-pass filtered (i.e., high frequencies were degraded). Sergent then varied the task so that one condition required the use of higher frequency information than the other. When the task was to determine whether the face was male or female (a relatively easy discrimination that typically does not require higher frequency details), performance favored the left visual field whether the stimuli were clear or blurred by low-pass filtering. When the task was to identify the face, a right visual field advantage emerged for clear faces but not for low-pass filtered faces.

In other words, the right hemisphere relied more on low-frequency information to categorize even clear faces, whereas the left hemisphere relied on high-frequency information to identify them. Sergent (1986) pointed out that the prevalence in normal subjects of an advantage for left field performance in face processing may be due to the brief presen-

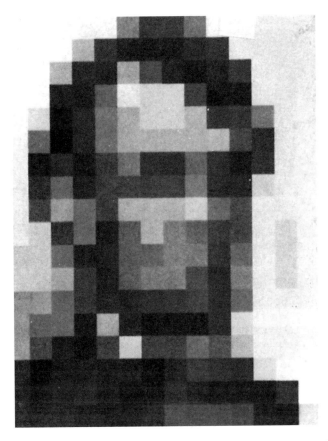

Figure 3.24 A luminance-averaged version of a famous face. The face is more easily perceived to be Abraham Lincoln when vision is blurred, which allows the lower frequency information to dominate. (From Harmon, 1973.)

tation of the stimuli, which was required to prevent eye-movement confounds. High frequencies are far more sensitive to degradation of this kind than are low frequencies.

One emphasis in the DFF theory is that the hemispheres are not specialized to process parts and wholes per se. Rather, the computations used by each hemisphere in perceiving the organization of visual displays are structured differently and will affect part/whole analysis—whether in objects or in faces—differently. That conclusion remains to be directly tested by studies that address the question of how we identify a face as a face (as opposed to a bowling ball) rather than how we identify a face as a particular individual or as familiar. The DFF theory would predict that a right visual field advantage would occur when the individual features of the face are most relevant for the task, but that a left visual field advantage would occur when something like the hairstyle or facial shape is most relevant. Also of interest would be a task requiring categorization of famous faces according to the relatively high or low spatial frequencies of distinguishing features. The predication would be that identification of faces with distinguishing features in the higher frequencies would produce a right visual field advantage, whereas faces with distinguishing features in the lower frequencies would produce a left visual field advantage.

SUMMARY

The experimental record from studies with healthy normal subjects supports the conjecture that hemispheric laterality in vision is linked to the relatively high and low spatial frequencies used to perform a task. The evidence from neurological patients, evoked potential studies, and imagining studies converges to support this conjecture. The anatomical locus of the difference has been associated with ventral posterior cortex. The critical areas appear to be early extrastriate cortex and its interactions with temporal-parietal cortex and, although not yet tested adequately, perhaps more anterior temporal cortex as well.

We also presented evidence showing that the differences in performance emerge after the sensory signal. For instance, if a stimulus is presented in peripheral vision, where low frequencies are better represented than high, then the global form is identified more readily than the local form on the basis of retinal position. If a stimulus is presented foveally, the local form may be identified before the global form. Thus, one cannot always expect faster response times for a global, as opposed to a local, form presented in the left visual field; nor can one expect faster response times for a local form, as opposed to a global form, presented in the right visual field. Such a predication would be expected only if some baseline measure were first used to demonstrate equal visibility of the two levels. In that way, the DFF theory predicts that when the global level is favored by sensory mechanisms the global advantage should increase when the right hemisphere is involved, and the global advantage should decrease when the left hemisphere is involved. When the local level is favored by sensory mechanisms the local advantage should increase when the left hemisphere is involved and decrease when the right hemisphere is involved. The evidence we have discussed in this chapter supports these predictions.

Finally, we have discussed how the DFF theory can account for alternative theories of hemisphere laterality in vision. For instance, the categorical/coordinate distinction may be a result of using higher or lower spatial frequency information to solve some problems. That example is particularly important because it shows how a qualitative difference, such as categorical versus coordinate judgments, may be based on a quantitative difference during encoding on a dimension such as spatial frequency. This is not to say that all theories of hemisphere laterality that postulate a qualitative difference can be accounted for by the DFF theory, but it does suggest that we might want to look more deeply at dimensions that may contribute to the qualitative appearance of the output.

In this chapter we have shown that the DFF theory can account for a variety of functional visual asymmetries for both simple and complex stimuli. Some investigators have argued that hemispheric differences are due to higher order processes, but it is not enough to leave the issue there. We have argued that hemispheric differences can arise from the initial use of relative frequency information that biases perception. Nevertheless, an adequate theory must include a mechanism by which absolute frequency, the form initially encoded in the visual system, is transformed into relative frequency. The DFF theory proposes that the transformation occurs through the attentional filtering mechanisms involved in spatial selection. The role of hemispheric differences in spatial attention will be the topic of the next chapter.

4 Attention and Visual Laterality

People respond selectively in order to achieve desired goals. Children enter the school playground and join a selected group of friends. A shopper shuffles through items on a clothing rack in search of a print blouse with long sleeves. The aging baby boomer scans the radio channels and stops when she hears a classic Beatles' tune. The people in all of these examples use attention volitionally. We want something, and we focus attention to find out where it is. Or, we see something and focus attention to find out what it is or what its parts might be.

Attention is not always volitional. It is often captured by external events such as loud noises, bright lights, or moving objects. Regardless of whether attention is directed by internal goals or by external events, selective attention is fundamental for survival. Without attention we would be overwhelmed by the dazzling array of perceptual inputs, unable to decide where to look and when to move in order to accomplish our goals. We are constantly directing and shifting the focus of attention in everyday life to perform even simple tasks.

The spatial scale of perceptual information can also be rapidly altered by shifts of attention. We can look at a scene using a broad attentional aperture to one or a few objects or parts in the scene. While relaxing on the porch, we may immerse ourselves in the expanse of the fields and distant hills. We may focus on a tractor on the horizon, only to be attracted by the movements of an ant crawling along the veranda railing. We experience such attentional changes as readily as we feel a change in the wind or orient to the sounds of a siren.

What is required to guide attentional selection in space? One necessity is a relatively accurate concept of space. We need a spatial representation of the three-dimensional world in which we live. This may sound trivial, but it is not. We need a higher level of representation than is given by the two-dimensional mosaic of the retina or by spatial representations in primary visual cortex. Knowledge of the spatial layout of the external world is required to volitionally guide attention to locations and divide it over smaller or larger regions of space.

Our experience is that we attend to space "out there." Yet spatial maps of out there are only internal mental representations computed by the nervous system. In order to selectively attend to locations in external space, we must select "locations" from an internal representation of that space. Those internal representations must bear some isomorphic relationship to the external world (see Palmer & Kimchi, 1986). The space to the left must be represented as opposite to the space to the right, and the space that is farther away must be represented relative to space that is closer. In that way space has an inherently relative quality. A location *to* the left is not *at* the left except in relation to some position to the right.

Fortunately, spatial representations that enter awareness have reasonable similarities to the spatial reality of the external world. When those internal maps fail, the consequences can be grim. For example, in the disorder of Balint's syndrome, described in chapter 1, the patients' representation of spatial information is altered or lost. In a limited way, those patients retain the ability to recognize an object but they fail to know where the object is located and they can't seem to move their attention to other objects (Coslett & Saffran, 1991; Friedman-Hill et al., 1995; Rafal & Robertson, 1995; Robertson et al., in press). They may have no clue whether an object such as a cup is on a table or suspended in mid-air. Such selective loss of spatial information limits their actions as one might expect: an object such as a cup may be readily recognized, but it cannot be picked up if its location in the external world is unknown.

Other internal representations of space appear useful for normal attention as well. In chapter 2 we discussed evidence demonstrating that attentional selection can operate on features such as spatial frequency. When subjects expect a grating of a given spatial frequency, stimuli at higher or lower frequencies are not detected as readily as are ones near the expected frequency. Similarly, we can expect to see a particular color or hear a particular sound. Selective attention can operate on both the internal spatial representations and on the internal representations of features that form the basis for object recognition. In other words, the attentional mechanisms that modulate the strength of sensory input can also be used to build spatial and nonspatial representations.

When attending to the big farmer in figure 2.3, we attend to a relatively large object in the scene. When we shift the focus of attention to the small farmer the scale of our attentional focus is reduced. That shift alters our expectations of the scale for other objects that might be present in the scene. If we look for a cow to accompany the little farmer, we readily focus on the small cow and exclude the large cow because of its disproportionate size. The spatial scale is expected to remain proportionally constant for objects within each scene. That is, we expect spatial consistency. The proportions must be derived from the representation we have of space as a whole; that is, from the representation of the three-dimensional structure and the placement and size of objects within that space.

We can think of the selection process in at least two ways. In one view, we choose to attend to a particular region of an internal representation of external space. We will refer to this representation as perceived geometric space, to convey that the representation includes information that is roughly isomorphic to the spatial geometry of the external world.

How might an attentional search occur over perceived geometric space? One possibility is that attention may be narrowed through modulation of cells representing particular regions, in order to highlight information from the selected region (Moran & Desimone, 1985). Many theorists appeal to the metaphor of attention as a spotlight, a mechanism that can be adjusted to span a selected region of space (Eriksen & St. James, 1986; Eriksen & Yeh, 1985; LaBerge & Brown, 1989; LaBerge & Buchsbaum, 1990). Perceptual processing is then assumed to be more efficient because information within the highlighted region is amplified at the cost of information outside the highlighted region. For example, if we want to identify the local elements of a hierarchical stimulus we might narrow the spotlight so that its scope matches the size of the local elements. The global shape exceeds the size of the spotlight, and its effect on perception should be reduced.

Alternatively, we can think of attention as an amplification of the information that is necessary to identify selected objects. Applied to hierarchical stimuli, this second view would posit that attention might amplify the relatively low frequency information in the perceptual input when the task requires the identification of the global shape or the relatively high frequency information when the task requires the identification of the local shape. Attention in that form would be analogous to applying a filter over the perceptual input. A low-pass filter would amplify low frequencies by filtering out the higher frequencies; a high-pass filter would amplify high frequencies by filtering out the lower frequencies. The filtering operation could be applied across the geometric representation of the entire scene. It would serve to highlight information at some spatial scales over others and it would encourage size constancy across the visual scene.

Both attention to spatial resolution and to spatial location can facilitate the ability to select objects in the visual world. We can choose to attend to larger or smaller regions of space by adjusting the size of our attentional window, and we can adjust the location of attention. We can also adjust attentional focus to attend to spatial resolution defined by differences in spatial frequency. Less time is required to find a target in a visual display when we know the correct region to attend to and also the appropriate size and resolution of the information to be selected. Such selection processes are helpful across species. A bird can rapidly find a small seed among larger pebbles if it knows where to restrict its search or if it knows the appropriate size and shape of the seed (Shettleworth, 1983). The search may fail if the animal expects the seed to be larger than the background objects, regardless of whether or not the bird is looking in the right place.

In this chapter, we lay the foundation for the discussion of different mechanisms of spatial attention and how they may interact to contribute to functional hemispheric asymmetries in visual processing. The review focuses on five critical points and assesses how each contributes to the lateralization of spatial cognition:

1. Selection by spatial location and spatial resolution operates on internal representations that use different descriptions of space. The DFF theory suggests one way in which spatial resolution guides attentional selection.

2. Selection occurs for absolute spatial locations and relative spatial locations as well as for absolute spatial frequencies and relative spatial frequencies.

3. As with attention to spatial locations, attention to spatial frequencies can be volitionally controlled or automatically captured.

4. Attention to spatial frequency and spatial location are both primarily associated with parietal lobe function but work in concert with different areas of the brain, creating different functional systems. Nevertheless, the principle of relative measures is critical in determining how selection occurs.

5. Some syndromes that are more closely associated with damage to the right hemisphere, such as unilateral visual neglect, may be due to a combination of deficits in attention to spatial location with the right hemisphere's bias for representing the lower frequency information required for global processing.

ATTENTION TO GLOBAL WHOLES AND LOCAL PARTS

The basic premise of the DFF theory is that the hemispheres are biased to respond to the *relatively* higher and lower spatial frequency information in a stimulus pattern. We have argued that there must be some type of attentional mechanism that selects the proper range of spatial frequencies to feed into the asymmetrically skewed hemispheric filters. If this were not the case, the hemispheres would be biased only to absolute frequencies. In other words, the spatial frequency—defined by the number, size, and spacing as projected onto the retina—would predict when the left hemisphere would prevail and when the right hemisphere would prevail. In a hierarchical figure, there would be some optimal size below which the left hemisphere would be more involved and above which the right hemisphere would be more involved. That is, absolute frequencies would predict that hemispheric effects would switch at some optimal size. As discussed in previous chapters, this conclusion has not received much support.

"Global" and "local" refer to relative values, and hemispheric differences are predicted in terms of those values (Lamb et al., 1990). That fact requires the existence somewhere along the processing pathway of a mechanism that converts absolute to relative values, just as there must be a mechanism that converts absolute retinal location to the relative locations used for a volitional visual search. There should exist a mechanism that acts as a medium between sensory registration of absolute values on the one hand and identification of global/local differences on the other.

What areas of the brain might be involved in selectively attending to the relevant spatial frequency spectrum? In order to address this question, we tested patient groups using an adapted version of procedures introduced by Kinchla, Solis-Macias, and Hoffman (1983). They showed hierarchically organized patterns to young healthy adults and varied across trials the probability, and thus the expectancy, that a target would appear at the global or local level. All patterns were shown centered on the screen at the point of fixation. When global targets were expected, performance was better for global than for local targets. When local targets were expected, performance was better for local than for global targets. As the probability schedules changed there was a consistent and direct trade-off between levels of both sensitivity measures and response times (figure 4.1).

We adapted those methods in a study with brain-injured patients and matched control subjects. As shown in figure 4.2, a group of patients with

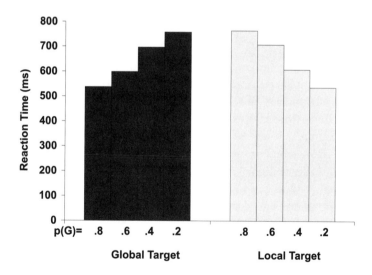

Figure 4.1 Mean reaction time for identification of global and local targets under different probability schedules. p(G) = probability of a global target in a block of trials. As p(G) decreases reaction time increases for global targets and decreases for local targets. (Adapted from Kinchla et al., 1983.)

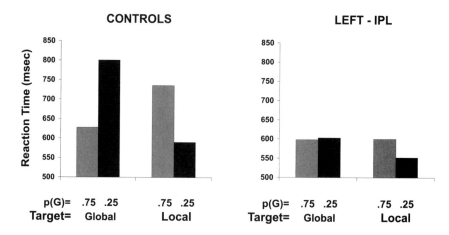

Figure 4.2 Mean reaction time for identification of global and local targets under different probability schedules in a group of patients with left parietal damage (Left-IPL) and a group of age-matched controls. p(G), probability of a global target in a block of trials.

lesions in the left inferior parietal lobe did not show the normal trade-offs (Robertson et al., 1988; 1991).

The stimuli were hierarchical letter patterns, and one stimulus appeared in the center of the screen in each trial. At the beginning of the experiment each subject was assigned two target letters, one of which was present in each trial. The target could be global or local, and the subjects had to identify the target as quickly as possible. The other level contained one of two nontargets on each trial. In one block of trials targets were equally likely to be global or local. In another block of trials the targets appeared at the global level 75% of the time and at the local level 25% of the time. In a remaining block, the targets appeared at the local level 75% of the time and at the global level 25% of the time.

Our study replicated Kinchla et al. (1983) in that the age-matched control subjects showed a symmetrical trade-off between global and local response times depending on whether a global or local target was expected in a block of trials (figure 4.2). Patient groups with temporal-parietal lesions showed the same trade-off as the normal controls, although the patients' trade-off was accompanied by the expected overall global or local bias depending on the side of the lesion. Patients with left temporal-parietal damage were faster to respond to global targets, and patients with right temporal-parietal damage were faster to respond to local targets when the target level was equally probable (i.e., baseline). When global targets were more likely, reaction time increased for global targets and decreased for local targets over baseline. When local targets were more likely, reaction time increased for local targets and decreased for global targets over baseline. Those trade-offs were present and not significantly different from those of normal controls.

In direct contrast to the temporal-parietal groups, patients with parietal damage had reduced trade-offs. Indeed, there were no reliable differences in the baseline measure between this patient group and normal controls. The left parietal group identified the targets at both global and local levels as fast as normal controls, but they did not show the normal trade-off in performance as target level probability changed. Possible floor effects or trade-offs between speed and accuracy that could have produced the pattern of results were ruled out. The effects were replicated in a second study (see Rafal & Robertson, 1995).

One possible explanation for the lack of trade-offs in the parietal group is that subjects did not notice the increased or decreased frequency of a target at either level. That explanation is not sufficient, however. In the replication study, the patients were asked at set intervals about the frequency of global or local targets in a block of trials. They clearly knew the probability schedules, but they were not influenced by them in the way that the normal and the temporal-parietal groups were.

Those findings are consistent with our hypothesis of the existence of a mechanism that controls how attention is allocated to levels of spatial structure. As with the data discussed in chapter 3, these data also show a double dissociation between deficits in allocating attention to different levels and in identifying global or local forms. Temporal lobe damage affects baseline performance in discriminating global from local shapes, whereas parietal lobe damage affects attentional measures. For reasons that are not yet clear, patients with left parietal lobe damage showed this abnormality, whereas right parietal patients did not. The group of right parietal patients was somewhat more variable and smaller than the left. However, a functional imaging study reported by Schneider (1993) found a similar difference in normal subjects. This difference could reflect many things, including greater functional separability between dorsal and ventral systems on the left than on the right, attentional control outside inferior parietal lobe on the right, or perhaps a weaker ability of the right hemisphere to allocate attention to hierarchical patterns.

Attention to Objects and to Space

Is attention directed to spatial locations or to objects? This has been a hotly debated issue in the attention literature. Objects appear at locations in space, which makes it difficult to know when attention is directed to the objects themselves and when it is directed to the positions occupied by the objects. This issue has become especially important given the discovery of two processing pathways through the cortex. Both animal and human data have supported the division of labor between a dorsal system that runs through occipital-parietal areas and responds to spatial information, and a ventral system that runs through occipital-temporal areas and responds to objects and their features (e.g., color, shape, brightness) (Newcombe & Russell, 1969; Ungerleider & Mishkin, 1982, 1994).

Consistent with the existence of two streams of processing, damage to both temporal lobes in humans produces deficits in the ability to perceive and identify objects, whereas damage to both parietal lobes produces deficits in the ability to locate objects and move attention between them (see De Renzi, 1982; Farah, 1990; Heilman & Valenstein, 1985). The degree of interaction between the two processing streams has become an area of active interest. Recent work has demonstrated that the spatial information associated with parietal lobes is also critical in the ability to correctly bind together object features, such as color and shape, size and shape, and motion and shape (Bernstein and Robertson, submitted; Friedman-Hill et al., 1995; Robertson, Treisman, Friedman-Hill, & Grabowecky, 1997). Those findings suggest that there are functional interactions between the spatial attentional processes of the dorsal stream and the nonspatial feature representations of the ventral stream. A recent PET study has provided additional support for the presence of interactions between the dorsal and ventral streams when feature integration is required (Corbetta, Shulman, Miezin, & Petersen, 1995).

An interesting laterality issue regarding the object versus space debate comes from the work of Robert Egly and his colleagues. Their work involved an elegant modification of the popular spatial-cuing task. Egly et al. (1994) presented two rectangles side by side, and subjects were required to press a button as soon as they detected the target (the filling in of one end of one rectangle; figure 4.3). Prior to the onset of the target, a cue (the brightening of one end of one of the rectangles) was presented. In the majority of trials the target location was validly cued. There were two types of invalid conditions. For one type the target appeared at the

INVALID CONDITION

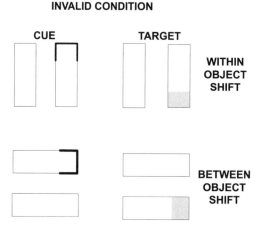

Figure 4.3 Examples of stimulus conditions used to examine within object shifts of attention versus between-object shifts. (Adapted from Egly et al., 1994.)

uncued end of the cued rectangle, which required subjects to shift attention within an object. In the second type of invalid trial the target appeared in the other rectangle, which required subjects to shift attention between objects. In both invalid cue conditions the target and cue were the same distance apart in the display but they were either in the same rectangle or in different rectangles, as shown in figure 4.3.

Normal subjects showed the typical spatial-cuing effect: targets at the valid cued location were detected faster than were targets at uncued invalid locations. In addition, there was a difference in detection time when the target appeared in an invalid location within the same object compared to when it appeared in an invalid location in a different object. Invalid targets in the same object as the cue were detected faster than invalid targets in a different object. Egly et al. concluded that attention is both object- and space-based. Object-based effects have been reported in other studies (e.g., Duncan, 1984; Baylis & Driver, 1992; Kramer & Jacobson, 1991), and neuropsychological studies have also suggested that attentional disorders can be manifest in both space- and object-based frames of reference (e.g., Behrmann & Moscovitch, 1994; Calvanio, Petrone, & Levine, 1987; Driver & Halligan, 1991).

Turning to the laterality issue, Egly, Rafal, Driver, and Starreveld (1995) have proposed that the two hemispheres may play different roles in utilizing the two reference frames for attentional selection. They have suggested that, while both hemispheres guide attention in space-based reference frames, attentional processes for object-based representations are associated only with the left hemisphere. Their laterality hypothesis was developed in part to account for the results obtained when a split-brain patient was tested with the rectangular cuing task represented in figure 4.3. In this study the procedure was modified so that, in each trial, the entire stimulus was restricted to one visual field. That is, both rectangles were placed on either the left or right side of fixation so that both the cue and target were always projected to the same hemisphere.

As was observed in normal subjects, the commissurotomy patient was fastest when the target appeared at the cued location. That result was found for both visual fields. The critical results occurred in invalid trials. When the stimuli were projected to the left hemisphere, the object-based effect was present: invalid targets that appeared within the same rectangle were responded to faster than were invalid targets that appeared in the other rectangle. The magnitude of the object-based effect was comparable to that observed in normal subjects. In contrast, there was no object-based effect when the stimuli were projected to the right hemisphere. Reaction times in invalid right hemisphere trials were essentially equal regardless of whether the cue and target occurred within the same rectangle or in different rectangles. Egly et al. (1995) concluded that attentional orienting of the left hemisphere is both object- and spaced-based, whereas attentional orienting of the right hemisphere is space-based, meaning that boundaries between objects can be ignored.

While theirs is an intriguing hypothesis, it is important to note that the DFF theory offers an alternative interpretation consistent with the idea that the two hemispheres provide asymmetric representations of the spatial frequency content of a stimulus. Consider what would happen if we low-pass filtered the two rectangles in figure 4.3. The edges defining the two rectangles would become fuzzy. Indeed, if our frequency cutoff were sufficiently low, we would no longer have an image of two rectangles; the two objects would blur into a single square-like blob. Within such a representation there would be no distinction between within-object and between-object shifts of attention. The two conditions would be functionally identical.

The application of the DFF theory to the commissurotomy data, then, is straightforward. The left hemisphere, with its amplification of relatively higher frequencies, is better suited to represent the two rectangles as objects (i.e., as the local elements of the stimulus). Object- and space-based attentional effects are possible with that type of representation. The local elements or objects are more weakly represented, however, in the lower frequency representation that is derived by filtering within the right hemisphere. Any object-based effect should be reduced or absent, at least when the object level is defined by the two rectangles. Attentional processes within the right hemisphere may also operate within both object- and space-based reference frames. But with the right's lower frequency representation, the object would be defined more by the global shape of the square formed by the two rectangles. Rather than emphasize qualitative differences in the frames of reference used by the two hemispheres to shift attention, the DFF theory suggests that the asymmetric filtering operations of the two hemispheres differentially define the objects contained in a scene. Attention may be object-based in both hemispheres, but attention in each hemisphere is tuned to objects at different levels of resolution.

Egly et al. (1994) also tested patients with unilateral parietal lobe lesions on a cuing task with the paradigm shown in figure 4.3. In accord with previous work (Posner, Early, Reiman, Pardo, & Dhawan, 1988), patients responded more slowly to invalid targets in the contralesional hemifield than to invalid targets in the ipsilesional hemifield. Such a result is often referred to as indicating deficits in disengaging attention. The additional object-based costs were also magnified for contralesional targets, especially in patients with damage to the left parietal lobe. Such results would, on the surface, appear to be at odds with the frequency-based account that we applied to the split-brain study. Assuming that the left hemisphere lesions forced the patients to reply on the low-frequency representation derived by the right hemisphere, one could predict a reduced object effect following left hemisphere damage. However, for most of the patients in this study the damage was restricted to regions superior to the critical temporal-parietal regions associated in the DFF theory with the second asymmetric filtering stage. Those more posterior regions would be expected to impair the first filtering operation, which is associated with directing attention to the relevant information; without the conversion to relative frequencies, the asymmetric filters would be required to work on the absolute frequency alone. Perhaps the increased object costs in the left hemisphere patients is another manifestation of a problem in directing attention. The left hemisphere patients may have become "stuck" on the object that contained the cue, but only when targets appeared in their contralesional fields.

Ultimately, the answer to questions about object-based attention depends on what we mean by an "object." This question has no clear answer, despite decades of attempts to provide one. Is the brightening of one end of a rectangle an "object" in figure 4.3? Are the two rectangles together an object? Is each rectangle an object?

It is likely that all of these can be perceived as objects, but they are objects at different levels of spatial resolution and/or at different spatial locations. This is not to imply that object-based attention does not occur. The evidence favors two different modes of attentional processing. But it should be kept in mind that the problem is inherently circular if we define an object by what we as observers perceive an object to be (i.e., it has face validity). Any theory of object-based attention will eventually have to contend with this difficult issue.

Spatial Location, Spatial Frequency, and Spatial Size

We have argued that functional asymmetries in the perception of local parts and global wholes are linked to differences in how the hemispheres utilize spatial frequency information in organizing hierarchical stimuli. As mentioned in chapter 3, the differences are reflected in terms of relative frequency. Recall that laterality effects for global and local forms have been observed over a wide range of sizes and visual eccentricities, and the evidence supports our conclusion that the laterality effects are superimposed on absolute frequency registration.

The fact that laterality effects can be described in terms of relative frequencies is a fundamental reason for proposing two stages of filtering. First, there is a filtering stage in which the relevant frequency range is selected by the system. That stage is followed by a second filtering stage in which the selected information passes through skewed filters that are biased in different directions in each hemisphere. Thus, the first effects of selection in the DFF theory are due to a filtering operation on the initial primary representations of frequency. The first stage of attentional selection modulates absolute frequency registration by increasing activation over a selected range of spatial frequencies. As will be seen below, which range is selected can depend both on stimulus information and on the task the subject is required to perform.

A primary goal, then, is to show that attention to local parts and global wholes can be linked to the selection of a restricted range of spatial frequency inputs. It is important to keep in mind that attentional allocation in perceived geometric space can also affect ability to identify local and global forms (see Brown & Kosslyn, 1995). Those two ways of attending—in terms of geometric space or in terms of stimulus spatial properties such as spatial resolution or size—can both operate at the same time (Robertson, Egly, Lamb, & Kerth, 1993). Knowing where to attend can facilitate identification of both the global and local forms, whereas attending selectively to a particular spectral region can favor identification of one level over the other. For example, attending to low-frequency information will selectively favor the analysis of the global form.

It should be noted that some theories of spatial vision suggest that the perception of coordinate space is computed from the spatial frequency spectra (De Valois & De Valois, 1988; Watt, 1988). In that view, there is no distinction between different types of spaces. Instead, spatial representations are a function of the information about object locations, which is derived from computations based on features. Spatial frequencies, orientations, contours, and the like appear spatially dispersed because basic visual functions perform a Fourier analysis or something similar, using those features as the basic perceptual building blocks. However, there is increasing evidence for multiple spatial maps (see Graziano & Gross, 1995). There is also evidence that subjects can attend to a spatial location and size before a stimulus appears. We are not taking a position on how spatial frequency contributes to the representation of those different maps, but we are arguing that at higher levels of analysis there is a distinction between the representation of spatial locations and spatial resolution (see Graham, Kramer, & Haber, 1985). Attention can be used to select locations and to adjust the window of attention in spatial coordinates, but it can also be used to select a particular scale of spatial resolution. (See Posner & Petersen, 1990, for a review of literature discussing the role of different neural structures in each type of spatial attention).

Under normal circumstances attention to different types of spatial features is hard to separate, but in the laboratory it is possible to show that attention to spatial resolution affects performance whether a stimulus is shown in an expected location or in an unexpected location (Robertson, 1996). The following section begins by discussing simple forms of stimuli and proceeds to a discussion of more complex forms.

Attentional Spotlights and Attention to Spatial Frequency

We begin with a simple stimulus and task used in visual psychophysics: the detection of sinusoidal gratings, a task that has appeared throughout the previous chapters (see figure 2.4). When there is no expectancy for a particular size of grating, people are faster to detect and discriminate low-frequency gratings than high-frequency gratings (see De Valois & De Valois, 1988). Similarly, except for very low frequencies, visual sensitivity is greater for low than for high spatial frequencies. However, attention can alter those effects. Sensitivity increases for stimuli in the neighborhood of an attended frequency region and decreases for more distant frequencies (Davis, 1981; Davis & Graham, 1981).

Consider two mechanisms that could account for such results. Subjects may directly attend to spectral cues by amplifying information at certain frequencies. Alternatively, they may alter the size of the region of space over which attention is allocated. That is, they may change the size of their attentional spotlight. Suppose that an observer were cued to expect a high-frequency grating. In order to take advantage of the cue, the observer could narrow the attentional spotlight to span only a small region of space. As can be seen in the pattern on the right in figure 4.4, such a narrow focus could slow the detection of a low-frequency grating since there would be little variation in brightness within the attended region. Indeed, the threshold for detecting the low-frequency grating could be raised to the point that a contrast change would not be detected at all within the attentional spotlight (e.g., if the grating in figure 4.4 were shifted slightly to the left or if attention shifted slightly to the right). Only the mid-luminance region of a single cycle falls within the attended region in the pattern on the right in figure 4.4; the alternation of dark and light stripes occurs outside the attended region. In the pattern on the left, the periodicity can be seen even though the size of the attentional spotlight is the same as in the pattern in the right.

Suppose that the observer were cued to expect a low-frequency grating. The attentional spotlight could be widened, as depicted in figure 4.5. In that case, the differences in response times to high- and low-frequency

Narrow Attentional Spotlight

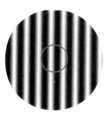 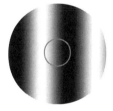

High Frequency   Low Frequency

Figure 4.4 A small attentional window (represented by the circles within each grating) interacts with the type of information within the window. Many cycles are present within the attentional window in the high-frequency grating (left) but not in the low-frequency grating (right).

Wide Attentional Spotlight

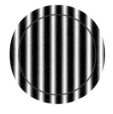
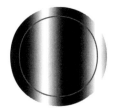

High Frequency   Low Frequency

Figure 4.5 A large attentional window (represented by the circles within each pattern) contains more cycles in each grating than are contained within the attentional window in figure 4.4.

patterns would be more subtle. Any spotlight size that spanned at least one cycle of the expected pattern would encompass more cycles of a higher frequency stimulus. Detection of high-frequency gratings could even be enhanced with a large spotlight, since there would be additional opportunities to detect the cyclic alterations of dark and light.

However, it is likely that there is an associated cost when attention is spread over a large area (Eriksen & St. James, 1986; Eriksen & Yeh, 1985; LaBerge & Brown, 1989). The idea is that we have a fixed amount of attentional resources. All attentional resources can be directed at a small region of space, or they can be dispersed over a larger region. When they are dispersed over a larger region, fewer resources are available per unit area.

To continue with the spotlight metaphor, the beam contains a fixed amount of energy that may be used to strongly highlight a smaller region, or it may be diffusely spread over a larger region. For instance, when we use an adjustable flashlight to look for a lost key in the grass, a narrow, powerful beam increases the ability to discriminate the key from the surrounding grass. However, a wider beam allows more ground to be covered. In choosing either option we run the risk of failing to detect the key, and we must decide which option best fits the circumstances. Increasing the size of the beam results in a loss of higher frequency resolution, whereas decreasing the size of the beam results in a loss of lower frequency resolution.

Returning to figures 4.4 and 4.5, it is easy to see why detection of a high-frequency grating could be poorer when the attentional spotlight is wide. Although more cycles will fall within the spotlight, each will be more weakly represented than when a fewer number of cycles fall within a narrow focus of attention. These examples demonstrate why attentional allocation to regions in space are difficult to separate from attention to spatial resolution.

These critical issues will be discussed throughout this chapter. Brown and Kosslyn (1995) have argued that the hemispheric differences found with hierarchical patterns are due to differences in the size of the region attended to by each hemisphere. In their view the hemispheres differ in the size of their attentional spotlights, with the right having a larger beam (more like figure 4.5) than the left (more like figure 4.4). The issue has not been satisfactorily resolved, and the preceding discussion makes it is easy to see why.

One way to approach the problem is to show that experimental variables have different effects on attention to the parameters that define perceived geometric space than they have on attention to parameters that define spatial resolution. Studies examining both types of spatial attention have been reported, and they support the existence of both types of spatial perception mechanisms. For instance, Robertson, Egly et al. (1993) manipulated the probability that a target would appear at the global or local level of a hierarchical letter pattern. In their study a cue was presented just prior to the appearance of a hierarchical stimulus. Either a large or small region of space was cued. The cues were correlated with the target stimulus such that global targets usually followed a cue to a large region of space, while local targets usually followed a cue to a small region of space. Subjects were told to report which of two predesignated target letters was present in each trial, regardless of whether it was global or local and whether it was cued or not. Cues were presented in half of the trials and were absent in the other half. The effects of the cue were analyzed by comparing response times in cued trials to those obtained in the uncued trials.

Their second manipulation varied the probability that the target would appear at either the local or global level over a block of trials, regardless of whether the target was cued or not. For one block of trials the target was at the global level in 66% of the trials. For another block of trials the target was at the local level in 66% of the trials. The methods were rather involved, but a representational scheme of the procedures is presented in figure 4.6.

As had been found previously (Kinchla et al., 1983; Robertson, Lamb, & Knight, 1988), probability manipulation over a block of trials had a significant effect on response latencies. When global targets were more frequent in a block of trials, global identification was facilitated while local identification was slowed. This effect occurred whether or not there was a cue. When local targets were more frequent in a block of trials, the reverse pattern of results was observed. Local identification was facilitated while global identification was slowed.

In contrast, the cuing manipulation operated within each trial, but the effects of the cue on local and global performance did not show symmetrical costs and benefits. When a large region of space was cued, both global and local identification improved over time (stimulus onset

Cued Trial

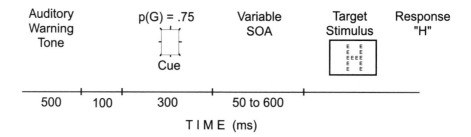

| Auditory Warning Tone | p(G) = .75 Cue | Variable SOA | Target Stimulus | Response "H" |

500   100   300   50 to 600

TIME (ms)

No Cue Trial

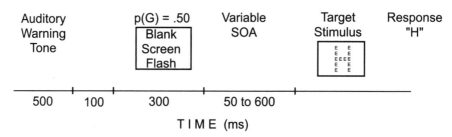

| Auditory Warning Tone | p(G) = .50 Blank Screen Flash | Variable SOA | Target Stimulus | Response "H" |

500   100   300   50 to 600

TIME (ms)

p(G) over block = .66

Figure 4.6 Stimulus parameters for a cued and no-cue trial in the Robertson, Egly, et al. study (1993). The subjects' task was to determine which of two predesignated target letters appeared in the target stimulus (In this case *H* is a target and *E* is a distractor). In one block of trials a cue trial predicted a global target with a probability of .75 (p(G) = .75) and in another it predicted a local target with a probability of .75. In the no-cue condition neither type of target was more probable (p(G) = .5). A grey screen flashed for 300 ms to signal that the probability of a global or local target was equal. In a block of trials with p(G) = .75 cued trials and p(G) = .50 no-cue trials, like those shown here, the overall probability of a global target, independent of the cuing conditions, was .66. SOA = stimulus onset asynchrony.

asynchrony or SOA) relative to the no-cue condition. When a small region of space was cued, however, only local identification improved over SOA. These improvements became more pronounced as the interval between the cue and target stimulus increased. There was no effect of the cue when the stimulus was presented just 50 ms after the cue, but by 450 ms robust cuing effects were present.

Together, the effects of cuing and of probability manipulations over a block of trials are consistent with the hypothesis of multiple attentional systems (Posner & Petersen, 1990). One system produced symmetrical costs and benefits that were set before the trial began and were constant over SOA. The other system was dependent on the cue and did not produce symmetrical costs and benefits. When the cue in a given trial predicted a global target, then benefits for both global and local targets were observed, consistent with an attentional spotlight set wide. When the cue predicted a local target, then benefits for only local targets were observed, consistent with a narrow attentional spotlight. Those benefits took over 300 ms to emerge and are consistent with control of attentional allocation over perceived geometric space. The benefits occurred within a trial. Attention to levels preceded the onset of the cue or target stimulus and produced symmetrical cost versus benefit trade-offs. The effects lasted across trials.

Attention, Global and Local Levels, and Spatial Frequency

The DFF theory proposes a selection process that precedes asymmetric filtering. The strongest evidence in support of this hypothesis is that the relative level of a stimulus is the critical factor in revealing hemispheric differences. Laterality effects associated with response speed in identifying local and global targets are based on relative spatial differences and not on absolute differences.

We have tended to discuss hierarchical stimuli as if the different levels of such complex stimuli map directly onto high and low spatial frequencies. This is clearly an oversimplification. After all, a hierarchical stimulus does not look like a grating. A global shape does not contain both information at the lower region of the spectrum and the local elements at nonoverlapping frequencies. With hierarchical stimuli the spectral content of the local elements is completely contained within the spectrum of the global pattern. This situation means that global patterns contain a larger range of frequencies than local patterns contain. The frequency components of the global form include a fundamental and higher harmonics, as shown in figure 4.7. Regardless of the overall size of the pattern, however, the fundamental frequency of a global form is lower than the fundamental frequency of a local form. It is this frequency relationship that is theoretically related to our relative spatial frequency proposal.

According to the DFF theory subjects should attend to relatively lower frequency information when identifying a global form than when identifying a local form. One of the most direct tests of that hypothesis comes from a dual-task study in which subjects performed a grating-detection task while identifying letters in hierarchical patterns (Shulman & Wilson, 1987). The gratings were sine waves (see figure 2.4) with a single spatial frequency value of either 0.5, 2.0, or 8.0 cycles/degree. The gratings were presented at a low contrast to ensure that subjects would have difficulty seeing them and would make errors on a proportion of the trials. The gratings were presented either before, after, or simultaneously with a hierarchical pattern. Subjects were instructed to identify a target letter in the hierarchical stimulus and to report the presence or absence of a grating.

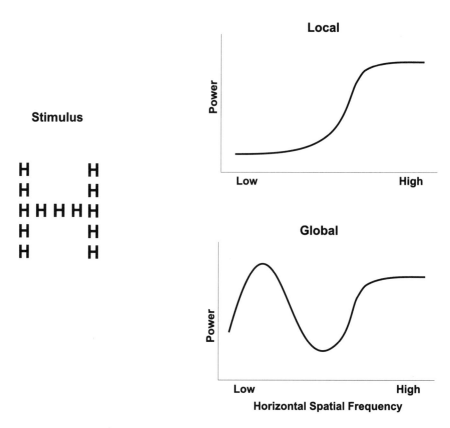

Figure 4.7 A simple schematic of relative power at high and low spatial frequencies for a local *H* and a global *H*. The global letter contains the higher frequency information of the local elements.

In separate blocks of trials the targets for the identification task were at either the global or local level. Subjects were informed of the manipulation and told that if they could, they should direct attention solely to the relevant level for each block of trials. The time between the presentation of the hierarchical pattern and the grating varied between −100 ms to 200 ms. All stimuli were shown in the center of a screen.

The results supported the hypothesis that attention directed to one or the other level of a hierarchical pattern affects the ability to detect a higher or lower frequency grating. When attention was directed to a global target low-frequency gratings were detected better than when attention was directed to a local target. When attention was directed to a local target high-frequency gratings were detected better than when attention was directed to a global target. Attending to a global target improved detection for lower but not for higher frequencies, even though the range of frequencies in the global target included the higher spatial frequencies of the whole pattern.

It is interesting to note the symmetry in those results. Attending to the global level increased sensitivity to low-frequency gratings, and attending to the local level increased sensitivity to high-frequency gratings. Local targets required subjects to attend to the relatively higher frequency information describing the hierarchical patterns.

It is again possible that the effects could be due to attentional shifts along the frequency dimension or to changes in the size of an attentional window over perceived geometric space. There are at least two important parallels in the differences between high- and low-frequency gratings and between local and global targets in hierarchical patterns. One parallel is the difference in the fundamental frequency: the global patterns have a lower fundamental than local patterns. A second parallel is the area over which the basic element extends: the overall shape defines the basic element at the global level, and each component part defines the basic element at the local level. For gratings, the bars constitute the basic element, which is the part that will be repeated cyclically. Thus, the basic element subtends a smaller area of space for local targets and for higher frequency gratings than it does for global targets and lower frequency gratings (see figures 4.4 and 4.5).

Subjects in the Shulman and Wilson study may have attended to a smaller region when looking for local targets, and that smaller "window" would facilitate performance on the high-frequency gratings. Adjustment of the size of their windows to distribute attention over a larger area of space when looking for global targets could disproportionately favor lower frequencies.

In order to distinguish between the two possible explanations for the subjects' performance it was necessary to vary the frequency information in the hierarchical patterns without changing the size of the basic elements or disrupting the hierarchical structure. In order to do this Robertson (1996) placed contrast-balanced dots on a screen to create a hierarchical stimulus. Contrast-balanced dots essentially remove the lower frequency information from the pattern by averaging over luminance, but the size and hierarchical nature of the overall pattern remains because each contrast-balanced dot can be arranged to form a pattern—in this case, a pattern with global and local forms or letters.

Each contrast-balanced dot is constructed by increasing the central pixel of a 3×3 array of pixels by a selected amount. The remaining 8 pixels are then decreased by a proportional amount (figure 4.8). Thus, the background luminance of the display and the mean luminance averaged across the 9-pixel region are equal. The dots can then be arranged on the screen to form larger patterns, creating hierarchical patterns (figure 4.9). Even though the procedure essentially eliminates the lower frequencies in the pattern, local shapes arranged into global shapes still can be perceived. Both the global and local letters can be resolved (although somewhat more slowly). Perception of both global and local levels must be accomplished through the use of the higher frequencies, because these are all that are available in the stimulus. (A Fourier analysis of

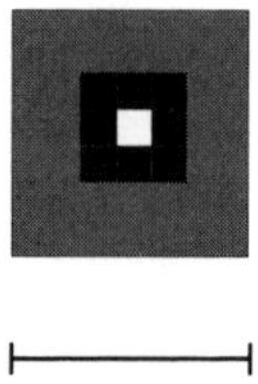

⊢————————⊣

X̄ Luminance = 0

Figure 4.8 Example of a contrast-balanced dot used to construct hierarchical letter patterns. The central pixel's luminance (white square) is increased and the eight immediately surrounding pixels' luminance (black squares) is decreased so that the average luminance of the two types of pixels equals the luminance of the background (grey square). The procedure creates a mean luminance of 0 across the unit of space.

stimuli constructed from contrast-balanced dots showed that the energy in spatial frequencies below 3 cycles/degree was eliminated.)

We will refer to patterns created from contrast balanced dots as high-frequency patterns and to the typical Navon patterns as mixed-frequency patterns. Perceptually, one of the high-frequency patterns does not stand out from the background as well as a mixed-frequency pattern. Note that in both high and mixed patterns, both global and local shapes extend over equivalent regions of space. Contrast balancing affects the spatial frequency spectrum in a hierarchical pattern, but does not affect either the overall size of global and local forms or the pattern's hierarchical structure. Thus, coordinate size and spatial frequency can be unconfounded. Importantly, global and local letters are still perceived. The inference that recognition of the global form is dependent on low-frequency information is supported by the fact that a global advantage found with normal hierarchical patterns is reduced or eliminated with the contrast-balanced high-frequency patterns (Hughes et al., 1990; Lamb & Yund, 1993).

Robertson (1996) examined how subjects modify their attention when presented with contrast-balanced stimuli. Under normal conditions sequential priming effects are observed with hierarchical patterns (Robertson, 1996; Robertson, et al., 1993; Ward, 1982). In other words, attending to one level in one trial affects performance in the next trial. Reaction times are shorter when the target appears at the same level on successive trials compared to when the target level changes. Is this priming effect also found when the stimuli alternate between contrast-balanced high-frequency patterns and typical mixed-frequency patterns?

Consider first the prediction if attentional selection is linked to the spatial frequency of a target level. Since the high-frequency stimuli require the analysis of high-frequency information for both local and global targets, there should be no general carryover effect (i.e., priming) when the target appears at the global level on successive trials. That is, if

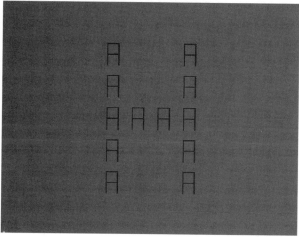

Figure 4.9 Examples of contrast-balanced high-frequency patterns and of a more typical mixed-frequency hierarchical pattern. The contrast cannot be controlled in the photograph as shown here, but the figure still gives an impression of how a stimulus created from contrast-balanced dots appears. The global and local forms are readily apparent.

level-specific priming is due to directing attention to a target through its fundamental frequency value, then level-specific priming effects would be expected to disappear when the prime was a high-frequency contrast-balanced pattern and the probe was a typical mixed pattern. In contrast, if attention involves an adjustment of the size of the attentional spotlight, then priming effects should persist and be the same for high-frequency and for mixed-frequency patterns. Suppose the target on a probe trial with contrast-balanced dots is at the global level. The spotlight would have to be expanded to identify this target.

In Robertson's experiment, subjects had to decide which of two targets was present; the target for a particular trial could appear at either the local or global level. The primary analysis focused on priming effects observed for the mixed-frequency stimuli as a function of whether the stimulus in the preceding trial was high frequency or mixed frequency.

Note that the task did not vary for the two different types of stimuli. For the subjects, the only relevant response was the identity of the target in each trial. The target could be at either the local or global level for both the probes and the primes, and subjects reported which target letter was present, not whether it was global or local.

The results were consistent with the predictions of the spatial frequency hypothesis (figure 4.10): attentional selection in a normal hierarchical pattern is based on spatial frequency information. When mixed-frequency patterns appeared in successive trials, reliable level-specific priming effects were obtained. A change in the target itself did not affect level priming. As found previously (Robertson, Egly et al., 1993; Ward, 1982), subjects were faster to respond when the target was at the same level in the prime and probe trials whether or not the shape itself changed. However, the effects were reduced and unreliable when contrast-balanced, high-frequency stimuli served as the primes.

It should be noted that when high-contrast-balanced patterns follow high-contrast-balanced patterns, priming effects are more specific to the target shape at the target's particular level (e.g., a global *H* followed by

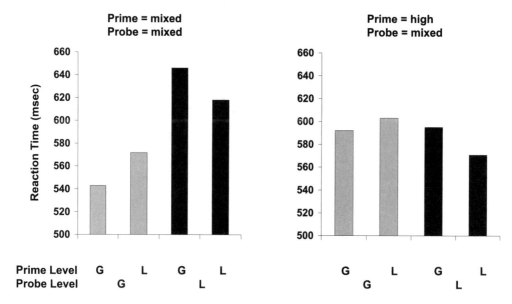

Figure 4.10 Mean reaction time for a group of normal young subjects to identify global (G) and local (L) probes following global or local primes. Primes were either the more typical mixed-frequency hierarchical patterns or contrast-balanced high-frequency patterns. Note that when both prime and probe were mixed patterns (left), response times were faster when the target appeared at the primed level than at the unprimed level. When the prime was a high-frequency pattern and the probe was mixed (right), those differences either were reduced or disappeared.

a global *H* produces significantly more priming than a global *H* followed by a global *S*). When the spatial frequency of the two levels cannot be used to discriminate levels, task performance relies on some other type of analysis that produces some object-specific priming. Under those conditions general level-specific priming (i.e., priming that occurs whether or not the shape or location changes) is either reduced or disappears altogether (Lamb & Yund, 1996; Robertson, unpublished data).

In sum, it was the spatial frequency of the target more than the area over which the target extended, that was the object of shifts in attention. In the Shulman and Wilson study, the effect of such shifts was observed within a trial with a short interval occurring between a grating and a standard mixed-frequency hierarchical pattern. Focusing on one level led to an increase in sensitivity for spatial frequencies of similar value. In the Robertson (1996) experiment, the effects of focusing attention carried over from one trial to the next across the 1 second interval. (Carryover has been found to occur across intervals of up to 3 seconds without reduction.) Attention continued to favor frequency values that were the most useful in selecting the target level in the preceding trial.

ATTENTIONAL SELECTION FOR LOCATIONS

The study of the representation of space has often been eclipsed by interest in the study of the representation of objects. Object perception intuitively seems more complex, whereas space seems to be a given—perhaps all the more reason to suspect it may require an enormous amount of computational power.

As was emphasized by William James (1890), attentional selection is selection for some *thing*. It is objects, sets of objects, or parts of objects that we seek. In this view, we attend to spatial locations because objects reside at some place in the world. Other theories suggest that we construct a representation of space by comparing the locations of objects. A strong version of this view is that the representation of space is essentially an epiphenomenon of object perception. In other words, there is no need to propose a spatial map independent of a representation of the layout of objects.

There are certain phenomena, however, that are difficult to reconcile with this view. For instance, we can attend to locations on homogeneous surfaces in expectation of a visual stimulus. In the laboratory the surface is often the computer screen. Although it can be argued that the computer screen constitutes an object (distinct from the surrounding background), attending to a location within the screen is quite different from attending to one level in a hierarchical pattern or to one object to the right of another. There is no obvious boundary for the "part" on the screen when we choose to attend to, say, a location in the upper left quadrant.

This position may be made clearer with a more ecologically justified example. If we scan the sky for a passing plane, we can attend to one location and wait for the plane to appear. We may move our attention about within this space. We can scan across the sky from left to right. We can even shift our attention to closer or farther locations within a single line of view. If we attend to distances that are too close, we may fail to notice the passing plane. It may blend in with the unattended background. The sky may appear as a surface, but it acts as a background to invisible layers of space between the sky and the perceiver. Spatial attention operates in this three-dimensional world. This may seem like an obvious and trivial point, but our visual system evolved to work within a three-dimensional world. If we lived in a five-dimensional world, our representation of space would have to be different.

The importance of perceived geometric spatial locations (i.e., the representation of space as we know it) for attention is also underscored by neurological syndromes showing that there are important hemispheric differences in spatial attention that can affect awareness itself. For example, spatial attention deficits are more severe following damage to the right hemisphere than they are following damage to the left hemisphere (Heilman, Watson, & Valenstein, 1985). Patients with right hemisphere damage are more likely to show symptoms of unilateral visual neglect to the left side of space than patients with left hemisphere damage to the right side of space. Although neglect is also sensitive to variables related to objects and object arrays (Behrmann, et al., 1994; Driver & Halligan, 1991; Grabowecky, Robertson, & Treisman, 1993; Ladavas, 1987), the most prominent feature of the syndrome is a deficit in attention to all or part of the contralesional side of space. It appears that spatial knowledge of the contralesional part of space disappears and that spatial attention can no longer be volitionally directed into that space.

Deficits in Attending to Locations of Space

We acknowledge that the DFF theory cannot account for all visual laterality effects. The mechanisms that underlie lateralization of global and local levels of spatial structure interact with other mechanisms that may represent the extent of spatial information and the location of objects in the world. In fact, it is that type of spatial information that researchers have most often cited as demonstrating lateralized spatial effects. The topic of this section is a discussion of the hemispheric differences that may exist and how they might interact with computations of the DFF theory to produce clinical differences in visual spatial processing.

The costs and benefits that are found when attention is directed to spatial locations are analogous to the costs and benefits that are found when attention is directed to levels of spatial structure. In the most common paradigm used to study spatial attention, a target appears at one of two spatial locations (figure 4.11) and a cue provides advance

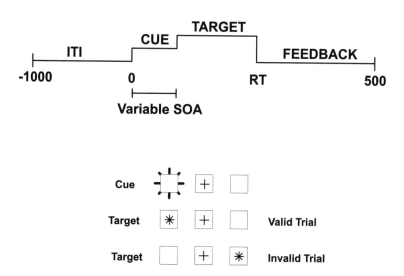

Figure 4.11 Schematic of stimulus parameters in a typical cuing task (Posner, 1980). The cue is the brightening of one of the three boxes in the display. The target (*) follows at a variable time and is located either in the cued box (valid trial) or the uncued box (invalid trial). The subjects' task is to press a button as soon as the target appears. They are told to fixate the central plus sign throughout the trial. Feedback informs the subjects of early responses (responses that occur before the target appears). A small proportion of catch trials (when no target appears) is generally included to discourage early responses. SOA = stimulus onset asynchrony; RT = reaction time; ITI = interstimulus interval.

information about the location of the upcoming target. The cue can be exogenous (i.e., appearing in the location where the target will soon appear), or it can be more abstract (i.e., a central arrow pointing in one direction). The common assumption is that exogenous cuing produces automatic orienting, whereas a more abstract cue like a central arrow requires volitional control. The cue need not be visual. It may be a tone predicting a target in one direction. People are faster to detect a target at the cued location than at the uncued location under both exogenous and endogenous conditions (Posner, 1980; Posner, Walker, Friedrich, & Rafal, 1984).

That task has proven quite useful in the study of spatial attention (for reviews, see Hillyard, Mangun, Woldorff, & Luck, 1995; Posner & Petersen; 1990; Rafal & Robertson, 1995). Studies with both healthy and neurologically impaired populations have led to the conclusion that attentional shifts within space do not reflect a unitary mechanism but rather entail the successful coordination of a composite of component operations that are anatomically distributed. Attention must not only be deployed to a cued location, it must also be disengaged from its current focus before it can move elsewhere. This situation has been likened to that of a spotlight moving across a surface. Other theorists have argued that a better metaphor for spatial attention would be a three-dimensional volume with different and competing levels of activation over space

(LaBerge & Brown, 1989). In both views there is a prominent role for the representation of geometric space.

One set of neuropsychological studies (Posner et al., 1984) has focused on the role of the parietal lobe in directing spatial attention. It has been argued that lesions to that brain region produce an impairment in the ability to disengage attention from a previously attended location, and that the impairment is most pronounced with right hemisphere damage. That deficit in disengaging attention is observed when attention is initially directed to an ipsilesional side of space and a target appears in a contralateral location (figure 4.12). In the cuing task described just previously, patients with parietal damage showed a disproportionate delay when the target appeared in the contralesional side of space following an invalid cue in the ipsilesional side of space. This particular response profile was different from that obtained with other patient groups (reviewed in Rafal & Robertson, 1995).

The problem was not so much one of responding to cues in the contralesional hemifield. When the cue and target both appeared on the contralesional side there was a relatively small increase in response latencies compared to similarly valid trials in which both cue and target appeared on the ipsilesional side. The major problem occurred in trials in which the cue was invalid and the target appeared on the contralesional side.

When the cue appeared it initially drew attention toward the location in either the ipsilesional or contralesional side of space. But when attention was drawn to the ipsilesional side the effect was as if the patient had

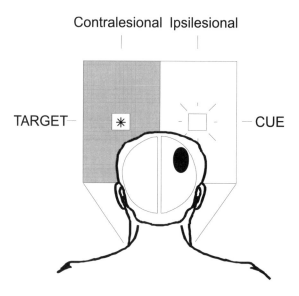

Figure 4.12 Example of a cue appearing in the ipsilesional field and a target in the contralesional field of a patient with right hemisphere damage. Shading is not actually present in the display. It represents the field affected by the lesion.

become stuck at the cued location, and the patient had great difficulty disengaging attention to shift to the actual target location. In contrast, when the contralesional side was cued and the target appeared on the ipsilesional side, the costs were greatly reduced. Although the pattern held with both left and right hemisphere damage, the problem was especially acute in patients with insult to the right hemisphere.

In a sense, the cuing task creates a laboratory model of what clinicians test when they examine patients for unilateral visual extinction, which is sometimes thought of as a less severe form of neglect (though this point is controversial). To verify that a patient with extinction can see both sides of space, the clinician may wiggle a finger in either the ipsi- or contralesional visual field while the patient looks directly at the clinician's nose. Patients with extinction are able to detect a solitary stimulus in either the left or right visual field. However, when there is more than one stimulus present—for example, when the clinician wiggles fingers on both hands at the same time—then the patient with extinction fails to detect the contralesional stimulus. That pattern was also found using the cuing task in patients with a moderate to severe amount of unilateral visual neglect, and the pattern was found to correlate well with the degree of neglect (Morrow & Ratcliffe, 1988).

Other attentional tasks have also been used with patients with unilateral visual neglect, and they have been consistent with reports using the cuing task. Those other tasks produced data that support the idea that at least one component of visual neglect is difficulty in disengaging attention from the ipsilesional side of space (for a discussion of other components of neglect, see Rafal and Robertson, 1995).

Eglin, Robertson, & Knight (1989), for example, demonstrated that a search for a target appearing on the contralesional side of a cluttered array was slower to begin when ipsilesional distractors were present than when they were not. One set of stimuli used a target that had features in common with the distractors (a conjunction target, as shown in figure 4.13). In healthy subjects the time required to find a conjunction target increases in a linear fashion with the number of distractors (Treisman & Gelade, 1980). That linear increase in reaction time has been replicated many times in the cognitive literature and is considered to be indicative of an attention-demanding, serial search process (see Treisman, 1988). Basically, attention is believed to be deployed to each item or group of items in the field until the target is found.

One interesting finding reported by Eglin et al. (1989) was that patients with unilateral neglect began their search for a target on the contralesional side as easily as on the ipsilesional side but only when no distractors appeared on the ipsilesional side (see middle display of figure 4.13). However, when items were added to the ipsilesional side (see lower display of figure 4.13), the patients acted as if they were stuck on one side. It often took them 10 to 20 seconds to continue on to the

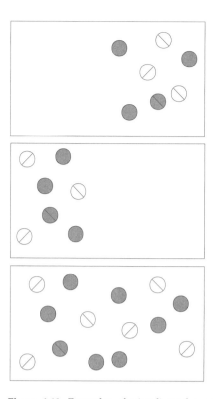

Figure 4.13 Examples of stimuli used to study visual search in patients with unilateral visual neglect. The stimuli were actually red dots (represented by grey circles) and blue dots with lines through them (represented by white circles). One red dot also contained a line, and this red dot was the target. In the top example the entire display is on the ipsilesional side for a patient with right hemisphere damage. In the middle example the display is on the contralesional neglected side. In the bottom example the target is on the contralesional side and there are bilateral distractors. Adapted from Eglin et al., 1989.

contralesional side to look for the target if they did not find it on the ipsilesional side.

Those results are relevant for our discussion of spatial representations. Patients with unilateral neglect act as if the space to their contralesional side does not exist, but only when nothing attracts attention to the ipsilesional side of space. They typically show little or no awareness of the contralesional side of space and behave as if half of the world had ceased to exist. Such patients may underestimate the width of a door and run their wheelchairs into a wall as they try to pass through. They may underestimate the length of a horizontal line or draw all the numbers of a clock on the ipsilesional side of a circle (figure 4.14). Note that in this latter example they continue to demonstrate knowledge that a clock has 12 numbers. They merely compress the numbers onto one side of space presumably because the other half is not part of their conscious awareness. Without awareness of contralesional hemispace they are unable or

Example of clock drawing of patient with neglect

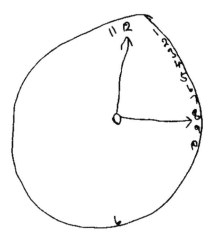

Figure 4.14 The observer drew the circle representing the clock face and asked the subject to draw in the numbers on the clock face. (From Robertson & Marshall, 1993.)

unmotivated to direct their attention in that direction. Dramatic examples such as these occur only in the most severely affected patients.

Consistently, most patients with unilateral neglect can be cued toward the contralesional side of space when nothing exists to attract their attention to the ipsilesional side of space. Under those conditions attentional resources are not demanded by the ipsilesional side. The patients often appear to cue themselves to look toward the left, and awareness of spatial extent into the contralesional field follows. All of those problems are more likely in patients with right hemisphere lesions than in those with left hemisphere lesions. In patients with left hemisphere lesions awareness of the global extent of the field is less affected than in patients with right hemisphere lesions.

Frames of Reference and Deficits of Spatial Attention

Patients with unilateral neglect do not simply neglect information that is projected to their damaged hemispheres (e.g., a person with right hemisphere damage and left neglect) Rather, patients can be seen to neglect information to the left of some *midpoint* of a scene or object even when all the information is projected to the intact hemisphere. Again, that kind of deficit requires the transformation of absolute spatial locations as defined by the retina or hemispheres into relative locations.

Given the decussation of the visual system, it might seem like a relatively easy task to model how space is represented. The left side of the fovea is mapped onto the right side of the visual cortex and vice versa. Furthermore, the upper visual field is mapped onto the ventral portion of striate cortex, while the lower visual field is mapped onto the dorsal portion in a remarkably isomorphic fashion (Tootell, Silverman, Switkes, & De Valois, 1982). However, neurophysiological experiments have revealed multiple spatial maps at various levels in the visual system, from the retina through higher cortical areas (Andersen, 1987; Graziano & Gross, 1995). A simple model of spatial representation might be based on the idea that a cue facilitates processing in those cells with receptive fields that encompass the cued location. This model could account for the benefits observed when the target is presented at the cued location. When a cell is activated by a cue, a subsequent target may be seen sooner because it is in the receptive field of neurons that respond to that location. When a cell is outside the cue-activated area, a subsequent target may not be primed. In the language of cognitive psychology, if spatial attention constitutes a fixed resource then drawing attention to one location would produce a cost in detection at another location.

However, such a model would postulate a single mechanism underlying both the benefits and costs associated with spatial cues. Behavioral and neuropsychological data are at odds with such a single-mechanism account, however. Benefits and costs can be affected by different experimental manipulations, suggesting that one process is responsible for benefits and that another process contributes to costs. One hypothesis is that a generalized inhibition arises at uncued locations, especially for locations in the opposite side of space. An alternative hypothesis holds that activation in the cued hemisphere increases the noise level in the uncued hemisphere.

There are at least two problems with such simple direct-access models in accounting for the data from brain-damaged patients. The first problem is that, when we look at single-cell activity in higher visual areas such as the parietal lobe, activity is not solely limited to stimuli in the contralateral hemifield for all neurons. The size of receptive fields increases dramatically as information flows anteriorly (Gattass, Sousa, & Covey, 1985). Many cells in the parietal lobe have large enough receptive fields to respond to visual information across the midline.

The second problem with direct-access models of spatial representation is that the effects of attention are not only defined by viewer-centered space (i.e., retinal right and left), but also by environment-centered space. When we move about, either by moving our eyes, head, or body, the positions of objects in the environment are perceived to remain constant. When we lie down the spatial positions of the environment do not recline with us. The ceiling is still perceived as above us and the floor below us. Even a vertically oriented sinusoidal grating viewed in a dark room from a prone position would continue to be perceived as upright. Our perceptual experience of space remains constant despite variations in the retinal image and the flow of stimulation over it.

The preceding discussion makes clear that there may be several different frames of reference or coordinate systems in which spatial attention may operate. Spatial maps may be viewer-centered, with left and right defined by the person's line of site. They may also be environment-centered, with left and right defined by salient landmarks in the natural world. A variant of this would be object-centered or scene-centered space. Left and right may be relative to a particular object or to an array of objects (a scene) within the environment.

Several studies have shown that attentional disorders such as neglect or extinction can be manifested in both viewer-centered and scene- or object-centered representations of space. Ladavas (1987) modified the basic cuing task so that both the cue and the target occurred in the same visual field. For instance, a cue that appeared in the left visual field would be followed by a target that appeared either at more eccentric or less eccentric locations in the same visual field (middle panel in figure 4.15).

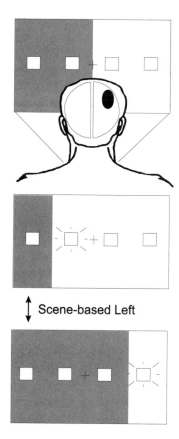

Scene-based Left

Figure 4.15 In the upper example the neglected side of the display (represented in grey) is coincident with the left visual field (the plus sign represents fixation). In the two lower examples the neglected side is relative to the display and is defined in object- or scene-based coordinates. Left and right are relative to the cued side, not to eye fixation (the plus sign).

In that example both the target and the cue were on the left side of fixation and were projected to the right (damaged) hemisphere. In scene-centered coordinates a more eccentric target was located in the contra-lesional direction away from the cue, but one closer to fixation was located in the ipsilesional direction. In effect, Ladavas's procedure produced two centers. One was defined relative to the subjects' eye position by the fixation point at the center of the display. The other was defined relative to the location of the cue, presumably at the center of attention.

For patients with right hemisphere lesions, deficits in spatial attention were found to reflect both frames of reference (Ladavas, 1987). Reaction times were slower when the target occurred to the left of the cue, regardless of whether the cue (and target) were in the contralesional left side of space or the ipsilesional right side of space (see, also, Gazzaniga & Ladavas, 1987). In addition, the subjects were slower to detect targets in the left visual field regardless of whether they were at the cued or uncued location.

Other studies of patients with neglect or extinction have also emphasized the contribution of different reference frames in spatial attention (Behrmann et al., 1994; Calvanio et al., 1987; Driver & Halligan, 1991; Farah, Brunn, Wong, Wallace, & Carpenter, 1990; Grabowecky et al., 1993), as have more recent studies of normal subjects (Logan, 1995; Robertson, 1995a).

Calvanio et al. (1987) asked patients with right-sided lesions and neglect to identify a letter presented in one of four quadrants in a display. The letters were always upright in the display, and the patients were either sitting upright, lying on their side rotated 90 degrees to their left, or lying on their side rotated 90 degrees to their right. As expected, when the patients were upright they made numerous errors when the letters were presented in the two left quadrants of the display, and their performance was nearly perfect when the letters were presented in the two right quadrants. When the patients performed the task while lying on their side, neglect was found in both viewer-centered and environmental coordinates (figure 4.16). Performance was best when the letters appeared in the right visual field and on the right side of the display. Poorest performance occurred when letters appeared in the left visual field and on the left side of the display. For the remaining two quadrants error rates were located between the two extremes. On some trials the environmental reference frame dictated which side would be neglected, and on other trials the viewer-centered reference frame dictated which side would be neglected.

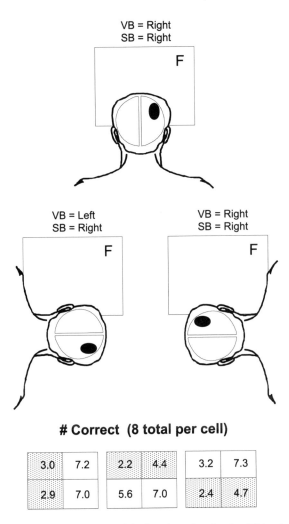

 # Correct (8 total per cell)

3.0	7.2	2.2	4.4	3.2	7.3
2.9	7.0	5.6	7.0	2.4	4.7

Figure 4.16 Example of the location of a stimulus (F) in viewer-based reference frames (VB) and scene-based reference frames (SB) under different conditions of head rotation. The data on the bottom are the mean number of stimuli that were correctly identified by a group of patients with left neglect due to right hemisphere damage. The shaded areas represent the neglected side in viewer-based coordinates. (Adapted from Calvanio et al., 1987.)

Importance of Coordinate Spatial Maps in Guiding Attention

Visual neglect of one side of space can occur in various coordinate systems, each of which defines different properties of the visual display. Reaction-time data in rotation studies with normal subjects are consistent with the idea that attentional selection can occur in spatial maps other than those defined by the retina (Logan, 1995; Robertson & Lamb, 1988, 1989; Robertson, 1995a; Rhodes & Robertson, 1996). There must be a rather high level of spatial abstraction for such selection to occur. One of the basic requirements is that one side of space is defined relative to another. That is, the right side of an object or scene implies an opposite or left side. Logically, neglect of the left side of an object implies some knowledge of the spatial extent of the whole object that contains a right side.

Neglect is not limited to a simple problem of one hemisphere being overly activated or directly inhibited. Rather, the selection process may be biased in coordinate systems that are defined by the environment, the object, the scene, or the retina. The spatial reference frames are perceived at some level, but one side of each reference frame may be neglected. Neglect is of relative locations, not absolute locations.

If coordinate two-dimensional space is represented symmetrically in striate cortex, then the selection bias toward the right or left in scene- or environmental-based coordinates must occur in space as it is represented at higher levels in the visual system. There is no reason for this space to remain viewer-centered and every reason for it not to remain so centered. For activities of normal daily life, we would not want to be limited to the space defined by the retina.

As with other spatial features such as spatial frequency, attentional selection occurs on sets of internal representations, producing relative scales. The important theoretical point of this discussion is that space is represented in different internally represented dimensional fields. The representation of space is not a slave to retinally defined coordinates with their right and left visual fields. There are many different representations of space, and each can be used to guide visual attention. When unilateral damage occurs, neglect of contralesional information can often be seen at each of the levels of spatial representation.

The problem facing us is not simply to describe the translation of the two-dimensional representation of space on the retina and striate cortex to a three-dimensional representation of objects in the external world (Marr, 1982). A further question is how multiple spatial representations combine to result in a unified perception of space. It is that unified representation that can make visual processing more efficient and allow us to combine visual information with internal goals in order to make our actions constructive.

If we conceive of space as an abstract internal representation in dimensional space, then several benefits follow. First, it is less difficult to entertain the idea that attentional selection is made not of objects in an external Euclidean world but of represented objects in the internal representation of geometric space. Second, how selection occurs in coordinate space and frequency space can be posed in similar ways (e.g., with reference to relative values). Third, hemispheric differences in processing one spatial value relative to another must distinguish among different types of spatial representations and how they interact with attentional mechanisms.

SPATIAL ATTENTIONAL MECHANISMS AND RIGHT HEMISPHERE DOMINANCE IN UNILATERAL NEGLECT

The preceding discussion focused on general issues regarding spatial attention. We now return to a fundamental concern in the consideration of hemispheric asymmetries as they relate to spatial attentional function. In particular, why do disorders of visual-spatial attention appear more pronounced following damage to the right hemisphere than following damage to the left hemisphere? This difference is most obvious in the acute period following onset of a neurological event. Patients with left hemisphere damage are not as likely to manifest clinical signs of neglect (Ogden, 1987).

As the preceding chapters have discussed, patients with right hemisphere damage are also more likely than those with left hemisphere damage to miss global aspects of patterns. It is quite possible that left-sided neglect after right hemisphere damage reflects a bias in orienting to the contralesional field combined with a global processing deficit. That idea has been most thoroughly discussed by Halligan and Marshall (1994). After reviewing a large number of studies of unilateral neglect they concluded that the visual behavior of patients with neglect due to right hemisphere damage could be attributed to the persistence of a left hemisphere processing system that amplified local over global information. That persistence could be assumed to dominate performance, especially if the lesion had damaged a different system designed to process global information.

A variety of evidence suggests that, in processing a visual scene, there is an initial analysis of global information. That analysis appears to occur at a preattentive stage. For example, patients with neglect continue to demonstrate an internal representation of the spatial extent of a visual display (Grabowecky et al., 1993), as well as a representation of basic grouping and shape properties such as symmetry (Driver, Baylis, & Rafal, 1993). Indeed, the fact that neglect can be object- or scene-based indicates that the global shape is represented below the level of awareness. In order to ignore one side of a display, in other words, the middle of the display must be established.

Halligan and Marshall (1994) revealed the presence of residual global perception in the face of neglect in an elegant manner. They showed a patient a display of a large square. The sides of the square were formed by a series of small *A*s. When asked to describe the form, the patient said he saw a square. However, when asked to draw a line through all of the *A*s, the patient only marked those on the right side of the page (figure 4.17). Thus, the patient comprehended the overall geometric shape, but when directed to attend to the local elements, he was no longer able to attend to information from the left side of space that was needed to define the global shape.

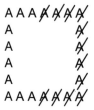

Figure 4.17 A patient with unilateral visual neglect was asked to cross out all the *A*s in the stimulus. She stopped at about the center of the display. (Adapted from Halligan & Marshall, 1994.)

Albert's Line Crossing Test

Instruction: Cross out lines at corners   Instructions: Cross out all lines

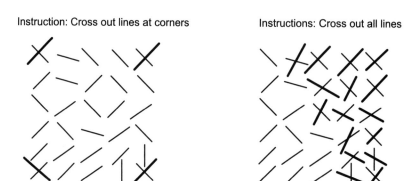

Figure 4.18 Performance of a patient with neglect when given instructions that encouraged attention to the global layout (left) compared to instructions that encouraged attention to the local elements (right). (Adapted from Halligan & Marshall, 1993.)

Similarly, another patient (Halligan & Marshall, 1993) showed a dissociation on two types of a line-cancellation task (figure 4.18). When asked to draw a mark through all the lines, the patient responded only to those on the right side of the page. When asked to draw a mark through the lines in the corners of the page, however, the patient succeeded in marking all four corners.

Seemingly bizarre dissociations such as those led Halligan and Marshall to conclude that the global configuration of the figure was processed by these patients. However, the damage to the right hemisphere did not allow a sustained representation of the global form when local processing became necessary. Attention could be directed to the global pattern when attention was not directed to the local elements. The global representation, in a sense, became submerged during local responses. The left hemisphere, with its preference for local information, continued to function to detect the small *A*s but only on the one side of the stimulus, since the right hemisphere could not sustain a global representation indicating the global extent of the stimulus explicitly.

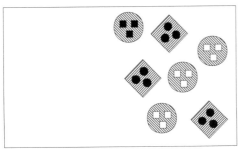
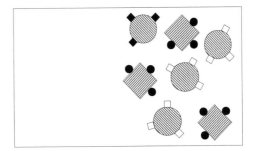

Local Elements   Attached Elements

Figure 4.19 Examples of stimuli used to study the effects of local elements on visual search in patients with unilateral visual neglect. The stimuli were large blue squares and orange circles with smaller orange squares and blue circles as elements. The target was a large blue square with small orange circles, representing the conjunction of shape, color, and size. (Adapted from Eglin, 1992.)

Eglin (1992) approached the problem differently. She presented large blue and orange dots in a display that required an attentional visual search for a conjunction target (figure 4.19). Subjects were required to locate the target, and their response times were recorded under various conditions that varied in terms of distractors and irrelevant elements scattered around the target. Those elements either were located between the larger dot distractors and the target, were attached to them, or were placed within the dots to create new local forms within each dot's global outline. A delay in searching the neglected side of the display was most pronounced when the irrelevant elements formed local objects within the dots, moderate when the irrelevant elements were attached to the dots, and weakest when the elements were randomly scattered around the display.

Right hemisphere damage increases the likelihood that attention will be unable to shift in the contralateral direction from one object to another. The likelihood is especially high when those objects contain information at a more local level (or at a relative frequency around the same location). From this perspective, neglect following right hemisphere damage can be viewed as a combination of the intact left hemisphere's preference for local (relatively high-frequency) processing combined with a bias toward the ipsilesional (intact) side of the visual field.

The DFF theory was not conceived to answer the question of why more severe neglect occurs with right hemisphere damage than with left hemisphere damage. Nevertheless, we can speculate that preattentive global processing of spatial extent and grouping can be accomplished by patients with unilateral neglect. That type of processing may be based on absolute spatial frequency analyses, which remain relatively intact (Spinelli & Zoccolotti, 1992). The absolute as well as relative size of the display has been consistently shown to influence the magnitude of observed neglect (Eglin, Robertson, Knight, & Brugger, 1994).

We can further speculate that preattentive global analysis provides information about the spatial extent of the stimulus display and can thus bias attentional orienting into the left or right side of a display. Response to the relative global properties may be disrupted in those patients because the mapping between primary visual input and higher-order visual representations may be disconnected. If such a disconnection occurs awareness of the global form may become either weakened or nonexistent. Under such conditions attention is more likely to become stuck on local elements on the intact right side of the visual display.

Alternative Explanations

Other accounts have been offered for the prevalence of spatial attentional deficits with right-sided lesions. One theory has already been discussed. Brown and Kosslyn (1995) suggested that the hemispheres differ in their contributions to adjusting the size of the attentional window. They claim that the right hemisphere monitors the output from neurons with larger receptive fields than does the left hemisphere and that larger receptive fields contribute to wider attentional distribution over space. However, we have shown that hemispheric differences for global and local patterns occur even when the stimuli change in overall visual angle. The fact that that can happen was also confirmed in a recent imaging study (Fink et al., 1996).

Brown and Kosslyn also suggest that the attentional window interacts with perceptual properties, but in their case the claim is for perceptual saliency. They assume that global properties are generally more salient than local properties and that a larger attentional window favors perception of those properties. Identification of local properties is facilitated by use of a smaller attentional window, which compensates for reduced saliency. As a result of the interactions between the saliency of parts of the stimuli and attentional demands, a larger area of metric space is affected when right hemisphere damage occurs than when left hemisphere damage occurs. (Note that their model is viewer-centered, and we have already shown that global/local differences by hemisphere occur even independent of the retinal or environmental location of the stimulus as a whole. Further, note that the assumption of global precedence has been repeatedly questioned).

Brown and Kosslyn (1995) tested their theory using right or left visual field presentation in a series of experiments with young, healthy subjects. The stimuli were either hierarchical letter or object patterns (figure 4.20). The subjects' task was to report which of two possible targets was present in each trial. For instance, the jacket in figure 4.20 might be designated a target and the sweater a distractor.

PICTURES   **LETTERS**

Experiment 1

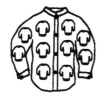
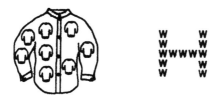

Experiment 2

Experiment 3

Figure 4.20 Examples of hierarchical object and letter stimuli used by Brown and Kosslyn (1995).

Contrary to what would be predicted if there were a general hemi-spheric asymmetry in the processing of local and global information, the two types of stimuli did not yield the same pattern of results across the three experiments. For the pictures, there was a general trend for a level-by-visual-field interaction; local targets were detected more rapidly when they were presented in the right visual field and global targets were detected more rapidly in the left visual field. For the letters, that interaction was only reliable in Brown and Kosslyn's third experiment, where the effect was due to faster responses to global patterns when they were presented in the left visual field. Moreover, global reaction-time advantages were only observed for the letter stimuli. In contrast, reaction times for the pictures were faster for local targets. Note that one discriminating item in the pictures was whether a central strip of buttons was present or not—a very local and high spatial frequency feature.

Because of the different profiles for the letter and picture stimuli, Brown and Kosslyn concluded that hierarchical level could not explain the visual field differences. Rather, they argued that visual saliency, com-

bined with the demand for spatial attention, provided a more parsimonious explanation. When discriminations were more difficult, more attention would be required.

In one sense, their account is a more elaborate version of a theory
proposed many years ago by Heilman and Van Den Abell (1980). They
suggested that the right hemisphere responds to visual input from both
sides of space, while the left hemisphere responds primarily to input from
the right visual field. Their hypothesis has received some support. For
example, PET measurements of brain activation have shown a greater
increase in activation in the superior parietal lobe of the right hemisphere
whether attention moved to the left or to the right, whereas greater
activation in the left hemisphere was found only when attention moved
to the right (Corbetta, Miezen, Shulman, & Petersen, 1993).

Moreover, neurochemical differences between the hemispheres have
been found that may underlie the hemispheres' differential contributions
to attentional processes. There appears to be a greater amount of
dopamine in the left hemisphere than in the right and a greater amount
of norepinephrine in the right hemisphere than in the left. Tucker and
Williamson (1984) suggested that the relative abundance of norepinephrine in the right hemisphere is associated with greater arousal.
Damage to this system has a disproportionate affect on arousal, perhaps
leading to the more severe neglect seen in right hemisphere patients.
However, none of those factors can explain why global patterns are
favored by the right hemisphere and local patterns by the left hemisphere. Lowered arousal should affect responses at all levels, not one
level more than another. In addition, the fact that a hierarchical stimulus
projected to the intact hemisphere produces the same global or local
deficit as when the same stimulus is projected to the damaged hemisphere in stable patients with unilateral damage questions theories based
on processes taking place within the hemisphere of input.

A different account of unilateral spatial neglect, offered by Kinsbourne,
centers around the idea that in normal function the left hemisphere is
more aroused than the right in humans. That proposed difference in
arousal is assumed to be due to the large emphasis humans place on
language, which is typically controlled by the left hemisphere.

Kinsbourne (1975) proposed an opponent-process model of laterality
to explain how spatial attention is divided between one side of space and
another. According to his theory the two hemispheres compete for activation through inhibitory connections between homologous right and left
hemisphere regions. Kinsbourne argues that because the left hemisphere
is more involved in language and because our behavior is presumed to
be so strongly mediated by language, there is thus a left hemisphere
advantage in the competition due to activation. The advantage stimulates
attentional systems associated with the left hemisphere, resulting in a
rightward bias of attention in normal individuals. Such a bias has been

observed with various reaction-time and signal-detection measures (Efron, 1990; Egly & Homa, 1984; Kinsbourne, 1975, 1987; Reuter-Lorenz, Kinsbourne, & Moscovitch, 1990; Yund, Efron, & Nichols, 1990). When brain damage occurs in the right hemisphere the normal bias becomes accentuated because the left hemisphere is virtually unopposed. Such accentuation results in the abnormal orienting pattern seen in patients with unilateral visual neglect.

Kinsbourne also suggests neurobiological mechanisms that could support his theory. There are strong ipsilateral connections between the parietal lobe and the superior colliculi (Sprague, 1991) as well as inhibitory connections between the two colliculi. A schematic is shown in figure 4.21. Kinsbourne argues that because the left hemisphere is generally more aroused, it more strongly activates the left colliculus, which produces stronger inhibition from the left superior colliculus onto the right

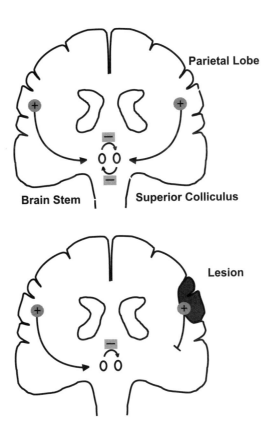

Figure 4.21 Drawing of hypothesized inhibition and activation channels that underlie the appearance of unilateral neglect. The superior colliculi are mutually inhibitory (–), and that inhibition is modulated by activation (+) from parietal neurons. When a lesion occurs in the parietal lobe, as in the bottom drawing, inhibition of the contralesional superior colliculus is reduced or lost as shown. The normal opponent inhibitory processes between the two superior colliculi, which are represented in the upper drawing, are disrupted, resulting in excessive eye and attentional movements into the ipsilesional field.

than from the right superior colliculus onto the left. As a result, the left colliculus dominates and attention is biased to the right even in neurologically healthy individuals.

Kinsbourne proposes that when damage to the right hemisphere occurs, activation of the right superior colliculus is substantially decreased, which results in less inhibition on the left colliculus and an exaggeration of the rightward bias (see the schematic at the bottom of figure 4.21). When damage to the left hemisphere occurs, the activation of the right superior colliculus is increased, which produces increased inhibition to the usually more dominate left colliculus. The left hemisphere would still be relatively active, however, due to the effort needed in trying to generate and understand language.

This elegant theory offers both neurobiological and functional explanations for the prevalence of right-sided neglect. In its current formulation, however, it is limited. The theory accounts for attentional differences in viewer-centered spatial coordinates (which perhaps occur in automatic orienting). However, there is no obvious way for the theory to account for neglect in other frames of reference, at least for those types of neglect that dissociate retinal and environmental space by rotating either the subject or the display. For example, the demonstration by Calvanio et al. (1987) that neglect can occur in upright environmental coordinates when the subject is lying down is not easily explained by the model of collicular function represented in figure 4.21. Similarly, the bias in normal subjects to attend to information on the right of a rotated display is not predicted by Kinsbourne's theory.

A recent set of data collected by Rhodes and Robertson (1996) may have some bearing on the problem. They examined exogenous and endogenous (reflexive versus voluntary) attentional cuing in different frames of reference and found that only endogenous attention showed a rightward bias. Exogenous attention showed no bias to the left or right side. Furthermore, the rightward bias in endogenous cuing followed the reference frames that were rotated either 90 degrees to the right or to the left. In other words, endogenous cuing was present within reference frames that could be dissociated from retinal coordinates and thus from the hemisphere of input.

Perhaps reflexive orienting is viewer-centered and is controlled by mechanisms similar to those that Kinsbourne has suggested, and perhaps voluntary orienting is environmental- or scene-based and is controlled by different neural systems that represent more abstract versions of space. It might be possible to find some patients with neglect who show only viewer-centered neglect and others who show only environmental-, object-, or scene-based neglect. Such subjects could help determine which neural structures may be involved in different forms of neglect.

There is at least one common theme between Brown and Kosslyn, Marshall and Halligan, Kinsbourne, and our own account. There are distributed multiple component processes that contribute to spatial attention and its use in perceiving objects. Unilateral visual neglect appears in different forms depending on the location of the lesions (see Rafal & Robertson, 1995). Data from studies over the past decade have shown that direct-access models have difficulty accounting for all forms of neglect, and that the parietal lobes are involved in a rather high level of spatial representation. The right parietal lobe may be more involved in selecting the range of absolute locations that will be converted to the relatively right and left sides of scenes, objects, or the environment. The left parietal lobe may be more involved in selecting the range of absolute spatial frequencies (and perhaps other spatial dimensions as well) that will be converted to the relatively global and local levels in a stimulus pattern. The parietal lobes may work together in that way to represent spatial properties of the external world and to guide attention through the visual field from one location to another but also from one level of an object to another.

SUMMARY

In this chapter we discussed two different types of spatial attentional mechanisms. One distributes attention over a range of spatial frequencies and the other over an area of space that theoretically can be represented through a system of spatial coordinates. Attention can be allocated through either or both. The DFF theory is limited to spatial frequency analysis, but that does not mean that other lateralized spatial effects do not exist. Both forms of attentional orienting have been linked to functions of posterior visual cortex and, more specifically, to parietal areas of the dorsal processing pathway. Many clinical symptoms of unilateral visual neglect may well be a reflection of the interaction between those spatial attentional systems and their influence on object perception systems.

5 Auditory Perception

Theory building in the behavioral sciences is strengthened by the use of converging operations. That is especially true in an interdisciplinary field such as cognitive neuroscience, where the goal is to relate behavior to brain function. As seen in the preceding two chapters, a variety of methodologies have been used in the study of both normal and brain-injured people to build a strong case for the asymmetric representation of spatial frequency information. In this chapter, the focus is on auditory perception. In particular, we examine the usefulness of the DFF theory in accounting for laterality effects in a number of disparate task domains.

COMPUTATIONAL GOALS IN AUDITION

Before turning to audition it is important to consider again the computational advantages that may be conferred by hemispheric specialization. In vision, the research described in the preceding chapters focused on problems of object recognition and spatial cognition. Our basic premise has been that information is represented at multiple scales and that the derivation of asymmetric representations allows that information to be extracted in an efficient manner. The emphasis in the right hemisphere on lower spatial frequency information allows an assessment of the global shape of an attended object; the emphasis in the left hemisphere on the higher frequency content facilitates the identification of the details. Note that when attention is directed to a scene that contains many objects, then a representation of spatial frequencies does not only facilitate object identification, but also proves useful for determining where the objects are located. Thus, a frequency-based representation can solve many critical computational problems in vision. Spatial frequency analysis by itself, of course, cannot contribute to many other computational problems in vision. For example, additional processing mechanisms are needed to perceive color or depth.

The computational goals in audition are more subtle. For certain goals, the issues are similar to those in vision. For example, sounds contribute to the identification of objects. Toddlers quickly learn to associate moos with cows and barks with dogs. Moreover, the physical properties of an object can be readily discerned by the sounds produced when that object collides with another. While our eyes may not always be able to distinguish whether the siding on a house is cedar or nicely painted aluminum, a rap on the surface quickly provides the answer. Similarly, we are pleasantly surprised when a drinking glass slips from our grasp, but bounces off the floor with the telltale sounds of plastic.

Object localization is another computational arena in which there are parallel goals in vision and audition. In both modalities, animals are equipped with remarkable capabilities to represent the layout of the environment. Species differences may be substantial: whereas sighted humans are hesitant when walking in the woods on a cloudy night, animals such as the owl and bat can identify and localize a potential meal with exquisite sensitivity (Konishi, 1993).

In other domains the computational goals for audition are somewhat unique. We are not only interested in determining what is producing a sound and where it is located; we also need to process the content of the sound. Audition is a medium for communication. This is, of course, most obvious in speech perception. Whereas oral communication for some species may not extend beyond simple determination of which member is vocalizing and a rough analysis of the content of the vocalization (Cheney & Seyfarth, 1990), speech perception requires a much finer analysis of the signal. Only slight acoustic differences in the sounds of speech allow us to distinguish one word from another, and the sound frequencies that underlie those differences are widely distributed. Moreover, the message conveyed by words is highly context dependent: the same sequence of words takes on vastly different meanings depending on the speaker's tone of voice (Lehiste, 1970).

Another prominent domain of audition is music, and here again the computational needs are complex. The melody of a piece is dependent not only on the notes in a sequence, but also on the timing, accent, and sequence with which those notes are played. Moreover, the aesthetic qualities of an orchestral piece derive not merely from our appreciation of the melody line, but rather from the complex interactions of the different instruments.

Given the complex uses of auditory information, laterality research in audition has tended to focus on comparing the contributions of the right and left hemispheres to the performance of different tasks. Many researchers in the field have appreciated that the perception of speech and music probably involve the operation of a set of processors, each devoted to analyzing a particular aspect of the stimulus (e.g., Kosslyn & Koenig, 1992; Peretz & Morais, 1993). Nonetheless, the emphasis has been on identifying those processors from the perspective that they are specialized for performance in task-specific domains.

Perhaps the best example of the focus on task domains can be seen in the enthusiastic reception of Kimura's initial work with the dichotic-listening task. Not only did those studies introduce the first paradigm for studying laterality effects in neurologically healthy subjects, but it provided a novel source of evidence for the role of the left hemisphere in language (Kimura, 1961a). Of course, there were initial concerns that the right ear advantage might reflect more general factors—perhaps the left hemisphere was simply more aroused or had greater access to response selection mechanisms. However, those concerns were alleviated when subsequent research demonstrated a left ear advantage for melody perception (Kimura, 1964; Bartholomeus, 1974). The most straightforward interpretation was that the right hemisphere was specialized for processing musical information. In keeping with the neurological traditions of the time, the brain was partitioned in terms of how different regions were specialized to perform particular tasks.

Problems with this approach soon emerged. Ear advantages (and visual field differences) were not only small and sometimes difficult to replicate (Bryden, 1982; Efron, 1990), but they also varied as a function of a number of factors such as the specific characteristics of the stimuli, musical aptitude (Gaede, Parsons, & Bertera, 1978), or experience (Bever & Chiarello, 1974). For example, it was difficult to fathom how musical processing could shift from the right hemisphere to the left hemisphere in skilled listeners. Could the music module somehow migrate across the corpus callosum as people became more skilled (see, also, Paquette, Bourassa, & Peretz, 1996)?

Such findings indicated that a task-based approach failed to capture the appropriate level of description for characterizing the fundamental differences between the two hemispheres. A more reasonable account of the shift in laterality effects that occurs with experience would be that skilled and unskilled listeners are focusing on different sources of information. Thus, there is a need for a finer-grained analysis of the component operations involved in music and language, similar to what we have seen in the study of object perception. Such considerations provided the motivation for development of the DFF theory. The frequency hypothesis is proposed as a general computational asymmetry that is utilized across task domains. In this chapter, we assess how well a theory based on the asymmetric representation of sound frequency information provides insight into the laterality effects that are observed in multiple auditory tasks.

Before turning to the review of audition, it is important to consider the analogy between spectral representations in audition and vision. With sound, spectral information arises due to dynamic processes: different frequencies are created by variation in the rate at which the sound-emitting object alters the local air pressure level. A tuning fork at 100 Hz oscillates with a period of 10 ms, whereas a tuning fork at 500 Hz oscillates with a period of 2 ms. In vision, spatial frequencies refer to static properties: the spectral composition of a visual scene is defined at a particular point in time.

Nonetheless, the DFF theory is premised on the assumption that, at central levels of processing, those two types of signals share a similar representational format. As noted in chapter 2 the key idea is that, as in vision, auditory representation is converted into a place code in which the component frequencies of a complex sound are represented by different neural elements. Thus, at that level of representation there is a commonality in how spectral information is represented in both vision and audition. For a given time sample, the spectrum of a sound is represented by the activity in neural units tuned to limited frequency bands. The asymmetric hemispheric filters postulated by the DFF theory are assumed to operate on those relatively static representations in which the signals that vary across time have converted into a place code.

In most natural situations, such as listening to speech, the central representations of sound are in constant flux. Similarly, visual perception is not a static process (Freyd, 1987). Not only do objects move about in the world, but the retinal input is altered as we move our eyes and head. Important information is provided by those temporal variations, whether they are related to the spectral transitions that characterize speech signals or to the flight of a moving object. Frequency information can also be described in the temporal domain. In chapter 6, we review evidence suggesting that the left hemisphere is specialized for processing rapidly changing signals (Tallal et al., 1993). Thus, there may be a third domain in which the two hemispheres differ in terms of how they process frequency information. However, as described in this chapter, there are numerous asymmetries in auditory perception that do not readily follow from a hypothesis based on the idea that the two hemispheres differ solely in terms of temporal sensitivity. Rather, those phenomena suggest that the representations of the spectral content of an auditory signal are amplified asymmetrically in the two hemispheres.

DIRECT TESTS OF THE REPRESENTATION OF SOUND FREQUENCY INFORMATION

It has been more than a decade since Sergent first proposed that the two cerebral hemispheres differ in how they process spatial frequency information (1982). Thus, it is not surprising that a relatively large literature exists in support of his hypothesis. In audition, the results of Ivry and Lebby (1993) provide the first direct test of an extension of a frequency-based hypothesis to audition. Converging evidence, therefore, is minimal at present.

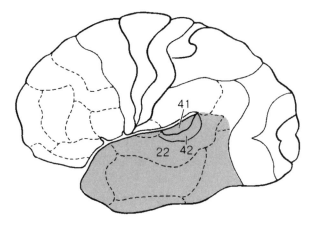

Figure 5.1 A lateral view of the cerebral cortex that highlights the prominent neural regions for auditory perception. The temporal lobe is shaded and the numbers refer to the Brodmann areas of primary auditory cortex (area 41) and secondary auditory cortex (areas 22 and 42). The right hemisphere contains homologous regions.

Frequency Judgments in Patients Following Temporal Lobe Surgery

Laterality research has greatly prospered through the study of patients with neurological disorders. Chapter 3 describes how this area of research not only provided converging evidence for the basic mechanisms of the DFF theory, but also allowed insight into the neural systems that perform those operations. We have recently begun to apply the same strategy in the study of hemispheric asymmetries in audition.

In our initial neuropsychological research into this problem (Ivry & Lebby, in press), we chose to focus on the temporal lobe (figure 5.1). That region constitutes approximately 20% of the neocortex (Jouandet et al., 1989) and includes primary auditory cortex (Brodmann area 41), which is the first cortical area innervated by subcortical auditory sensory pathways. Just inferior to primary auditory cortex are located the so-called secondary auditory regions (Brodmann areas 22 and 42). Surrounding tissue in both the parietal and temporal lobes contains cells that respond to auditory stimuli, although the activity in those cells may not be strictly tied to audition.

In addition to their general theoretical interest in the temporal lobes, neurologists have focused on the region because of its role in epilepsy. For many epileptics the focal point of seizure is the temporal lobe. The large and oscillatory increase in brain activity begins in the temporal regions and then spreads through the rest of the brain, leading to an abrupt cessation of normal cognitive activities. As noted previously, epilepsy can be controlled in most cases by medication. In severe cases surgical procedures are required. One form of treatment, severing the corpus callosum, is described in chapter 1. Seizures are thought to be reduced following this treatment because the epileptic activity cannot spread to the contralateral hemisphere and a reverberating loop is thereby aborted. A second form of treatment involves the resection of the temporal lobe and adjacent limbic structures. The goal here is to surgically eliminate the tissue thought to be the source of seizure activity. Candidates for such surgery must have a well-localized generator site centered in one hemisphere or the other. This treatment method is currently employed extensively throughout the world. Approximately 90% of patients experience a dramatic reduction in seizure activity.

There are few reports of cognitive deficits resulting from the surgery itself. At first blush, it may seem surprising that removing as much as 6 cm from the anterior portion of the temporal lobe produces little change in cognitive function. However, it must be kept in mind that those patients have suffered chronic, severe seizures. It is likely that the excised tissue was highly dysfunctional even prior to surgery. And indeed, it is rare that temporal lobectomy patients are normal in terms of cognitive abilities prior to surgery. A sizable percentage are mentally retarded. For others, the deficits are more subtle and become apparent only during the course of refined neuropsychological studies.

A number of research groups centered at hospitals at which the surgery is performed have explored differences in auditory perception between patients who have had left versus right temporal lobe surgery (see Zatorre, 1988; 1989). Some of their findings are discussed in subsequent sections. First, we describe a recent study (Ivry & Lebby, in press) in which a small number of lobectomy patients were tested on a modified version of the auditory laterality task introduced by Ivry and Lebby (1993).

The patients for the study were recruited through the Epilepsy Surgery Program at the University of California in San Francisco. Eight patients, four with right-sided surgery and four with left-sided surgery, were included. All the patients were tested postoperatively. Figure 5.2 shows a schematic that indicates the approximate extent of the resections, which included the anterior portion of the temporal lobe and underlying limbic

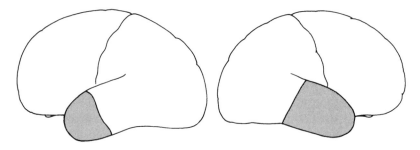

Figure 5.2 Sketch of temporal lobe resections for the left hemisphere and right hemisphere patients. The shaded region indicates the approximate average extent of the resected tissue.

structures. A typical resection for left-sided patients excises 4.5 cm of lateral cortical tissue. For right-sided patients the resection generally extends for 5 cm or more along the lateral surface.

The patients were given a complete neuropsychological assessment. For our research we only included patients with IQ scores within the normal range. In informal assessments the patients did not present any evidence of hearing loss. Each patient was tested at least six months after surgery. By that point in time they had recovered from the effects of surgery and had enjoyed a number of months of seizure-free life.

The stimulus frequencies used in the study are presented in the bottom panel of figure 5.3. Each stimulus was composed of a single pure tone. We chose to use less complicated stimuli since, in our previous research, we found that use of a distractor tone was not necessary to produce the

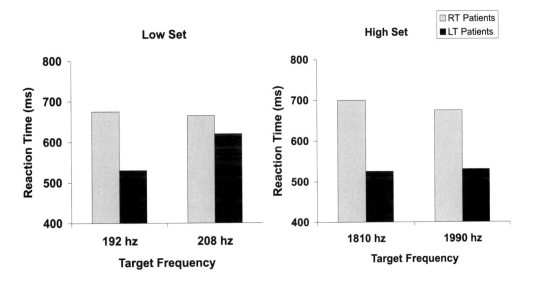

	Irrelevant Tone	Target Tone	Correct Response
Low Set	1900	192	Low
	1900	208	High
High Set	200	1810	Low
	200	1990	High

Figure 5.3 (Bottom panel) Stimulus sets used in the temporal lobectomy study. The stimulus sets were smaller and the range of target frequencies greater than those used in Ivry and Lebby's research (1993) with normal subjects (see table 2.1). Note that the stimulus sets were smaller and the target frequencies were more distinct. Moreover, the stimuli were presented binaurally. (Top panel) Response time as a function of the target frequency. RT and LT patients refer to the groups of patients with right hemisphere lobectomy and left hemisphere lobectomy, respectively. The predicted ear-by-group interaction is most evident with the low tones. The advantage shown by the patients with left hemisphere lobectomies is attenuated for the higher frequency 208 Hz tone.

laterality effect (Ivry & Lebby, 1993, Experiment 4). Note that we also reduced the number of stimuli in each set and increased the magnitude of the frequency differences between members of each set. Both modifications were done to make the task easier for the patients. Moreover, we wanted to obtain sufficient observations with each stimulus while keeping the testing session relatively brief so that the patients would not become fatigued.

The most important modification for the patients, though, was that the stimuli were presented binaurally. A critical assumption in our research with normal subjects is that monaural stimuli are predominantly processed in the contralateral hemisphere. That assumption is not required in lesion studies. The stimuli were presented to both ears simultaneously and, presumably, projected to both hemispheres. We were therefore able to see if differences in performance occurred as a function of the side of the lesion.

The results are in accord with predictions derived from the DFF theory (figure 5.3, top panel). Subjects with left-sided lobectomies responded faster to the lower frequency tones, whereas subjects with right-sided lobectomies responded faster to the higher frequency tones. Despite the small number of subjects, the group-by-relative-frequency interaction was statistically reliable. Although figure 5.3 shows the interaction to be most evident with the low set of tones, there was no statistical difference between performance on the two tone sets. Thus, the data are in agreement with the results obtained with normal subjects, in that there is no evidence of laterality effects in terms of absolute frequency.

Two of the subjects were tested over multiple sessions in order to assess the replicability of the results. The data for those patients are presented in figure 5.4. Again, the predicted interaction was obtained.

Further testing is needed to explore the observed asymmetries. Our early results are still encouraging and important for a number of reasons. First, they provide converging evidence that the two hemispheres differ in how they process frequency information. Since the stimuli were presented binaurally, it is difficult to account for the observed asymmetry without assuming that it reflects differences in cortical processing.

Second, the results suggest that the asymmetric representations of frequency information are derived in those cortical regions that are involved in auditory processing. Presumably, the lesioned regions were important in deriving the asymmetric representations. Removing tissue from one side confers an advantage for processing in the intact hemisphere. Biases in the representations in the intact hemisphere are thus evident in the reaction-time profiles. For example, the performance on auditory tasks by patients with left hemisphere lesions is assumed to be dominated by right hemisphere processing. Since the right hemisphere amplifies lower frequency information, the subjects respond faster to the relatively low-frequency targets.

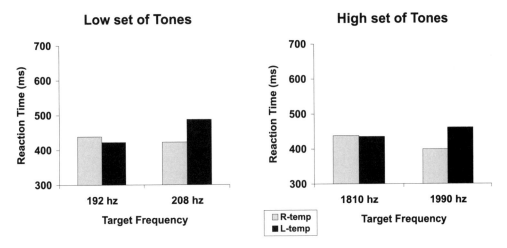

Figure 5.4 Results for two patients tested over multiple sessions. The patient with a left hemisphere lobectomy is faster in classifying the lower frequency target for each set, an effect that presumably is due to the intact right hemisphere. The opposite pattern is observed for the patient with a right hemisphere lobectomy.

It is important to compare our results to those obtained in patient studies of visual asymmetries. There, the critical neural structure is the temporal-parietal junction. That area is quite posterior to the surgical foci in the temporal lobectomy patients. Although it is possible that the temporal-parietal region is also damaged in epileptics due to long-term seizure activity, a more probable working hypothesis is that the neural mechanisms producing the laterality effects in vision and audition are separable. Hemispheric asymmetries in representations of frequency information are observed in both modalities, but the implementation of the parallel asymmetry is likely carried out by modality-specific mechanisms. Indeed, in studies with normal subjects correlations between auditory and visual laterality measures are typically quite low (see Hellige, 1993).

Laterality Effects in Pitch Perception

Our tasks used a discrimination paradigm, in which the experimenter defined which sounds were to be judged "low" and which sounds were to be judged "high." The subjects were forced to apply an arbitrary criterion based on frequency differences. More typical in the study of laterality effects in auditory perception, however, has been the use of pitch-perception tasks.

Pitch describes a psychological experience. It is the perceived fundamental sound associated with an auditory stimulus. The pitch of pure tones corresponds to the frequency of the tone, since all the energy of the signal is concentrated at that frequency. Conversely, there is no pitch associated with white noise, since the energy is equally distributed across a wide range of frequencies. Between the two extremes lie most auditory stimuli: complex tones containing both a fundamental and harmonics of the fundamental. In most natural situations the pitch of such complex sounds corresponds to a physical entity. The pitch is the fundamental frequency of the stimulus.

For example, in speech the pitch of a speaker's voice is determined by the rate at which the vocal cords open and close as air is pushed up from the lungs. Sound is produced by those glottal pulses and is created by the turbulent oscillation between phases in which the passage of air is unconstricted and phases in which the passage of air is blocked. The fundamental frequency, or pitch, of the speaker's voice corresponds to the rate of vocal cord oscillation. The speech signal, however, contains many overtones of the fundamental frequency, due to the resonant properties of the vocal tract.

A speaker's pitch is primarily determined by the length of the speaker's vocal tract (figure 5.5). For males, the normal rate of oscillation

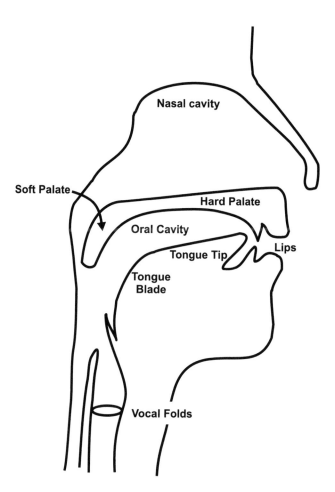

Figure 5.5 The primary components of the articulatory tract. The speed at which the vocal folds open and close determines the pitch of a person's voice. That speed is primarily a function of the length of the articulatory tract. (Adapted from Foss & Hakes, 1978.)

is between 80 and 200 Hz. For females, the normal rate is higher, due to the comparatively shorter length of the vocal tract; the range extends over 400 Hz. Those normal rates can be altered by many factors. When a speaker is stressed the voice tends to rise, due to an increase in the rate of oscillation. When a speaker is drunk the speech articulators are slowed and the speaker's pitch decreases (Pisoni & Martin, 1989).

Nonspeech sounds may also have a pitch. Again, in many situations the pitch corresponds to the fundamental component of the physical stimulus. To make an A-major chord, a pianist strikes the A, E, and C-sharp keys. A complex sound is generated, composed of not just the frequencies associated with the vibrating strings linked to those keys, but also of the harmonic frequencies (octaves) of those notes. The pitch of the root of the chord is heard at 440 Hz, which is the frequency at which the A key vibrates.

However, an interesting illusion is apparent when only the E and C-sharp keys are struck. Instead of changing to correspond to the frequency associated with the E key the pitch remains the same, as if

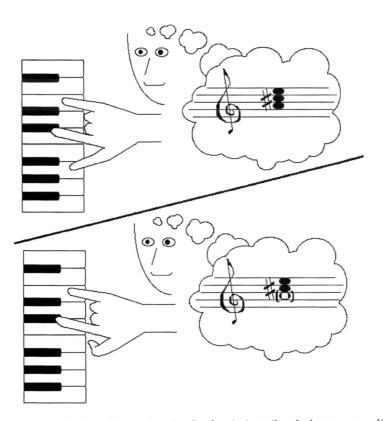

Figure 5.6 To produce an A-major chord a pianist strikes the key corresponding to the root of the chord and the two keys corresponding to the third and the fifth (top panel). when the pianist only strikes the keys corresponding to the third and the fifth (bottom panel), the perceived pitch is also at the frequency of the root. Although the two sounds are not heard as identical, the perceived pitch remains unchanged.

the entire chord had been played (figure 5.6). The power of the illusion is compelling. Indeed, it is exploited in one of our favorite modern conveniences, the telephone. Phone companies find it efficient to use transmission lines that attenuate frequencies below about 500 Hz. Nonetheless, the pitch of a voice sounds similar over the phone as it does in person. The higher frequencies used in speech allow the caller's pitch to be extracted.

Audiologists have investigated ear asymmetries in pitch perception using a wide range of stimuli and tasks. Chapter 2 discusses the literature that indicates greater right ear sensitivity for mid-frequency tones (e.g., between 1000 Hz and 6000 Hz). In those studies a detection task was used, and the authors generally interpreted the results as indicating potential asymmetries in the sensitivity of peripheral frequency detectors (e.g., Previc, 1991).

Suprathreshold matching tasks have also been used to compare pitch perception in the two ears (Van den Brink, 1969). In those experiments the listener was presented with 400 ms sounds that alternated between the ears and were separated by a silent interval of 1.6 s. The frequency of the right ear signal was adjusted in small steps by the listener until a match was achieved with the frequency of the left ear signal. The frequency of the left ear stimulus ranged from 250 to 5000 Hz. Based on the DFF theory, and its proposal that the left hemisphere amplifies the output from relatively higher frequency detectors than those amplified by the right hemisphere, we might expect that the right ear stimulus would be set to a lower frequency than the left ear sound. Thus, for two sounds to be perceived as equal in pitch, the right ear sound would need to be lower in pitch.

The data reported by Van den Brink (1969) do not support that prediction. For most frequencies tested there was a small difference in frequency between the matched pairs, a phenomenon called diplacusis. The magnitude of the difference was generally less than 1%, although in some conditions it reached 2%. However, the direction of the difference was not consistent between subjects. Of the five subjects tested two tended to set the right ear frequency lower than the left ear frequency, one tended to set the right ear frequency higher, and the other two did not have a consistent bias. The differences do not appear to reflect measurement error, since the results for a given subject were replicated across testing sessions separated by many years. The failure of the DFF theory to account for the data are unclear. Diplacusis may result from minute asymmetries in the peripheral detectors of the basilar membrane of the inner ear. Note that, unlike the task used by Ivry and Lebby (1993), the matching task requires minimal memory and decision processes, and thus diplacusis may not reflect the operation of central processing.

With more complex tasks the evidence suggests a dominant role for the right hemisphere in pitch perception (Gordon, 1974; Sidtis & Volpe, 1988). In one study, patients with unilateral lesions restricted to either the right or left hemisphere were tested along with control subjects on a set of tasks requiring the analysis of spectral information (Robin, Tranel, & Damasio, 1990). In a frequency-discrimination task three tones were presented in succession, separated by an intertone interval of 500 ms. The frequency of the first tone was always 440 Hz. The frequency of one of the comparison tones matched the target tone and the other was different. The subjects' task was to identify which of the two comparison tones was different than the standard 440 Hz frequency. Difference thresholds were obtained by adjusting the frequency of the different tone. For patients with left hemisphere lesions and for control subjects the difference threshold was quite small, averaging under 2 Hz. In contrast, the patients with right hemisphere lesions were severely impaired, requiring a mean difference of almost 60 Hz in order to consistently select the correct comparison tone. The asymmetry was even more striking on a pitch-matching task in which the subjects were presented with a 440 Hz square wave and asked to adjust a pure tone until the two tones matched in pitch. Whereas there was little frequency difference between the matches produced by the left hemisphere and control groups, the mean frequency difference for the right hemisphere group was more than 500 Hz! Zatorre and Samson (1991) have also found that patients with right temporal lobectomies perform poorly on pitch-matching tasks with complex tones, especially when a series of irrelevant tones are interpolated between the target and comparison tones.

The relevance of all these studies to the DFF theory is difficult to assess. One plausible interpretation is that, since pitch roughly corresponds to the lowest perceived frequency of a sound, the right hemisphere involvement in such tasks is in accord with the predictions of the DFF theory. In some of these examples, however, pure tones were used. We have argued that both hemispheres can represent the full range of frequencies. With pure tones the spectral representation would be concentrated within detectors tuned to the frequency of the stimulus. On same versus different judgments the essential processing requirement is to determine whether two successive stimuli activate the same set of detectors. It is not clear why a system biased to represent low-frequency information would be more accurate on such a task.

The pitch-matching tasks (Robin et al., 1990; Zatorre & Samson, 1991) are more readily accommodated within the framework of the DFF theory. In those studies the stimuli involved more complex sounds and thus provided activation across a range of frequency-tuned detectors. The low-frequency portion of the signals, the information critical for performing the task, would be expected to be represented with greater fidelity in the right hemisphere. Thus, we would expect—in accord with the results—that right hemisphere lesions would produce a greater disruption in performance, since the representation of the critical information is affected. Indeed, we would predict that as more (irrelevant) high-frequency information is added, the dominant role of the right hemisphere in pitch perception would become more apparent. That prediction is based on the assumption that, as the stimuli become more complex and span a wider range of frequencies, the asymmetrical representation of low-frequency information becomes amplified.

There are a couple of studies that support that prediction. Sidtis (1980) used a matching task with four different conditions. The difference between conditions was in the complexity of the stimuli. For each set the pitch of the stimuli ranged from 264 to 528 Hz (C_4 and C_5 on the major scale). In one set the stimuli were pure tones. In the plus-one and plus-two conditions either the first or first and second harmonics were added. In the square wave condition the stimuli consisted of the fundamental frequency plus all the odd harmonics.

A dichotic-listening paradigm was used to assess ear advantages for sound identification (figure 5.7). In each trial two sounds from a given set were presented simultaneously, one to the left ear and one to the right ear. Next, a binaural probe (a single stimulus presented to both ears) was played and the subjects had to judge if the probe stimulus matched either member of the dichotic pair. Although there was no difference in accuracy between the two ears on the pure-tone set, a consistent left ear advantage was found for the sets with overtones. The asymmetry became more marked as a function of the number of harmonics, with the left ear advantage reaching 9.8% for the square wave stimuli. As with other dichotic studies, Sidtis (1980, 1981) interpreted this laterality effect as reflecting hemispheric asymmetries. His inference is bolstered by converging neuropsychological evidence. The ear asymmetry became much greater in an epileptic patient following a callosotomy operation and was amplified in patients with right hemisphere lesions (Sidtis, 1988).

To account for the increase in performance asymmetries as additional harmonics were added, Sidtis (1980) proposed that the right hemisphere is specialized for analyzing harmonic information. He inferred that one capacity of the right hemisphere is for chord perception. To relate his inference to frequency, his view would be that the right hemisphere plays a more dominant role in the analysis of higher frequency information, or is more adept in representing sounds containing information over a greater spectral range.

However, an alternative—and essentially opposite—interpretation can be derived from the DFF theory. For all four sets of stimuli, we assume that the subjects' judgments are based on a comparison of the pitch of the binaural probe with the pitch of each member of the dichotic pair. Adding harmonic information increases the range of represented frequency information. Given the low- and high-pass properties of the right and left hemispheres, respectively, increasing the range will also increase the difference between the hemispheres in their representation of the fundamental frequency, which is the information critical for determining pitch. This idea is captured in figure 5.8. In the sine wave condition all

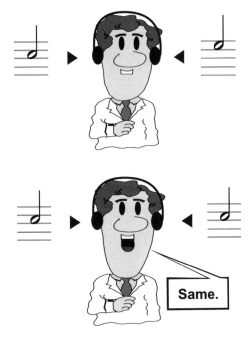

Right Hemisphere Auditory Perception

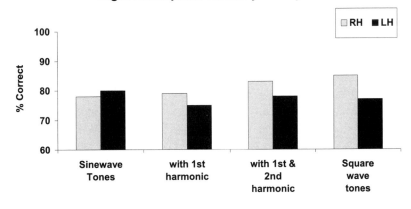

Figure 5.7 (Top panel) Schematic of the Sidtis (1980) experiment. In each trial the subject is dichotically presented with a pair of nonidentical sounds. After a brief delay a binaural probe stimulus is presented, and the subject indicates if the probe matches either of the two samples. The sounds are either pure tones or pure tones combined with various harmonics. (Bottom panel) A right hemisphere advantage becomes more pronounced as additional higher frequency components are added.

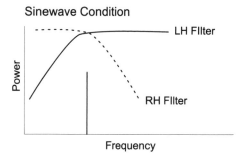

Sinewave Condition

Power

Frequency

LH Filter

RH Filter

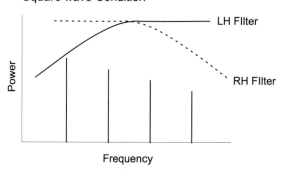

Square wave Condition

Power

Frequency

LH Filter

RH Filter

Figure 5.8 The account based on the DFF theory for the results of Sidtis (1980). In the pure-tone condition (top panel), the hemispheric filters are centered at the stimulus frequency and the effects of their asymmetric filtering operations is minimized. Adding higher frequency information shifts the position of the hemispheric filters to a higher frequency (bottom panel). Under those conditions, the representation of the critical, fundamental frequency is asymmetric because it is amplified by the low-pass property of the right hemisphere filter.

the information is carried at a single frequency. Thus, we might expect the attentional filter to focus on that region, and the center of the hemispheric filters would correspondingly be positioned near that frequency. In the square wave condition the information is distributed across a range of frequencies. Assuming that the attentional filter selects a wider range of frequencies, the hemispheric filters would now be positioned away from the fundamental and towards the higher frequencies. Such positioning would amplify the effects of the asymmetric filtering properties of the hemispheric filters.

Zatorre (1988) used a task that clearly required judgments to be based on pitch. For his experiment he exploited the missing-fundamental illusion. Subjects were presented with two successive stimuli, both of which were composed solely of harmonics without any power at the fundamental frequency (figure 5.9). Stimulus pairs were constructed so that both members had the same mean and range of frequencies but differed in terms of the fundamental frequency. For example, a stimulus derived from a fundamental of 200 Hz contained energy at the third through sixth

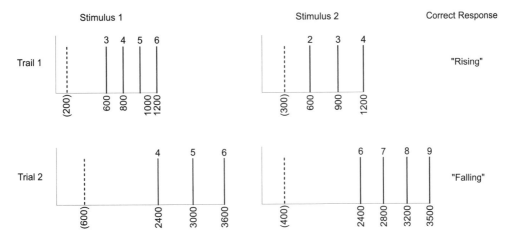

Figure 5.9 Examples of the stimuli used to assess pitch perception in patients with temporal lobectomies. In all of the stimuli the pitch must be inferred from the frequencies of the harmonics. The subjects judge whether the pitch is rising or falling when they successively hear Stimulus 1 and Stimulus 2. (Adapted from Zatorre, 1988.)

harmonics (600, 800, 1000, and 1200 Hz) and was paired with a stimulus derived from a 300 Hz fundamental that contained energy at the second through fourth harmonics (600, 900, and 1200 Hz). The subjects' task was to indicate whether they perceived an increase or decrease in pitch over the two sounds.

The subjects in Zatorre's experiment were temporal lobectomy patients. Because the missing fundamental is perceived when two harmonics are presented dichotically, it is assumed that there is a cortical origin for the illusion (Houtsma & Goldstein, 1972; Pantev, Hoke, Lutkenhoner, & Lehnertz, 1989). Zatorre was interested in whether there would be a difference in performance of this task between patients with right-sided versus left-sided lesions. The results showed a deficit in the performance of patients with right temporal lobectomies.

Zatorre interpreted the results as further implicating the right hemisphere in pitch perception (see, also, Paquette et al., 1996). We take a slightly different tack, suggesting that the right hemisphere deficit is due to the fact that the task requires the subject to abstract lower frequency information in order to perceive pitch. The stimuli were presented binaurally, thus making the full spectrum of information available to both hemispheres. However, lesions of the right hemisphere interfered with the subjects' ability to derive the missing fundamental from the physically present harmonics. Indeed, the DFF theory also provides an explanation for why the right hemisphere patients' deficit on the missing-fundamental task was more marked when the stimuli contained harmonics that were selected from a higher region of the spectrum (Zatorre, 1988). The inclusion of a higher set of frequencies shifts the range of represented frequencies away from the region of the fundamental. The shift makes it more difficult to detect low-frequency resonance, given that the intact left hemisphere filter attenuates low-frequency information.

In summary, the DFF theory provides a new interpretation of the prominent role of the right hemisphere in pitch perception. Rather than emphasize specialization in terms of a task, such as pitch perception, our theory focuses on the computational requirements needed to perform a task. The pitch of a complex auditory signal corresponds to the (implicit or explicit) fundamental, which is the lowest frequency of that signal. It is that region of the spectrum that is amplified by right hemisphere processing.

The Sidtis (1980) and Zatorre (1988) studies also serve as excellent examples of problems that surface in trying to interpret the laterality literature. Studies such as theirs were designed to explore hemispheric specializations for specific tasks such as pitch or chord perception. It is frequently difficult to determine the critical source of information that guides performance on such tasks. Lack of ability to specify the task-relevant frequency range means that the results are amenable to alternative interpretations. The reader may be easily frustrated by seemingly post hoc accounts that are designed to fit within particular theoretical perspectives, a dilemma that was made explicit in our discussion of Sidtis's work. The problem also surfaces when interpreting the findings of Zatorre (1988). One may as well argue that the right lobectomy patients were unable to perform well on that task because the lesions disrupted processing of high-frequency information. With a poor representation of higher frequency information, it would be difficult to infer the missing fundamental. Nonetheless, by stating a clear computational hypothesis, we hope future researchers will be able to design stimuli that can help unconfound alternative interpretations.

FREQUENCY BIASES IN MUSIC PERCEPTION

One of the universal cognitive capabilities of people is the ability to appreciate music. As the study of hemispheric specialization gained momentum, an early consensus emerged that the right hemisphere played a dominant role in that task domain. Support for the idea again came from dichotic-listening tasks with normal and patient populations (Kimura, 1961a, b; Shankweiler, 1966) as well as from the performance of temporal lobectomy patients on musical aptitude tests (Milner, 1962). In addition, the clinical literature includes striking examples of accomplished musicians who continue to compose following left hemisphere strokes that disrupted language abilities (Gates & Bradshaw, 1977; Luria, Tsvetkova, & Futer, 1965). The Russian composer Shebaline suffered two strokes that resulted in Wernicke's aphasia, a syndrome in which the ability to comprehend language is severely compromised. Nonetheless, his musical abilities remained intact (Sergent, 1993).

The early emphasis on the right hemisphere's role in music may have partly reflected the contrast between laterality effects in that domain and those observed in language tasks (Bartholomeus, 1974; Goodglass & Calderon, 1977; Kimura, 1964). As cognitive models of music perception and production became more sophisticated it became apparent that those tasks depended on a number of separable component operations, requiring the integrity of a distributed set of neural mechanisms (Peretz & Morais, 1993; Zatorre, 1984). The appreciation of music involves analysis of a combination of pitch, harmony, intensity, timbre, and rhythmic information. The study of neurological patients indicates that those analysis processes are associated with nonoverlapping neural systems. For example, whereas pitch perception is typically disrupted following right hemisphere damage, deficits in rhythm tasks have been reported in patients with left hemisphere lesions (e.g., Peretz, 1990; Robinson & Solomon, 1974). Moreover, the relative salience of different musical properties may change as a function of either the experience of the listener or the strategies used to perform the tasks. Such changes may account for the reversal between naive and expert listeners of certain laterality effects in music perception (Bever & Chiarello, 1974; Burton, Morton, & Abbess, 1989; Mazziotta, Phelps, Carson, & Kuhl, 1982; Peretz & Babai, 1992).

It would be foolish to expect the DFF theory to account for all the phenomena reported in the music perception literature. There are undoubtedly many component operations involved in music perception, only some of which depend on the representation of frequency information. Thus, much of the neuropsychological research on music perception is not relevant to an assessment of our theory, either because the methods are not clearly specified or because the manipulation of the independent variables is orthogonal to any predictions that can be derived from the DFF theory. Thus, our goal in this section is relatively modest. We focus on two compelling musical illusions and argue that a frequency-based account of hemispheric specialization provides new insights regarding phenomenal experience. The two illusions also provide independent evidence for the basic premise of the DFF theory, namely, that the two hemispheres are differentially biased in their representation of sound frequencies.

The Octave and Scale Illusions

A schematic of the simple stimulus sequence leading to the octave illusion is sketched in figure 5.10 (Deutsch, 1974). Two tones are presented dichotically. The frequencies of the tones are separated by an octave (e.g., 400 and 800 Hz). The stimuli alternate between the two ears so that at any point in time the high note is played in one ear and the low note is played in the other ear. In Deutsch's experiments the stimuli were 200 ms in duration and there was no interstimulus interval.

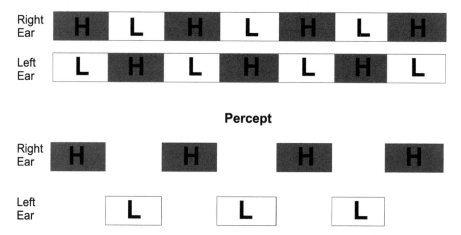

Figure 5.10 The octave illusion. The stimulus consists of a series of dichotic tones. The tones are separated by an octave and alternate between the two ears. The percept is marked by two illusions. First, at any point in time subjects report hearing only a single sound that alternates between the two ears. Second, the higher frequency is almost always localized to the right ear, and the lower frequency is localized to the left ear. (Adapted from Deutsch & Roll, 1976.)

The resulting percept is powerful and surprising. Listeners rarely hear both tones simultaneously. Rather, the most common percept is of a single tone that alternates in pitch and location. Most relevant to our present concern, the pairing of ear and pitch is not random. People generally hear a high note in the right ear alternating with a low note in the left ear. In the basic experiment the rapid alternation makes it difficult to temporally associate percepts with stimuli. It appears that the high note is heard veridically (i.e., when that stimulus is presented to the right ear), whereas the low note is perceived in the left ear when it is actually the high note that has been presented to this ear! That effect occurs even when a silent interval is inserted between successive events. The illusion is also apparent when the stimuli are presented over speakers (Deutsch, 1975). Again, the percept is of a single tone that is high in frequency when emitted by the speaker to the right of the listener and low in frequency when emitted by the speaker on the left.

In further studies Deutsch found that the illusion was based on the relative pitch of the two tones. Using frequency pairs of 200 and 400 Hz, 400 and 800 Hz, and 800 and 1600 Hz, the percept remained constant. For each pair the lower pitch tone was heard in the left ear and the higher pitch tone was heard in the right ear. The illusion was most consistent for right-handed subjects. Left-handers could also hear a sequence of single tones, but the localization of the low and high sounds was more evenly distributed between the two ears. Presumably, that difference reflects the less-consistent hemispheric organization for left-handers. The octave illusion can also be heard with sequences in which the frequency played in a given ear changes after every second or third event (Deutsch & Roll, 1976).

The most puzzling aspect of the octave illusion is that only a single tone is heard at a given point in time. This result is paradoxical, given our frequent experience of hearing different sounds simultaneously. The suppression of one stimulus appears to result from the octave relationship between the two stimuli. Indeed, when the stimuli are not harmonically related, two sounds are perceived. Deutsch has argued that the illusion shows a dissociation of mechanisms involved in localizing and identifying auditory stimuli. She proposes that the percept is localized to the ear that receives the high-frequency signal, but that the identity is given by the stimulus presented to the right ear. When the high tone is presented in the right ear the output of the two mechanisms are in accord with one another. However, the two are dissociated when the high tone is presented to the left ear. Because location is determined by the higher tone the sound is localized to the left ear in this situation. However, the percept is determined by the frequency in the right ear, and thus the subjects report hearing the low-frequency tone.

The DFF theory cannot account for why people fail to hear both tones simultaneously (nor can Deutsch's what versus where hypothesis). Nonetheless, the octave illusion does demonstrate a right hemisphere bias for perception of the lower frequency information in any stimulus pair and a left hemisphere bias for perceiving higher frequency information. One possibility is that the continuous stimulus sequence leads to a maintained representation of both frequency components in each hemisphere. Those representations would be expected to be asymmetric, reflecting the low- and high-pass filtering properties of each hemisphere. As the input changes there may be a corresponding change in the percept. The differential representation of the dominant frequency in each hemisphere may offer appropriate candidates for the alternating percept.

A different illusion, the scale illusion, further demonstrates biases in the perception of dichotic musical stimuli. An example of a stimulus and its percept is shown in figure 5.11. Ascending and descending scales are simultaneously presented, but the notes from each scale alternate between the two ears. Rather than a cacophony of fluctuating pitches in each ear, the percept is of two coherent streams, each forming a melody. One melody consists of a scale that initially descends and then ascends. The reverse is heard for the other melody. (Note that, in contrast to the octave illusion, the two streams are heard simultaneously. This even occurs for the beginning and final notes, which are separated by an octave.)

The most common percepts of the scale illusion conform to the predictions of the DFF theory. The stream composed of higher notes is localized

Stimulus

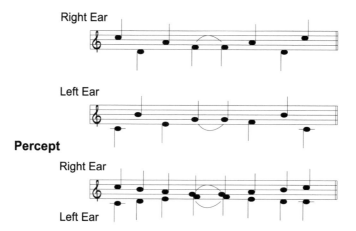

Figure 5.11 The scale illusion. The stimulus consists of dichotic tones. Together, the tones form an ascending and descending scale, although the components of each scale alternate between the left and right ears. Subjects group the tones into the two coherent scales. Of relevance to the DFF theory, the lower frequency tones of each pair are perceived to originate in the left ear; the higher frequency tones of each pair are perceived to originate in the right ear. (Adapted from Deutsch, 1985.)

to the right ear and the stream of lower notes is localized to the left ear. The frequency bias is most striking for the middle notes of the scales. At that point, each ear receives one note twice in succession and the left ear tone is one musical step higher than the right ear tone. Nonetheless, the percept for both notes is reversed so that the lower note is heard in the left ear and the higher note is heard in the right ear. The effect is also found with melodies that do not stream into two scales (Deutsch, 1985).

Based on the illusions reported by Deutsch, Gordon (1980) examined whether an ear bias would be observed for dichotic chords. The chords were composed of four notes, and frequency differences at the low end of the spectra were also present at the high end of the spectra. For example, the fundamental frequency and the highest harmonic note of a B-flat chord were both lower than the corresponding parts of a B-major chord. In separate experimental sessions subjects had to identify the side of presentation for the lower or higher chord. Subjects more accurately judged which ear received the lower chord when the target was presented in the left ear. The reverse was found when subjects had to judge which ear received the higher chord. Here, performance was better when the target was presented to the right ear. Thus, the bias seen in the octave and scale illusions with single tones is also evident with complex stimuli. Most important, all of those effects are consistent with the basic tenet of the DFF theory. In those studies, perceptual asymmetries for processing musical stimuli indicate a right hemisphere bias for low frequencies and a left hemisphere bias for high frequencies.

Changes in Laterality Effects with Experience and Strategy

On a more speculative note, the DFF theory may lead to new avenues for exploring one of the central controversies in the neuropsychology of music literature. In dichotic-listening studies, a left ear advantage has been reported for melody recognition (Bartholomeus, 1974; Goodglass & Calderon, 1977; Kimura, 1964; King & Kimura, 1972; Zatorre, 1979). The inference that the left ear advantage reflects asymmetries in hemispheric function is most convincing in studies with the same set of stimuli in which laterality effects reverse depending on task requirements. For example, Bartholomeus (1974) constructed short melodies in which a singer sang a series of digits at different notes. When the subjects had to report the digits, a right ear advantage was obtained, presumably reflecting the linguistic demands of the task. However, a left ear advantage was found when the subjects had to recognize the melodies (see, also, Goodglass & Calderon, 1977).

The left ear advantage for melody perception has not always been replicated, and the theoretical position that the right hemisphere is critical for melody perception appears to be tenuous (e.g., Bever & Chiarello, 1974; Peretz & Morais, 1980). One factor that appears to mediate ear differences in melody perception is the musical experience of the subjects. Inexperienced subjects tend to show a relatively great left ear advantage; musically skilled subjects either show no differences or a right ear advantage (Bever & Chiarello, 1974; Gordon, 1974).

Those reversals reemphasize an important problem faced by cognitive neuroscientists. We choose a task and seek to determine the brain structures that are required for the performance of the task (e.g., left or right hemisphere; parietal or temporal lobe). However, once some sort of localization is achieved, it is not sufficient to simply conclude that the identified neural structure is specialized for that task. Experimental tasks do not directly correspond to psychological processes. Early dichotic results may have suggested a specialized melody module in the right hemisphere (perhaps homologous to a specialized speech module in the left hemisphere). The divergent findings with more experienced subjects, however, indicate that this form of thinking is too optimistic. A more reasonable view is that the computational processes for melody perception are different for novice and for expert musicians, and those differences account for the reversal on the dichotic studies.

A variety of ideas have been put forth to account for changes in how novice and expert musicians process melodies. One hypothesis is that skilled musicians use a symbolic mediation strategy to process simple melodies, such as construction of images of musical scales (Grossman, Shapiro, & Gardner, 1981; Zatorre, 1989). An alternative argument draws a parallel with work in other laterality domains, positing that expert musicians use a more analytic strategy than do nonmusicians and that the left hemisphere is more adept at more analytic processing (Bever & Chiarello, 1974). A more recent variant on that idea is that analytic processing requires processing of the local elements of the melody. The holistic strategy employed by nonmusicians involves a crude analysis of the overall contour of the melody without elaborate processing of the individual elements (Peretz & Morais, 1987).

A more computationally explicit hypothesis can be derived from our theory. We suggest that the left ear advantage for melody perception in nonexpert musicians is related to the right hemisphere dominance for pitch perception. For nonexpert subjects melody is primarily perceived by attending to the fundamental frequency of the composition. Pitch differences can allow us to differentiate "Mary Had a Little Lamb" from "Twinkle Twinkle Little Star." On the other hand, due to their extensive training, accomplished musicians may attend to different aspects of the stimulus. For example, they may be more sensitive to the complexities of the melody, and their performance may be based on a representation that is richer than that given by a simple pitch contour. This hypothesis is related to notions of differences in analytic versus holistic processing (Peretz & Morias, 1980). The DFF-based hypothesis leads to the prediction that skilled musicians are more capable at processing higher frequency overtones than are nonmusicians.

SUMMARY

In this chapter, we engaged in an admittedly selective review of the laterality research in auditory perception. We sought to provide converging evidence for the hypothesis that the two cerebral hemispheres are asymmetric in how they represent sound frequency information. The right hemisphere is biased to represent relatively low regions of the sound spectrum, whereas the left hemisphere is biased to represent relatively high regions of the spectrum. Thus, in auditory perception we see principles of hemispheric specialization similar to those found in visual perception. In some of the studies the manipulations were designed to directly reveal such biases. In other cases, the biases were inferred through consideration of the computational demands of particular tasks.

That last point can not be overemphasized. If we restrict our analysis to the tasks we choose to study, then we are forced to develop models in which the brain is viewed as a hodgepodge of processing systems designed to solve particular tasks. Within that framework, the quest to link brain and behavior becomes focused on the task: what are the neural mechanisms required for pitch perception or for melody perception or for chord perception? Models such as the DFF theory offer the possibility of precisely stating the computational mechanisms that underlie hemispheric specialization on such tasks. As we have argued, pitch perception is not the unique domain of the right hemisphere, but rather is an emergent property of the fact that the right hemisphere is more adept at representing the lower frequency portion of a stimulus. Similarly, analyzing the subtle characteristics of a chord may require representations of the higher frequency portion of the signal.

In the next chapter, we turn to a discussion of language, which is the preeminent domain of hemispheric specialization. We argue that consideration of the computational requirements in speech perception also provides at least partial insight into the dominant role of the left hemisphere. Moreover, we argue that the DFF theory offers a novel view regarding contributions of the right hemisphere in speech perception.

6 Speech Perception and Language

The seminal task associated with hemispheric specialization is language. As described in chapter 1, that point was brought to the forefront of neurology by the observations of Broca and Wernicke in the nineteenth century. Disorders of language, or aphasias, are the cardinal sign of left hemisphere damage. Most patients with left hemisphere strokes suffer some form of aphasia, although in many cases the deficit may be transient. Aphasic signs are frequently absent following right hemisphere lesions, and if present are much milder and narrow in range. Further evidence of the asymmetric division of labor in language can be found in numerous studies with split-brain patients as well as with healthy subjects using both behavioral (e.g., Kimura, 1961a) and neuroimaging techniques (e.g., Posner & Raichle, 1994; Fiez, Raichle, Balota, Tallal, & Petersen, 1996).

LANGUAGE AS A COMPONENT PROCESS

While it is indisputable that the left hemisphere is dominant for language, the question of what exactly is lateralized remains. Consideration of the overall goals and requirements for language has led to a number of general accounts of the asymmetry. Some theorists have argued that the adaptive benefits of oral communication exerted sufficient evolutionary pressure to lead to mechanisms specialized for speech production (Lieberman, 1991). The speech production system is capable of producing a relatively limited set of sounds or articulatory gestures. One perceptual theory has argued that our speech perception system is similarly constrained, specialized to analyze speech signals so as to recover the articulatory gestures that were produced by the speaker (Liberman, Cooper, Shankweiler, & Studdert-Kennedy, 1967). In this view, the speech modules operate independently of normal auditory processes. If an auditory input bears basic characteristics of speech, then the speech processors will be engaged; if it does not, then the processing will be deferred to general auditory analyzers (Liberman & Mattingly, 1989). Other theorists have taken a broader perspective, arguing that the role of the left hemisphere in language reflects certain basic asymmetries in how information is handled by the two hemispheres. There are certain kinds of processing for which the left hemisphere may be more adept. For example, the left hemisphere may be more adept in the symbolic and sequential modes of processing that are needed to comprehend and produce language (Corballis, 1991; Kosslyn, 1987).

The study of neurological patients has demonstrated that language deficits can be quite varied. In the relatively rare cases of global aphasia, all aspects of language appear compromised. More often, the deficits are more limited. Comprehension problems may be restricted to one modality, as in acquired dyslexia. Language disorders do not always respect modality boundaries; rather, they may reflect deficits at more abstract levels of organization based on semantic relations and properties. In such disorders we see that narrow domains of knowledge may become muddled. Hart, Berndt, and Caramazza (1985) reported a patient who was severely impaired in comprehending the names of fruits and vegetables but showed intact comprehension for other classes of objects. Other patients show deficits selective for certain classes of words, such as verbs or nouns (Damasio & Tranel, 1993). Language deficits may be restricted to grammatical operations or to syntax. As was discussed in the review of music perception, it has become evident that language also requires the operation of numerous processes. The processes are distributed across a number of neural systems, not just the classic left hemisphere language areas named for Broca and Wernicke.

Moreover, certain language-comprehension tasks have implicated right hemisphere involvement. We believe that the DFF theory can account for some of those anomalous results because those tasks are dependent on information contained in the relatively lower portion of the speech spectrum. A corollary of our hypothesis is that for the most part speech perception requires the analysis of relatively high-frequency information, which may be one reason for the dominant role of the left hemisphere in speech perception.

Before turning to our review of the relevant literature, two general points must be emphasized. First, for the most part, the discussion will be limited to perceptual phenomena. We recognize that there are marked asymmetries between the two hemispheres in terms of their roles in speech production; indeed, much of the evidence suggests that the dominant role of the left hemisphere is even more pronounced on the output side (Corballis, 1991). Nonetheless, the extent of the DFF theory is limited to how the two hemispheres extract asymmetric representations of a common sensory input. At present, we focus on the implications of frequency-based asymmetries for speech perception tasks. Second, we have continually emphasized that, due to an attentional process that selects task-relevant information, hemispheric asymmetries are based on relative frequency rather than absolute frequency. The distinction between relative and absolute frequency becomes blurred in speech perception. The speech signal is distributed across a wide range of frequencies, and under normal listening conditions we exploit all of that information. Within the computational framework of the DFF theory, we assume that the aperture of the selection mechanism spans the full range of the speech spectrum. As such, absolute and relative frequency are confounded.

THE PERCEPTION OF PROSODIC INFORMATION IN LANGUAGE

In thinking about what is required to understand speech, our first intuition is to focus on how words are identified. We readily parse speech into constituent elements that correspond to phonemes, syllables, and words. The spectrogram of this fairly continuous auditory stream shows rapid fluctuations in the distribution of frequency information, which are the result of the rapid changes in the vocal tract that occur during articulation. Surprisingly, the pauses in this signal do not always correspond to transitions between words or syllables (figure 6.1). Yet our percept is of individual syllables and words, and it is our ability to recognize those units that allows us to comprehend the message of the speaker.

But comprehension requires more than simply matching auditory signals with stored representations of lexical items. Mere identification of the words contained in an auditory signal is insufficient to understand the linguistic intent of the speaker. The meaning of an identical sequence

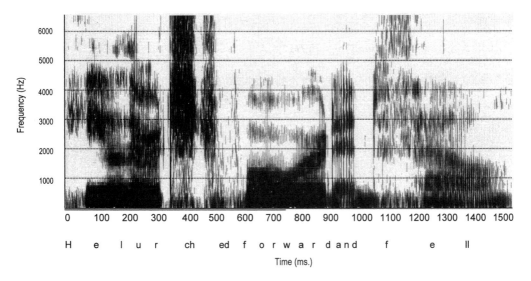

Figure 6.1 Spectrogram of the utterance, "He lurched forward and fell." The distribution of energy over time is depicted; the dark bands correspond to the formants of speech. Note that the periods of silence do not provide a reliable cue to the pauses between words or even between syllables. For example, there is minimal energy preceding and following the "ch" in the word "lurched."

of words can vary. "I am taking care of the children today," and "I am taking care of the children today?" require very different responses. In the first instance, the speaker is making a declarative statement. In the latter instance, a question is being asked. Languages such as English have adopted symbolic conventions in written language to make the distinction between statement and question clear. Comprehension of such distinctions in spoken language is accomplished with a parallel set of acoustic conventions that include systematic changes in the intonation contour across the speech stream. For example, English speakers generally raise their voices at the end of questions. Such acoustic conventions are referred to as prosody.

The perception of prosody has been described as dependent on the "melody of speech," the fluctuations in the pitch, rhythm, and stress (Monrad-Krohn, 1947). In addition to the distinction between declaration and interrogation, melodic changes can convey important information regarding the semantics and emotional meaning of a message. Listeners can readily discern whether the caregiver is pleased or exhausted by the prospect of taking care of the children by the prosody of the declarative statement. Prosody also contributes to the pragmatics of speech. If I say, "I am taking care of the children today," in response to a query about whether I would like to play tennis, it is clear to my friend that my domestic responsibilities preclude tennis. I may use prosody to express my disappointment at the lost recreational opportunity.

Evidence of Right Hemisphere Involvement in Prosody Perception from Dichotic-Listening Paradigms

Research over the past 25 years has convincingly demonstrated that the right hemisphere is dominant in the perception of prosody. Our hypothesis is that, unlike most language tasks, prosodic cues are primarily contained in the low-frequency portion of the speech signal. In particular, the pitch changes associated with prosody are reflected in variations in the fundamental frequency of speech (figure 6.2). Note that because the formants of speech are the nonattenuated higher harmonics of the fundamental, higher frequency information will change in a correlated fashion. Either low- or high-frequency cues may be used to analyze prosody. However, the intensity or power of the speech signal is greatest at the fundamental frequency and becomes attenuated at higher frequencies. For this reason, we suspect that the perception of prosody is dominated by low-frequency information.

The asymmetric utilization of frequency information can be shown with filtered speech. While listeners are unable to recognize the words contained in low-pass filtered speech (e.g., high-frequency cutoff around 500 Hz), they are still able to make accurate judgments concerning prosody. The perception of prosody (and semantics) is lost when only

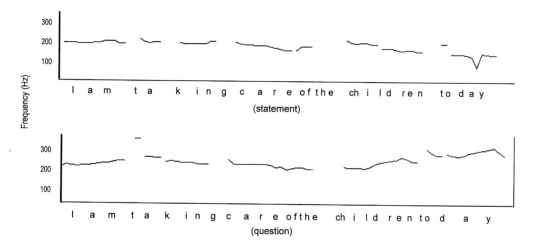

Figure 6.2 Pitch contour for two utterances of the sentence, "I am taking care of the children today." In the top panel the sentence is a statement; in the bottom panel the sentence is a question. Note how speaker cues the question format by making her pitch rise near the end of the sentence.

the higher formants are preserved (e.g., low-frequency cutoff around 1500 Hz).

Blumstein and Cooper (1974) used a dichotic-listening task to demonstrate the importance of the right hemisphere for perceiving intonation contours. The stimuli in their first experiment were four three-word sentences: a declarative ("It has come."), an interrogative ("Has it come?"), an imperative ("Hal, come here!"), and a conditional ("If he came, . . ."). The stimuli were low-pass filtered with an upper cutoff frequency of 510 Hz. The words were unintelligible in filtered form, but with training the subjects learned to identify the pitch contour. In each trial of the experiment, subjects were first presented dichotically with a pair of the four stimuli. They were then presented with a binaural probe that either matched one of the dichotic pair or was different from both. Subjects were more accurate when the probe matched the dichotic stimulus that had been presented to the left ear, indicating a right hemisphere advantage.

In a second experiment the speech sounds were replaced by sequences of nonsense syllables. When tested with low-pass filtered versions of the stimuli, subjects again showed a left ear advantage. Perhaps more surprising, the asymmetry held even when the stimuli were unfiltered. Thus, when the stimuli failed to activate lexical representations the subjects appeared to continue to focus on the pitch contours. The intact yet nonsensical phonological information failed to produce a right ear advantage. Those findings stand in stark contrast to results from typical dichotic-listening studies, which consistently show a right ear advantage when the task requires phonological analysis of either words or nonsense syllables.

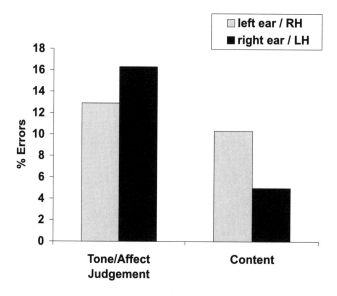

Figure 6.3 Results from a dichotic-listening study in which subjects had to report either the emotional tone of sentences or the content of the sentences. In the former condition subjects were more accurate in reporting the stimuli presented to the left ear. In the latter condition subjects were more accurate in reporting the stimuli presented to the right ear. Thus, the ear advantage was not a function of the stimuli per se, but of the stimuli and task combined. (Adapted from Ley & Bryden, 1982.)

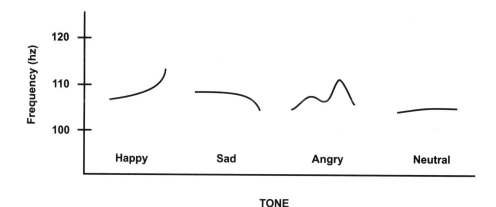

Figure 6.4 Schematic of the fundamental frequency used to convey the emotions of "happy," "sad," "angry," and "neutral." The pitch contours provide an important cue to the emotional state of the speaker.

Prosody not only supplements linguistic analysis but also plays a key role in conveying metalinguistic (e.g., emotional) information. Here, too, there is evidence for right hemisphere dominance. Ley and Bryden (1982) had speakers read sentences in four different tones of voice to convey different emotional states (happy, sad, angry, and neutral). When judging the emotional tone of the sentences, listeners were more accurate if the sentence was presented to the left ear (with a competing neutral sentence in the other ear). In contrast, the laterality effect for the same set of stimuli was reversed when the subjects were asked to report the content of the sentences (figure 6.3).

Such results have been interpreted as pointing toward the dominant role of the right hemisphere in the perception of emotion (Blonder, Bowers, & Heilman, 1991; Ross, Edmondson, Seibert, & Homan, 1988). On the other hand, as with other prosodic cues the different emotions are conveyed by predictable fluctuations in the pitch contour (figure 6.4). Indeed, one might argue that the right hemisphere bias to represent low-frequency information contributes to the importance of the right hemisphere in affective processing. The DFF theory provides a parsimonious computational account of ear differences in detecting pitch differences, based on the fact that the advantage of the left ear and right hemisphere on prosody tasks is similar for both affective and linguistic intonation contours (Shipley-Brown, Dingwall, Berlin, Yeni-Komshian, & Gordon-Salant, 1988). Moreover, recognition of individual voices is also more accurate for stimuli presented to the left ear (Kreiman & Van Lancker, 1988; also, Van Lancker, Kreiman, & Cummings, 1989). Individual differences between speakers are clearly manifest in pitch contours.

Neuroimaging Studies of Pitch Perception

A series of PET studies have further linked neural regions within the right hemisphere to pitch perception. Interestingly, the studies reveal similar laterality effects for pitch with both musical (Zatorre, Evans, & Meyer, 1994) and linguistic stimuli (Zatorre, Evans, Meyer, & Gjedde, 1992). In the linguistic study subjects listened to pairs of syllables under three sets of instructions. In the control condition they simply listened to the syllables and pressed a key after every other pair of sounds. In the phonological task subjects were instructed to respond only when the members of a pair had the same final consonant. In the pitch task subjects were instructed to respond when the fundamental frequency of the second syllable was higher than the fundamental of the first syllable. The study was constructed in this manner so that the stimuli, as well as total motor output, were equated across all three tasks.

By subtracting brain activity observed during the control condition from each of the other conditions, Zatorre et al. (1992) identified neural loci associated with each of the discrimination tasks. In accord with many other studies (e.g., Fiez, Raife, Balota, Schwartz, & Raichle, 1996), various regions of the left hemisphere were activated during the phonological task. However, during the pitch task the primary foci were located in the right hemisphere. Simply changing the task demands produced a reversal of laterality effects for an invariant set of stimuli. Within the framework of the DFF theory we would argue that one factor contributing to the reversal is that the two hemispheres differ in the fidelity with which they represent the critical information associated with each task. The phonological task may require the analysis of relatively higher frequency information; the pitch task is likely to involve the analysis of relatively lower frequency information. This is not to argue that the asymmetric representation of frequency information is the only contributor to the laterality effects. Asymmetries are also surely associated with other component processes required by the tasks (e.g., the retrieval of stored phonological labels).

It is important to note that the right hemisphere foci associated with pitch perception were in frontal cortex rather than in the temporal lobe regions linked to auditory perception. Perhaps the perceptual analysis of the stimuli was similar in all three conditions. The asymmetric activations may not reflect perceptual asymmetries but rather processes involved in response selection and preparation that access task-relevant information. The frontal activity in the right hemisphere during the pitch task may reflect greater access within this hemisphere to representations of low-frequency information. Grafton, Hazeltine, and Ivry (1995) provide another example of a PET study in which blood flow changes were restricted to the right hemisphere even when all responses were made with the right hand. Interestingly, in a PET study of melody perception, increased blood flow was observed in both prefrontal and auditory association cortex of the temporal lobe when subjects were required to remember the pitch of a stimulus over an extended period of time (Zatorre et al., 1994). Activation may be restricted to frontal regions when the response can be made immediately following stimulus presentation, with laterality effects reflecting which side provided the key information guiding the response. Delay tasks, on the other hand, may involve a working memory system between frontal cortex and the more posterior regions that provide the primary perceptual representations (Goldman-Rakic, 1992).

Converging Evidence from Neuropsychology

Neuropsychological studies provide a third source of evidence for right hemisphere involvement in prosody perception. Tucker, Watson, and Heilman (1977) compared patients with right and left hemisphere lesions on two tests requiring the perception of affect. None of the patients with right hemisphere lesions was aphasic. The patients in the left hemisphere group were classified as conduction aphasics, a disorder characterized by an impairment in phonological analysis despite relatively intact comprehension. Such patients can comprehend a sentence but are unable to repeat or parrot a series of sounds. The patients listened to sentences that were neutral in linguistic content but were spoken in one of four affective tones (angry, happy, sad, or indifferent). They were asked to judge the emotion conveyed by each sentence. The average percentage of correct responses for the right hemisphere patients was 32%. The left hemisphere patients (who would have difficulty repeating the sentences) were correct on 80% of the judgments. The asymmetry became even more marked on a discrimination task in which the subjects simply had to judge whether or not two successive sentences were spoken in the same tone of voice. On that test the left hemisphere patients' responses were nearly perfect (95% correct), while the right hemisphere patients performed at chance (see, also, Ross, 1981).

The neuropsychological research on prosody perception has tended to emphasize two important points. First, right hemisphere lesions can be more disruptive than left hemisphere lesions on certain language tasks. This clearly indicates that language processes are distributed and that the distribution is not restricted to the left hemisphere. Second, neuropsychological research has played a central role in theorizing about specialization for processing emotional information.

As noted above, variations in fundamental frequency provide a salient cue to emotional intent (e.g., Ross, Edmondson, & Seibert, 1986). If the prosody deficit were a consequence of a more general problem with processing affect, then the right hemisphere deficit might be restricted to prosody tasks involving emotional distinctions. Little data exist to assess that hypothesis. However, Blonder et al. (1991) examined the performance of right and left hemisphere patients on a range of prosody tasks. The stimuli for some of the tasks differed in terms of the emotional tone of the speaker's voice. For others the prosodic differences were emotionally neutral and involved the discrimination of interrogative versus declarative sentences. Patients with right hemisphere lesions were impaired on both tasks, although the deficit appeared to be more marked on the emotional judgments. Those data demonstrate that the prosody deficit is not restricted to the emotional domain.

It is interesting that right hemisphere lesions have not only been associated with deficits on tests of prosody perception, but have also been linked to deficits in the production of prosodic cues (Edmondson, Chan, Seibert, & Ross, 1987; Ross, Edmondson, Seibert, & Homan, 1988; Ross, 1981; Shapiro & Danly, 1985; Tucker et al., 1977). The speech of patients with right hemisphere lesions has been characterized as monotonous and unmodulated. Ross and Mesulam (1979) report a patient who had difficulty disciplining her children because they could not detect when she was upset or angry (she eventually learned to emphasize her speech linguistically by adding "I mean it!" to the end of her sentences). Correlations in hemispheric asymmetries between perception and production have been noted in many domains. One might suppose that the correlations result from disruption to a shared representation used in both perception and action. However, numerous instances in the literature show dissociations between perceptual and motor aprosodias. (Ross, 1981). An alternative hypothesis is that an asymmetry may develop to solve a restricted problem that is limited to either perception or production, but over time the asymmetry becomes exploited in other task domains. The relationship between asymmetries in production and perception is ripe for future investigation.

ASYMMETRIES IN PROCESSING LINGUISTIC INFORMATION OVER DIFFERENT TEMPORAL RANGES

In the preceding discussion of prosody, we suggested that the dominant role of the right hemisphere emerges because prosodic information is primarily contained in the lower portion of the acoustic spectrum. In this view, we continue to emphasize relatively static properties of the spectral representation of the speech signal. Although prosody must involve the analysis of changes in the fundamental formant, the critical information is carried in detectors tuned to the lower portion of the spectrum.

An alternative account could be developed by considering the temporal window over which prosodic cues are extracted. Prosodic cues are rarely limited to single words or syllables. Rather, they emerge over the course of a series of utterances that form a phrase or sentence (although prosodic variations can certainly be used in one-word sentences such as "What?" to indicate the speaker's intent). Prosody is reflected in the overall contour of the utterance: is the pitch rising to indicate a question or does it fall to connote a statement? Thus, one could argue that prosody is carried by variations occurring over low temporal frequencies.

In contrast, information regarding the linguistic content of a speech utterance is conveyed at much higher temporal frequencies. A typical syllable lasts for about 200–250 ms. Consider the spectrogram for the production of the syllable /bā/ as in "baby" (figure 6.5). The total duration of the utterance is 170 ms. During the initial 40 ms, the spectral structure of the formants undergo rapid changes. The initial acoustic changes reflect the rapid movements of the articulators as the lips part to produce the consonantal /b/ portion of the syllable. Following that transitory phase the formants remain relatively invariant, reflecting the stable configuration of the articulators during the portion of the sound primarily associated with the vowel. Note that while the steady-state characteristic of the vowel is readily apparent in the isolated syllable, the spectrogram of a continuous utterance is more labile. In the spectrogram of the last word in the phrase, "kiss the baby," there are changes in the

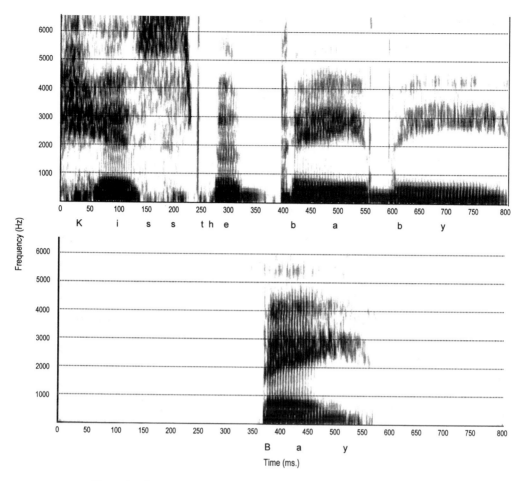

Figure 6.5 Spectrograms of the syllable /bā/, by itself and embedded in the sentence, "Kiss the baby." The formant frequencies change rapidly during the consonantal portion of the sound—the consonantal transitions. In contrast, the frequencies are relatively stable during the steady-state vocalic portions of speech.

vowel portion associated with the /a/ sound as the speaker prepares to utter the /b/ sound associated with the second syllable.

The Left Hemisphere as a Decoder for Rapidly Changing Acoustic Signals

It has been proposed that the dominant role of the left hemisphere in language may be the result of a specialized processing capability for that hemisphere in decoding rapidly changing signals (for reviews, see Tallal et al., 1993; Miller, Delaney, & Tallal, 1995). Coupled with the right hemisphere dominance in processing slow changes that can be associated with prosody, it is reasonable to propose that the basic laterality tenet of the DFF theory may generalize to the temporal domain. The left hemisphere may be biased to analyze high temporal frequency information and the right hemisphere biased to analyze low temporal frequency information.

Evidence that the left hemisphere is important for processing fast acoustic variations comes from a number of sources. First, a large body of literature shows a right ear advantage in dichotic-listening tasks with verbal stimuli. In the seminal research with this paradigm, Kimura (1961a) presented pairs of digits dichotically. Subjects were consistently more accurate in reporting digits presented to the right ear in comparison to those presented to the left ear. A voluminous literature has since emerged that essentially replicates that finding across a range of stimuli and languages. The literature has provided perhaps the strongest evidence from healthy subjects of left hemisphere language dominance. The right ear advantage is amplified in patients who have undergone a corpus callosotomy (Milner et al., 1968; Sparks & Geschwind, 1968). For example, one patient was able to report every digit and animal name presented to the right ear, but was unable to report a single item presented to the left ear.

One interpretation for that effect might be that the left hemisphere is more adept at remembering linguistic stimuli, perhaps resulting from a specialization for storing a mental lexicon (Damasio, Grabowski, Tranel, Hichwa, & Damasio, 1996). However, the right ear advantage is also found with nonsense syllables, backwards speech, and unfamiliar foreign languages (see Kimura, 1973). A crucial feature across those stimulus sets is that the right ear superiority is most evident with stimuli containing rapid changes in the acoustic spectrum, which would be found in nonsense syllables and in backwards speech. Furthermore, while the right ear advantage is most marked with relatively brief-stop consonants (i.e., sounds in which the airflow is briefly occluded such as /ba/ and /da/), the effect is minimal or disappears with isolated vowels (Cutting, 1974; Studdert-Kennedy & Shankweiler, 1970). Vowels are surely linguistic entities, but the time course over which the critical information is present is considerably longer than with stimuli containing consonants.

A second line of evidence implicating a left hemisphere specialization for processing rapidly changing information comes from the work of Tallal and her colleagues. Schwartz and Tallal (1980) compared the performance of normal subjects on dichotic-listening tasks using two sets of stop consonants like /ba/, /da/, and /ga/. The stimuli were generated on a speech synthesizer to allow the researchers to control the duration of the consonant transition. In one set the transitions lasted 40 ms; in the other set the transitions were extended over an 80 ms interval. The stimuli in both sets were easily identified when they were presented in isolation to either ear, but a right ear advantage during dichotic presentation was especially pronounced for the 40 ms set.

Tallal has also examined the performance of language-impaired subjects on tasks requiring the perception of sequences of rapidly changing acoustic stimuli. Adults with focal brain lesions in the left hemisphere were found to have difficulty identifying the order of successive pairs of stop consonants with 40 ms transitions. The deficit was less marked when the transitions lasted 80 ms, even though the overall length of each syllable was held constant by shortening the vocalic portion of the sounds in the latter set. Similar results have been obtained with children with developmental language disorders (Tallal, 1980).

The deficit appears to be related to processing brief signals rather than processing the rapid changes that may occur during the transitions. Tallal and Piercy (1975) constructed pseudospeech out of vowel-vowel syllables by splicing together short duration vowels (43 ms) onto normal vowel segments of 207 ms duration. For example, a brief long /e/ sound might precede a normal long /i/ sound. Within each part of the stimulus the frequencies of each formant remained constant. That type of stimulus was contrasted with consonant-vowel syllables in which the transitions were extended over 95 ms. By constructing the study in this manner the effects of segment duration and rate of acoustic change were unconfounded. The results indicated that the performance of language-impaired children was most disrupted when processing the vowel-vowel short duration sylla-bles in comparison to the consonant-vowel long transition stimuli.

Generalized Operation of the Left Hemisphere Rapid Decoder

Language-impaired subjects have also been found to have difficulty dis-criminating brief nonspeech auditory and visual stimuli (Tallal & New-combe, 1978; Tallal, Stark, Kallman, & Mellits, 1981; but, see Tallal & Piercy, 1973; Farmer & Klein, 1995). A deficit in processing rapidly chang-ing visual stimuli has also been suggested as a primary cause of devel-opmental dyslexia (for reviews, see Galaburda & Livingstone, 1993; Lovegrove, 1993). Interestingly, recent postmortem studies of the brains of dyslexic individuals suggest a selective loss in the thalamus of those visual neurons that are most sensitive to high temporal frequencies (Liv-ingstone, Rosen, Drislane, & Galaburda, 1991). Examination of tissue from the same brains reveals additional abnormalities in thalamic audi-tory neurons projecting to the left hemisphere (Galaburda, Menard, & Rosen, 1994). Thus, it has been proposed that the language problems in dyslexia may reflect a generalized problem in processing rapidly chang-ing signals.

Neuroimaging studies have provided new evidence that is consistent with the hypothesis that there is a left hemisphere specialization for processing high temporal frequency information, at least in the auditory modality. In one PET study (Fiez et al., 1995) a region in the left frontal lobe (Brodmann area 45) was activated when subjects listened to stim-uli with rapidly changing acoustic spectra (figure 6.6). Area 45 had previously been linked to phonological processing, and lesions that

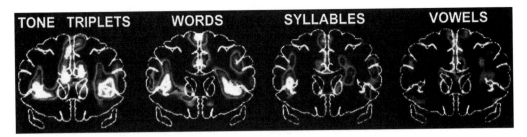

Figure 6.6 PET evidence in support of the hypothesis that the left hemisphere is essential for decoding rapidly changing acoustic information. The stimuli in all four conditions were 250 ms in total duration. For the tone triplets the stimuli were three 60 ms tones separated by a 35 ms interstimulus interval. Subjects responded whenever they heard a target pitch sequence. In the conditions involving vowels, consonant-vowel syllables, and words, subjects responded whenever they heard a target stimulus. The spectra for the vowels was fixed for the 250 ms interval, whereas it varied during the consonantal portion of the syllables and words. Compared to during rest, regional cerebral blood flow increased in the left frontal lobe during the tone, syllable, and word tasks, but not during the vowel task. Note the trend toward a similar effect in homologous regions of the right hemisphere, although that effect failed to reach significance. (Adapted from Fiez et al., 1995.)

encompass the area can produce Broca's aphasia and/or speech dysarthria. However, in the PET study activation within that region was found with both speech (syllables or words) and nonspeech stimuli (tone sequences). The area was not activated when subjects listened to vowels, which are speech sounds with much slower acoustic changes.

The evidence reviewed in the preceding pages led Tallal to suggest that there is a general left hemisphere mechanism for processing brief stimuli. In her view, this hemispheric asymmetry may be antecedent to the role of the left hemisphere in language. Speech perception requires processing of the rapid acoustic changes that occur during human articulation. A specialized mechanism within the left hemisphere evolved for processing high temporal frequency information, she hypothesized, and it was this advantage that paved the way for left hemisphere dominance in language processing.

As might be expected, that hypothesis has proven controversial. By proposing a generalized problem with processing rapidly changing signals, Tallal is arguing that language problems, both auditory and visual, are not specifically related to language. Many other theorists in this area have argued that such problems are domain specific (see Studdert-Kennedy & Mody, 1995); indeed, a traditional definition of disorders like dyslexia is that the language deficit can exist without generalized perceptual problems. Some people may have difficulty processing rapidly changing speech and nonspeech stimuli, but there are many cases in which the two deficits are dissociated. Thus, a pattern of co-occurrence may reflect deficits in independent processors (Studdert-Kennedy & Mody, 1995). Mody, Studdert-Kennedy, and Brady (in press) have recently argued that poor performance on Tallal's temporal-order task may reflect a problem with rapidly categorizing phonetically similar sounds. In support of their hypothesis they found that poor readers had difficulty discriminating between the sequences /ba/ /da/ and /da/ /ba/ but had no problem when the stimuli were highly discriminable (e.g., /ba/ and /sa/). With both sets of stimuli the phonetic information was condensed into a brief temporal window.

Recent remediation studies have also shown that if language-impaired children are given extensive training in making phonological discriminations they will show substantial improvements on a temporal-order task with rapidly changing formant transitions (Merzenich, Jenkins, Johnston, Schreiner, Miller, & Tallal, 1996; Tallal et al., 1996). Those results further suggest that the basic problem may involve making fine perceptual discriminations rather than doing rapid temporal analysis.

Nonetheless, two aspects of Tallal's work are especially relevant for the present discussion. First, her proposal for a left hemisphere specialization in processing high temporal frequencies may provide a third dimension of the generalized asymmetry in how the hemispheres process frequency information. Similar to spatial perception in vision and spectral perception in audition, the left hemisphere may be biased to process higher frequency information in the time domain. Temporal asymmetries could, of course, be manifest in either the visual or auditory modality (as well as in other sensory channels, such as that related to haptics), and might hold true for both linguistic and nonlinguistic stimuli. Indeed, the work of Peretz and her colleagues (Peretz & Morais, 1980; Peretz, 1990; Peretz & Babai, 1992) suggests such an asymmetry in music perception. For example, an advantage of the right ear and left hemisphere is seen when subjects are required to detect musical events that occur over a short time scale, whereas an advantage of the left ear and right hemisphere is manifest when the events require subjects to integrate information over a longer time scale.

Second, from the research reviewed in the preceding two sections, we can derive alternative accounts to account for the role of the right hemisphere in prosody perception. Within the framework of the DFF theory, a spectral argument posits that prosodic information is primarily carried by the lower frequency portion of the speech signal. Alternatively, within the framework of Tallal's theory, one may assume that the right hemisphere has developed an advantage in processing low temporal frequency variations to complement the left hemisphere specialization for high temporal frequency variations. The right hemisphere's role in prosody perception could then be attributed to the fact that prosodic cues are generally conveyed over a longer time period than are those required for the linguistic aspects of speech perception. Note that both hypotheses are consistent with the basic hypothesis of hemispheric specialization for frequency information. One argument focuses on spectral aspects of audition, the other on temporal aspects. Moreover, the two hypotheses are not mutually exclusive. A generalized right hemisphere specialization for processing lower frequency information, whether spectral or temporal, would suggest two reasons (at least) for asymmetries in the perception of prosody.

PHONEME PERCEPTION AND THE RIGHT HEMISPHERE

Those hypotheses regarding the role of the right hemisphere in prosody perception do not impinge upon the general hypothesis regarding left hemisphere dominance for language. Prosody is only one aspect of speech perception, and deficits in prosody perception may not be extremely disruptive to language functions. Prosody is best considered a paralinguistic phenomenon. While it contributes to our ability to use language as a communicative device, it does not have a direct impact on our ability to use and understand words. Thus, linking prosody to the right hemisphere does not mandate a strong revision of the general hypothesis that the left hemisphere is specialized for language. It only requires that the range of the left hemispheric specialization be narrowed to the phonological domain that is necessary for extracting lexical and semantic representations.

We now turn to more general implications of the DFF theory for speech perception. To account for the dominant role of the left hemisphere in language, theorists have argued for specialized speech modules (e.g., Liberman & Mattingly, 1989) or have offered general purpose models such as the temporal frequency hypothesis articulated by Tallal et al. (1993). In either type of theory the left hemisphere is assumed to play a special role in the perception of phonological information, at least for the rapid formant transitions that characterize consonants. However, the spectral emphasis of the DFF theory is also relevant here. Specifically, we hypothesize that for the most part acoustic cues in the speech signal for identifying phonemes, syllables, and words are primarily carried by the relatively higher sound frequencies.

The Distribution of Acoustic Information for Discriminating Speech Sounds

Consider the spectrograms of a variety of consonant-vowel syllables shown in figure 6.7. All of those sounds were generated by a single speaker. The syllables are individuated by their respective spectral characteristics. For example, during the first 50 ms the frequencies of the higher formants rise for /ba/ and fall for /da/. Note that for this pair there is little difference in the information in the lower frequencies. The lack of low-frequency differences is even more apparent in the spectrograms for /da/ and /ga/. For those sounds there are minimal differences

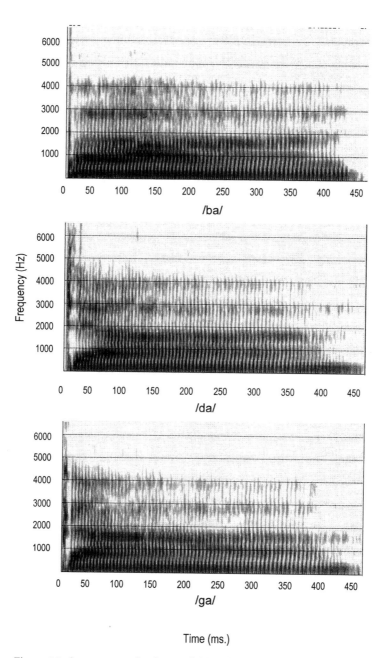

Time (ms.)

Figure 6.7 Spectrograms for three syllables: /ba/, /da/, and /ga/. The fundamental and first formant—blurred together in the spectrograms—are essentially identical for the three sounds. The sounds differ in terms of the formant trajectories during the initial consonantal portions of the sounds. For /ba/ the second formant rises, whereas it drops for /da/ and /ga/. The latter two sounds are distinguished in terms of the trajectory of the third and higher formants.

for the fundamental, first, and second formants. The primary spectrographic difference is found in the third formant. Indeed, intelligible synthetic versions of the sounds can be generated solely by varying information in the range of 1800–2700 Hz. Across the set there is little variation in the lowest frequency portions of the sounds, which is the portion associated with the fundamental frequency. That lack of variation reflects the fact that the depicted sounds are all voiced consonants. The vocal cords begin to vibrate at the onset of the sounds, and the fundamental frequency reflects the rate of vibration. In many languages, such as English, variation in pitch does not provide substantial phonetic information. Rather, phonetic distinctions are made by variation in the configuration of the oral articulators, which distort the higher harmonics of the fundamental and not the fundamental itself.

Given that variations in the relatively higher frequencies underlie most phonetic distinctions, the DFF theory offers a novel account for left hemisphere specialization for speech perception. We propose that the left hemisphere is more adept at processing the higher frequencies that are requisite for discriminating between speech sounds. When stated in this manner, we face a problem in making comparisons between two theories. The speech is special theory argues that the left hemisphere has evolved a specialization for processing certain types of inputs, namely speech (Liberman & Mattingly, 1989). Based on the DFF theory we argue that the left hemisphere is specialized for processing the relatively higher spectral cues in the speech signal and that this form of processing is necessary for speech perception. To differentiate the theories we need to look at examples in which phoneme differences and frequency differences are not confounded. That is, we want to look at hemispheric asymmetries in the perception of a phonetic feature that is correlated with acoustic events in the lower frequencies of the speech signal. The DFF theory predicts a more prominent role for the right hemisphere in perceiving that type of phonetic information. One phonetic feature that meets the criterion is voicing.

Before turning to an explanation of why the perception of voicing may depend on lower frequencies, we briefly review some of the articulatory events that underlie the production of consonants. Consider the schematic spectrograms for three consonants: /ba/, /da/, and /pa/ (figure 6.8). The spectrograms are simplified cartoons, showing the mean frequencies for the first four formants (F_0–F_3) across the duration of each syllable. They do not show the bandwidths of the formants or the higher frequencies. However, with appropriate bandwidths and higher formants at constant frequencies, subjects will readily perceive the three syllables if the trajectories shown in figure 6.8 are used to produce synthetic speech sounds.

Each of the three syllables begins with a stop consonant. Stop consonants, such as /b/, /p/, /d/, and /t/, derive their name from the fact

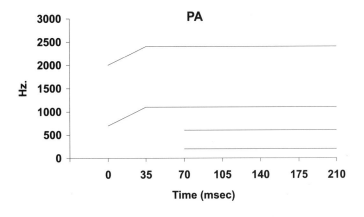

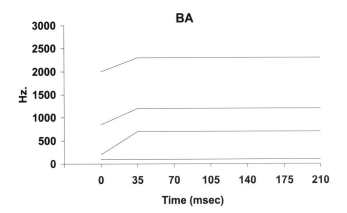

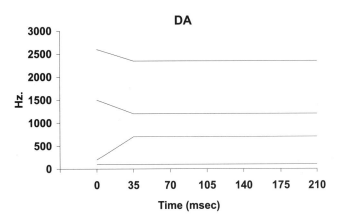

Figure 6.8 Schematic spectrograms for three syllables: /pa/, /ba/, and /da/. Only the center frequencies for the fundamental and first three formants are shown. The difference between the voice /ba/ and the voiceless /pa/ can be acoustically described by the presence or absence of power at the lower frequencies. The difference between the labial /ba/ and the alveolar /da/ can be acoustically described by the initial trajectories of the higher frequency formants.

that during articulation the flow of air from the lungs is constricted at some point within the articulatory tract. One prominent phonetic feature, the place of articulation, refers to the point at which that constriction occurs. For the labials /b/ and /p/ the lips must be brought together. For the alveolars /d/ and /t/ the airflow is blocked by the placement of the tongue just behind the upper teeth on the alveolar ridge. The sudden parting of the lips or lowering of the tongue releases the flow of air and results in the formant trajectories that differentially characterize labials and alveolars. As can be seen in figure 6.8, the initial frequencies for the second and third formants are higher for /da/ than for /ba/.

Voicing is a second prominent feature used to classify stop consonants, and refers to the timing between the articulatory release and the onset of the periodic vibration of the vocal folds in the larynx. In voiced stop consonants such as /ba/ and /da/ the release and vocal cord vibration begin at approximately the same time. In contrast, the production of voiceless stops such as /pa/ require that the release precedes the onset of vocal cord vibration. In figure 6.8 the voiceless feature is indicated by the fact that the fundamental and first formants are absent during the initial 70 ms of the syllable. The interval between the release and the onset of vocal cord vibration is referred to as the voice-onset time (VOT). For voiced sounds in English VOT typically ranges from −5 ms to +10 ms. For voiceless sounds the VOT is between +40 and +60 ms. While the exact values may differ between languages, the basic temporal distinction between voiced and voiceless sounds is found in all languages (Lisker & Abramson, 1964). Some languages, such as Thai, include a third category, the prevoiced stop consonants. For those sounds the onset of voicing precedes the oral release.

The psychological process or processes that allow a listener to differentiate voiced and voiceless stop consonants has been the subject of much debate. In a reflection of the label used to describe that feature—voice-onset time—many researchers have assumed that the psychological process analyzes the temporal properties of the sounds (e.g., Liberman, Delattre, & Cooper, 1958; but, see Ivry & Gopal, 1992). By that method, there would presumably exist a psychological process sensitive to the temporal delay between the onset of the sound and the onset of voicing (see, also, Phillips et al., 1995). If the interval is negligible then the sound is a voiced phoneme. If there is a significant asynchrony then the sound is a voiceless phoneme.

However, some studies have indicated that spectral correlates of VOT provide an important source of information (Stevens & Klatt, 1974; Summerfield & Haggard, 1974). To appreciate how spectral information may be used to distinguish voiced and voiceless sounds, consider the schematic spectrograms of the /ba/ and /pa/ in figure 6.8. The formant trajectories for the second and third formants, at least as depicted, are identical for both labials. Where they differ is in terms of the energy present in the fundamental and first formant during the transition. Reflecting the fact that the vocal cords begin to vibrate with the consonantal release for /ba/, lower frequency information is present at the beginning of the formant transitions. For /pa/, energy at the lower frequency is absent during the initial voiceless period.

Speech Perception Predictions of the DFF Theory

Given those frequency differences, a spectral hypothesis for determining voicing can be stated quite simply. If energy is present at the fundamental frequency at the onset of the sound, then the consonant is voiced. If the onset of energy at the fundamental is delayed, then the consonant is voiceless. That hypothesis rests on the assumption that perception of speech sounds involves a continuous spectral analysis over time (Stevens & Blumstein, 1981; Phillips et al., 1995). It should be noted that the auditory system may utilize both temporal and spectral information in the perception of voicing (Lisker, 1975; Stevens & Klatt, 1974; Summerfield & Haggard, 1974).

Figure 6.8 makes clear the relevance of the distinction between voiced and voiceless syllables for evaluating the present theory. Information regarding place of articulation is generally carried in the relatively higher frequencies of the speech signal. Thus, /ba/ and /da/ can be synthesized solely by varying the initial frequencies and trajectories of the second and third formants. Cues to voicing, in contrast, are available in the relatively lower frequencies of the speech signal. Indeed, voicing is a relatively unique feature in that a phonemic distinction can be determined by low-frequency information.

However, one caveat should be kept in mind. The spectrograms in figure 6.8 are simplified cartoons and do not reflect the distribution of energy in natural speech. Voiced and voiceless phonemes also contain spectral differences in the higher formants during the initial portion of the sound. The lack of a fundamental energy source during the voiceless period results in a more diffuse spread of energy during the transitions. Although those differences can be reduced with synthetic speech, natural speech does contain voicing cues across the spectrum. Unlike most phonemic contrasts, however, low-frequency differences do exist between voiced and voiceless consonants. That information may provide the critical cue for voicing or supplement cues extracted from higher frequency regions of the sounds. Cues to place of articulation are not available in the lower frequencies.

We can now state the critical prediction of the DFF theory regarding phoneme perception. The theory predicts that the right hemisphere is relatively more important in the perception of voicing than in the perception of place of articulation. The prediction follows because the low-frequency region of the spectrum carries cues to voicing. In contrast, our theory predicts that perception of the place of articulation depends on left hemisphere processing because the critical information is contained in relatively high frequencies. This latter prediction may also be derived from theories that assign a generic left hemisphere role in speech perception, either due to specialized speech processors or to a specialized processor for analyzing rapidly changing information. Given the similar time frame (e.g., <50 ms) for formant transitions and VOT, a left hemisphere mechanism for processing high temporal frequencies should be similarly required to determine both place of articulation and voicing.

Electrophysiological Evidence of Asymmetries in Speech Perception

To summarize, the DFF theory predicts an interaction between hemispheric involvement and speech feature (place versus voicing). The current literature provides, at best, weak support for that prediction.

The positive evidence comes from studies that measured evoked potentials during speech perception. Many of those studies converge with behavioral data indicating a left hemisphere specialization for speech perception. For example, when stimuli differed in terms of place of articulation, then electrophysiological correlates of categorical perception were found over the left hemisphere. Elmo (1987) created a /ba/–/da/ continuum of seven sounds by varying the frequency of the second formant. He presented two of the sounds in each trial and asked the subject to judge whether they were the same. Of primary concern were two types of trials in which the stimuli differed acoustically. For one type of trial, the same-phonetic condition, the percepts were identical (both /ba/ or both /da/). For the other type of trial, the different-phonetic condition, a comparable frequency difference led to different percepts (one /ba/ and one /da/). The focus of the study was to identify evoked potentials that were correlated with the subjects' categorical perception. That is, would there be a difference in the evoked responses in trials in which stimuli were judged to be from the same category in comparison to trials in which the stimuli were judged to be from different categories?

Evoked responses to the stimuli were obtained from electrodes placed at various sites on the scalp. The responses over both hemispheres differentiated trials in which the two stimuli were identical from those in which the two stimuli differed acoustically. Of greater interest is the finding that only the evoked response over the posterior left hemisphere discriminated between the same-phonetic and different-phonetic conditions (see also Wood, Goff, & Day, 1971).

A similar result was reported by Molfese (1978a; 1980). In that study the stimuli varied from /bae/ to /gae/, a distinction that can be synthetically created by varying the trajectory of the third formant. A single stimulus was presented in each trial, and the subjects indicated whether they heard the consonant as /b/ or /g/. Differences in the evoked potentials for the two sounds were detected from electrodes placed over temporal lobes of the left hemisphere. In contrast, the evoked responses from the right hemisphere failed to discriminate between the two percepts. Molfese (1978a) found similar effects with nonspeech sounds composed of a set of sinusoids, each at a frequency matching the primary formants. Again, the only difference in the evoked potentials were seen in the output from electrodes situated over the left hemisphere.

However, in other evoked potential studies, Molfese and his associates consistently obtained a right hemisphere marker for certain speech contrasts. Specifically, those other studies used stimuli that differed in terms of voicing (Molfese, 1978b; Molfese & Hess, 1978; Molfese, 1980). Molfese (1978b) created a stimulus continuum from /ba/ to /pa/ by using VOT of 0, 20, 40, and 60 ms. The first two sounds were perceived as /ba/; the latter two as /da/. Using a component factor analysis of the evoked potentials, Molfese (1978b) identified two factors that discriminated the two short VOT stimuli from the two long VOT stimuli. When applied to the potentials recorded over the left hemisphere, those factors failed to distinguish between the short and long stimuli. In other words, although subjects reported a clear perceptual division of the four stimuli, no electrophysiological correlates of the distinction were found from electrodes situated over the left hemisphere. Surprisingly, the perceptual distinction was correlated with differences in the evoked potential patterns recorded over the right hemisphere. That is, differences in the output from the right hemisphere electrodes were correlated with the perceptual transition observed between the 20 and 40 ms stimuli.

A similar right hemisphere electrophysiological correlate of VOT was obtained in studies with four-year-old children (Molfese & Hess, 1978) and infants less than five months old (reported in Molfese, 1980). Moreover, Molfese (1980) tested nonspeech sine wave stimuli designed to mimic the voice-onset feature. The sine wave stimuli consisted of two pure tones at 500 and 1500 Hz. The onset of the 500 Hz tone was set to occur either 0, 20, 40, or 60 ms before the onset of the 1500 Hz tone. Although the stimuli do not sound like speech sounds, the factor analysis again revealed that activity from right hemisphere electrodes corresponded to the boundary between the stimuli with short tone-onset times and the stimuli with long tone-onset times (TOT). Evoked potentials from left hemisphere electrodes varied across the four stimuli, but not in a manner that corresponded to the percepts. For example, stimuli with TOT of 20 and 40 ms led to one pattern of evoked responses, whereas stimuli with TOT of 0 and 60 ms led to a different pattern.

Left hemisphere evoked potentials correlated with place of articulation discriminations, and right hemisphere evoked potentials correlated with voicing discriminations. That finding is in accord with the basic hemispheric asymmetry assumed in the DFF theory. The interaction is hard to reconcile, however, with laterality theories that assume that the left hemisphere is dominant for all tasks that involve linguistic processing. Those theories also require modification to account for the comparable effects for speech and nonspeech sounds (Molfese, 1978a; Molfese, 1980), since only the former is linguistic. The DFF theory is not similarly restricted. It assumes that the same processing mechanisms are applied to all kinds of sounds. Functional asymmetries arise when tasks make differential demands on information contained at either relatively low or relatively high regions of the spectrum, as occurs during discrimination of voicing or place of articulation, respectively. It should be pointed out that, even though he consistently found a right hemisphere correlate of voicing differences, Molfese was unable to provide a theoretical interpretation of those results. The DFF theory offers a plausible explanation.

Behavioral Tests of the Predictions

One important caveat must be emphasized regarding the current extension of the DFF theory to speech perception. Although there are clear behavioral consequences associated with the involvement of the right hemisphere in processing prosodic information, there is no behavioral evidence implicating the right hemisphere in voice perception. Evoked potentials measure physiological events; it is not mandatory for such events to be directly related to the primary psychological processes that guide perception. It remains to be seen whether the right hemisphere correlates of a distinction between voiced and voiceless phonemes play a casual role in the perception of that phonetic feature.

Indeed, the available evidence suggests that the left hemisphere is important in both the perception of place of articulation and voicing. Whereas a lack of hemispheric asymmetry was reported for voicing (Zatorre, Blumstein, & Oscar-Berman, 1987), Shankweiller and Studdert-Kennedy (1967) found a right ear advantage in dichotic listening for consonant-vowel syllables that differed in either place or voicing. The DFF theory would have predicted a reduced or reversed effect for voicing. Contrary to that prediction, the voicing asymmetry was twice as great as the place asymmetry, although the difference was not significant. Moreover, in two other experiments (Basso, Casati, & Vignolo, 1977; Blumstein, Cooper, Zurif, & Caramazza, 1977) only left hemisphere patients showed aberrant categorical perception for stimuli that varied in VOT (/da/ versus /ta/). Patients with right hemisphere lesions were reported to perform similar to healthy control subjects, although the data were not provided in either study.

There are at least three possible interpretations of those results. First, contrary to the indications of the evoked potential studies the left hemisphere may be critical for the perception of voicing, reflecting a general dominance of the left hemisphere in speech perception. Perhaps the left hemisphere contains mechanisms that are sensitive to nonspectral cues that are important in discriminating voiced and voiceless phonemes. Second, although the right hemisphere may play a role in perceptual analysis of voicing, the tasks used in the behavioral studies perhaps introduced factors that also depend on left hemisphere processing. Speech perception surely involves more than a spectral analysis of the acoustic signal, and those additional processes may depend on left hemisphere processes. For example, accessing the verbal labels used in identification tasks may be impaired following left hemisphere lesions (Damasio et al., 1996).

Third, it remains possible that even voicing distinctions are carried by differences in relatively high-frequency information. As mentioned previously, in normal speech the absence of a fundamental frequency during the voiceless segment of a phoneme is also correlated with reduced power at the higher frequencies during that segment. Thus, a high-frequency distinction may also subserve the discrimination of voiced and voiceless sounds. Although that confound can be minimized with synthetic stimuli, VOT has been manipulated by removing energy at both the fundamental and first formant in the unvoiced interval (Basso et al., 1977; Blumstein, Cooper, et al., 1977). Perhaps the perceptual distinction between voiced and voiceless sounds depends on an analysis of energy around the first formant rather than the fundamental.

That last proposal is admittedly post hoc and has the potential of making it impossible to generate novel predictions regarding phoneme perception on the basis of the DFF theory. That would be unfortunate, since a new theory should lead to critical experiments that pit the newcomer against older theories. The DFF theory does lead to one critical prediction: place of articulation should be more dependent than voicing on the left hemisphere, since the former depends on relatively higher frequency information. Similarly, the right hemisphere should have a relatively greater contribution to perception of voicing than to perception of place of articulation. Experiments with brain-injured populations do not provide a strong assessment of those predictions. Experiments that used both left and right hemisphere subjects only tested voicing (Basso et al., 1977; Blumstein, Cooper, et al., 1977), whereas those that used both place and voicing stimulus sets only tested left hemisphere patients (Blumstein, Baker, & Goodglass, 1977).

There are at least two ways to test the predictions of the DFF theory regarding phoneme perception. First, left and right hemisphere patients could be tested on two sets of stimuli, one set that varied in place of articulation and one set that varied in voicing. Left hemisphere patients would be expected to perform more poorly on the place of articulation task than on the voicing task, and right hemisphere patients would be expected to perform more poorly on the voicing task than on the place of articulation task. Two studies provide support for the first half of that prediction. Blumstein, Baker, et al. (1977) report that left hemisphere patients make more errors when a phonemic discrimination must be made on the basis of a place difference instead of on a voicing difference. A similar comparison was not made for control subjects, probably because their performance was essentially perfect. Sidtis and Volpe (1988) also report that left hemisphere patients make more errors on a dichotic-listening task when the dichotic pair differs in place of articulation than when the pair differs in voicing. We are currently conducting similar studies with neurological patients to directly test the predicted interaction.

A second test of the DFF theory's predictions regarding phoneme perception would involve studies with normal subjects to examine whether the perception of voicing and place varied as a function of the ear that received the stimulus. A problem with many speech perception studies is that performance is nearly optimal. With suprathreshold stimuli, subjects are usually highly consistent in assigning speech stimuli to one category or the other.

To overcome that obstacle we conducted two studies in which suboptimal performance was obtained by presenting speech sounds in low signal-to-noise conditions (Ivry & Lebby, in press). Two speech continua were used. For the voicing continuum the VOT was varied from −10 to +80 ms, and subjects were required to identify the sound as either a /ba/ or /pa/. For the nine-item place continuum the trajectories of the second and third formants were covaried to create either rising or falling transitions over the first 35 ms. Subjects were required to identify those stimuli as either /ba/ or /da/. The speech sounds were presented monaurally over a cassette tape. To create suboptimal conditions white noise was presented in the other ear.

In the first experiment each subject was tested in two sessions, with the stimulus targeted for the left ear in one session and the right ear in the other session. The sessions began with a calibration phase, during which the amplitude of the speech signal was varied against a constant level of noise. One set of stimuli was employed during the calibration phase. Each block of trials within the calibration phase consisted of 36 stimuli comprising four presentations of the nine stimuli.

Identification tests with speech stimuli generally produce categorical functions: subjects choose one response category for stimuli on one side of the categorical boundary and the other response category for stimuli on the other side. We assumed that if the perceptual representations of the speech sounds were suboptimal, then subjects would deviate from normal categorical performance. That is, they would be inconsistent in how they labeled a particular stimulus. In some trials the stimulus would be assigned to one response category and in other trials it would be assigned to the second response category. We developed a score for inconsistency by determining the number of times each stimulus was assigned to its nonpreferred category (Ivry & Gopal, 1992). With perfect categorical perception that score is zero, since each stimulus is consistently assigned to the same response label (e.g., all /ba/ or all /pa/ for the voicing continuum). Inconsistent responses occur when the responses are divided between the two response categories. For example, if the third stimulus on the continuum is labeled /ba/ on six trials and /pa/ on two trials, then the inconsistency score for that stimulus is two. A final inconsistency score was derived by summing across the individual scores for each stimulus in the continuum. Weighted versions of this consistency measure are discussed in Ivry and Gopal (1992). They generally provide results similar to the basic measure.

During the calibration phase the intensity of the speech signal was adjusted after each block of 36 trials until the subject was making between four and six inconsistent responses. Within four calibration blocks all the subjects consistently assigned a stimulus to one category or the other in 83% to 89% of the trials. The amplitude was then fixed for the test trials with that ear.

A test block consisted of 72 sounds composed of eight presentations of each stimulus. For the first session subjects completed two test blocks with one of the continua and then two more test blocks with the other continuum. The phonemes were presented to only one ear per session. Following a new calibration phase the phonemes were presented to the other ear during the second session. In this manner, we sought to control for idiosyncratic differences in the sensitivity of the two ears. Half of the subjects began with the left ear and half with the right ear. The order of stimulus continua (voicing or place) was counterbalanced.

Figure 6.9 presents mean response functions for the four conditions. The functions are similar to what is found in standard categorical perception studies, with the exception that the functions are not as steep: the low signal-to-noise conditions increased the number of inconsistent responses.

Inconsistency scores were calculated individually and the means are presented in the top panel of figure 6.10. Of greatest interest is the significant interaction between the ear of presentation and the stimulus continuum. Subjects were more inconsistent in responding to stimuli from the place continuum when those sounds were presented to the left ear. However, the reverse was observed for the voicing continuum. Here, performance was more inconsistent when the sounds were presented to the right ear. Those results were replicated in a second experiment in which the stimulus intensity was fixed and, within each session, both ears were tested on a single continuum.

To summarize the results of those initial studies, the observed interaction was in accord with predictions derived from the DFF theory. Specifically, we predicted an advantage for the right ear and left hemisphere with the place continuum, since the critical information was contained in the relatively high-frequency region of the speech spectrum. More critical,

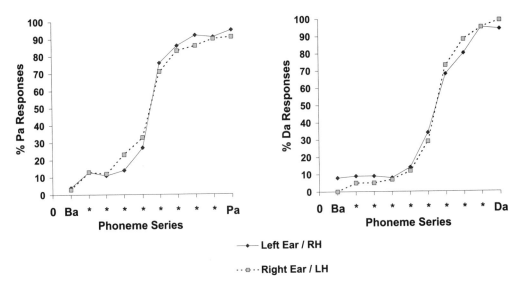

Figure 6.9 Mean response functions on the /ba/–/pa/ (left) and /ba/–/da/ (right) continua as a function of the ear receiving the stimulus. The functions are quite steep, which indicates categorical perception of those synthetic sounds. As VOT increases or as the initial frequency of the second and third formants is increased, subjects are more likely to label the sounds as /pa/ and /da/, respectively. (Adapted from Ivry & Lebby, in press.)

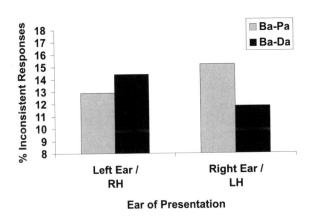

Figure 6.10 Mean inconsistent responses for the two continua as a function of the ear receiving the stimulus. Sounds from the /ba/–/da/ continuum were labeled more consistently when heard in the right hear, a result that is consistent with the hypothesis of a left hemisphere advantage in speech perception. However, the reverse was observed for the /ba/–/pa/ continuum. For those sounds, subjects were more consistent when the stimuli were presented in the left ear. (Adapted from Ivry & Lebby, in press.)

an advantage for the left ear and right hemisphere was predicted for the voicing continuum. With those sounds the phonetic distinction could be made on the basis of low-frequency information.

Those results are difficult to reconcile with alternative hypotheses regarding speech perception. Theories that hypothesize a specialized speech perception module in the left hemisphere may posit different mechanisms for certain phonetic subclasses (e.g., consonants and vowels), but in their current form they do not differentiate between hemispheric asymmetries in the perception of voicing and place of articulation. The results also appear to present difficulties for Tallal's hypothesis that consonant perception depends on a left hemisphere processor specialized for perceiving rapidly changing information. Although the temporal events spanned a longer period of time in the voicing continuum (e.g., a range of 90 ms) than in the place continuum (35 ms), the consonantal cues in both continua were given over relatively short time intervals. In natural speech the difference between voiced and voiceless sounds is much closer to the duration of the consonantal transition; for example, the VOTs for voiced and voiceless labials are around 5 and 50 ms. Although the current results do not argue against an extension of the DFF theory to the temporal domain, they do emphasize the importance of spectral information. Even within the domain of phoneme perception the right hemisphere may be important for discriminating speech contrasts carried in the low frequencies.

Before concluding this section we want to point out one other class of language phenomena that may prove useful in exploring the extension of the DFF theory to speech perception. In tonal languages such as Thai, Taiwanese, or Mandarin, variations in the fundamental frequency are used to signal different lexical items (figure 6.11). For example, in Mandarin the word *ma* can be spoken with one of four pitch contours: flat /ma/ meaning mother, rising /ma/ meaning hemp, falling then rising /ma/ meaning horse, and falling /ma/ meaning scold (Wang, 1976). Although such variations in the fundamental are correlated with

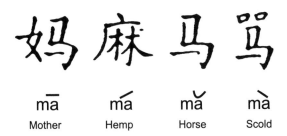

Figure 6.11 In tonal languages such as Mandarin, lexical information can be conveyed by variation in the fundamental frequency. The marks over the "a" in each word indicate the trajectory of the fundamental during the vocalic period of each word. (Adapted from Wang, 1976.)

variations in higher frequencies, native speakers of tonal languages are able to discriminate and identify words that are only cued by variations in the fundamental (Abramson, 1975; Gandour & Dardarananda, 1983). The DFF theory would predict that the right hemisphere would play a relatively important role in the perception of such tonal discriminations.

As with the studies of voicing, the available behavioral data do not support that prediction. Van Lancker and Fromkin (1973) report that native Thai speakers display a right ear advantage on a dichotic-listening task for tonal words. Moreover, the effect appears to be as great as it is for stimuli that contain different consonants. Similarly, Gandour and Dardarananda (1983) found that patients with left hemisphere lesions were poor in identifying words that only varied in tone. A control subject and a patient with a right hemisphere lesion were essentially perfect in identifying those words.

Nonetheless, the available data do not provide a sufficient test of the role of the right hemisphere in tone perception. Studies similar to those used in our tests of the voicing prediction are needed before any strong conclusions can be drawn. For example, more patients with right hemisphere lesions should be tested with tone stimuli. More importantly, experiments need to focus on comparing the relative importance of the right and left hemispheres in identification of lexical pairs that differ either in pitch or some other phonetic feature that is correlated with differences in high-frequency information.

SUMMARY

In this chapter we focused on the contributions of the right hemisphere in the perception of language. There is a substantial literature that points to an important role of the right hemisphere in the perception of prosody. The contribution of the right hemisphere to phoneme perception is more problematic. Our behavioral studies suggest that the right hemisphere may contribute to the perception of voicing, but additional studies are obviously warranted.

It remains clear that lesions of the left hemisphere lead to much more marked disturbances of language than do right hemisphere lesions. As it relates to perception, the DFF theory leads to the hypothesis that one reason for the dominant role of the left hemisphere is that many phonological distinctions require an analysis of cues contained in the higher region of the speech spectrum. In Western languages such as English the fundamental frequency provides little phonemic or lexical information. For such languages voicing represents a rare exception of a phonetic distinction that is correlated with events in the lower region of the spectrum. Thus, the left hemisphere bias to abstract high-frequency information may be central to the role of that hemisphere in representing the content of speech. In contrast, as shown by studies of prosody, the right hemisphere bias for representing low-frequency information is useful for establishing the context of speech. The evaluation of language functions typically (and rightfully) emphasizes assessment of a person's understanding of the content of speech. A loss of that ability is surely more debilitating than the prosodic disturbances observed following right hemisphere lesions.

Nonetheless, the review of speech perception tasks that depend on the right hemisphere demonstrates one advantage of the current approach for understanding hemispheric specialization over alternative theories that emphasize task or material differences. Normal speech perception requires the operation of both hemispheres. Indeed, the DFF theory is consistent with evidence suggesting that both hemispheres are capable of perceiving speech. As in the earlier analysis of visual perception, the DFF theory assumes that each hemisphere is provided with a full representation of the sound spectrum. Due to different filtering operations, however, the representations are asymmetric. Under many circumstances a right hemisphere representation that amplifies the lower region of the spectrum may prove sufficient for decoding phonological information.

We suggest that right hemisphere computational capability underlies the fact that speech perception remains possible when processing is functionally restricted to the right hemisphere. Patients with extensive lesions of the left hemisphere are able to comprehend oral language (e.g., Hugdahl & Webster, 1992). It is possible that that ability may reflect reorganization within the spared tissue of the left hemisphere. However, one PET study involving patients who had recovered from Wernicke's aphasia indicated that the recovery process was correlated with increased activity in regions of the right hemisphere homologous to those regions that are usually active in normal subjects during language comprehension (Weiller et al., 1995). Moreover, patients who have undergone a complete hemispherectomy of the left hemisphere are able to comprehend speech, as are split-brain patients, even when their performance is dependent on the isolated right hemisphere (Gazzaniga & Smylie, 1984; Zaidel, 1978). Theories that posit specialized mechanisms in the left hemisphere have difficulty accounting for such flexibility.

We recognize that there are limitations to how well the DFF theory can account for lateralization in language. First, the model is restricted to asymmetries in perception and does not offer any account of production asymmetries. Not only do humans show a strong asymmetry in terms of handedness, but the evidence suggests that speech production is even more lateralized to the left hemisphere than is speech perception (Gazzaniga, 1995; Kosslyn, 1987). Some theories attribute those two motor asymmetries to independent mechanisms (Previc, 1991), whereas others view them as reflecting a common precursor. For example, Corballis (1991) proposes a general purpose sequencing device in the left hemisphere that underlies the greater dexterity of the right hand in most individuals and the left hemisphere role in speech production. Alternatively, an asymmetry at the production level may trigger asymmetries in terms of how information is represented (Kosslyn, 1987). At present, we have little to add to this debate.

Even if we restrict our analysis to perception, reevaluation of the left hemisphere dominance in language leads to a classic chicken or egg conundrum. Our review emphasized that a fundamental asymmetry in the representation of frequency information can provide a unifying principle for incorporating a variety of laterality effects in vision and audition. However, we do not wish to imply that a generalized asymmetry in the representation of frequency information provided the initial seed for hemispheric specialization in language. Evolutionary pressures facing a species capable of using sophisticated oral communication may have led to an advantage in asymmetrically representing spectral information.

Adaptations survive when they confer an advantage in solving specific problems. It seems reasonable to assume that members of our ancestral species who evolved an efficient means for processing complex information would have enjoyed a reproductive advantage. One solution to the conundrum could be based on a system in which the two hemispheres derive similar yet nonredundant representations. That is, the asymmetric representation of frequency information might have evolved as a mechanism for improving the ability of human ancestors to comprehend vocalizations. On the other hand, the frequency asymmetry may have evolved for other reasons perhaps even unrelated to auditory perception. Exploitation of asymmetry for comprehending language may, in Gould's terms, provide a case of exaptation (Gould & Vrba, 1982). The current asymmetry in function may have originally utilized asymmetries that had arisen for other purposes. It is also possible that the similar asymmetries in processing frequency information across different tasks reflects a case of coevolution. For example, oral communication (or some other task) may have led to hemispheric asymmetries in audition, while different problems led to a coincidental specialization in vision. Exploring hemispheric asymmetries in the representation of frequency information in other species should prove a useful tact for addressing such issues.

7 A Computer Implementation of the Double Filtering by Frequency Theory

Computer modeling has established itself as a new and powerful tool in cognitive neuroscience. The information processing revolution that laid the foundation for cognitive psychology received its impetus from the development of the computer. There are obvious differences between the silicon chips of a computer and the neurons of organic creatures. Computers are extremely fast, serial, error-free under the right program, and subject to few processing limitations. Brains are considerably slower and noisier, involve massive parallel activity, and, to our chagrin, consistently demonstrate severe limitations in processing capability. Computers can access information that was stored 10 years ago as readily as data that were input only in the last minute. Humans, on the other hand, are not only unable to recall the phone numbers of their childhood friends, but frequently find themselves unable to remember a phone number heard just seconds ago.

Nonetheless, both the brain and the computer are impressive information processing machines, capable of representing massive amounts of information and performing transformations on the information to solve a variety of problems. Early efforts in artificial intelligence were primarily focused on developing computer programs capable of solving difficult problems such as playing chess or finding the optimal path between two locations (see Garay & Johnson, 1979). The emphasis was generally on using the programs as existence proofs to show that certain behaviors that might seem to be uniquely human could be performed by artificial systems. Some researchers did use those early programs as tools for understanding human cognition. But the comparisons were generally made at abstract levels, in terms of general principles that characterized the similarities between humans and computers.

Over the past 25 years the computer has emerged as a tool for developing and testing models of cognition that are increasingly neurologically

The lead researcher in the simulation work described in this chapter is Eliot Hazeltine, a graduate student at the University of California at Berkeley. We are very much indebted to Eliot for his efforts on this part of the project and for allowing us to present this preliminary report here.

constrained. Rather than simply using the computer to demonstrate that a machine can accomplish a particular task, researchers have turned to using computers to examine the processes that allow the task to be performed. In particular, computer programs are used as simulations of brain function, with the representations and computations designed to bear a close resemblance to the way the brain may actually perform the task. In this way, computers provide a viable tool for testing large-scale models of brain function.

In this chapter we present our initial efforts to develop a computer implementation of the DFF theory. The implementation is consistent with our hypothesis that a common architecture based on the asymmetric representation of frequency information can provide a parsimonious account of seemingly unrelated phenomena reported in the laterality research of visual perception. Before turning to this discussion we review Kosslyn's (1987) theory regarding hemispheric specialization in the representation of spatial relations. The review is important for two reasons. First, at a conceptual level, the two theories differ in their fundamental approach to hemispheric specialization. In Kosslyn's theory processing asymmetries emerge due to the fact that visually guided behavior relies on qualitatively different types of representations. In the DFF theory the two hemispheres derive similar representations, but those representations may differ in terms of their utility for performing various tasks. Second, through the process of implementing his theory, Kosslyn was led to argue that the two hemispheres represent frequency information asymmetrically. As we shall see, this work has provided a close convergence between his theory and the DFF theory.

DIVIDE AND CONQUER

Chapter 3 describes Kosslyn's (1987; Kosslyn et al., 1992) theory of hemispheric specialization. At the heart of the theory is the hypothesis that the two hemispheres are specialized to construct representations that serve distinct functions for spatial cognition. Processing within the left hemisphere yields categorical representations, which are useful for determining basic information regarding relative spatial relations such as above versus below or on versus off. Processing within the right hemisphere, on the other hand, is essential for abstracting precise topographical properties, or what he calls coordinate representations: Where is an object located in space? What is the distance between two objects?

In Kosslyn's view categorical and coordinate representations serve qualitatively different purposes (Kosslyn et al., 1989). Categorical representations are likely to be an important component of object recognition, at least when recognition processes operate in object-centered coordinates. For example, a defining feature of the human body is that the head is located above the legs. Coordinate representations are not essential for establishing such relations. The relative position of the head to the legs holds steady for infants and adults. However, coordinate representations are essential for action. We need to know exactly where a glass is located on the table in order to successfully pick it up (figure 7.1).

Superficially, one might suppose that the categorical/coordinate distinction would map more closely to the ventral versus dorsal or what versus where dichotomy of higher visual processing (e.g., Ungerleider & Mishkin, 1982) rather than to a difference between the two hemispheres. However, Kosslyn (1987) argues that the construction of both categorical and coordinate representations are linked to the dorsal pathway in correspondence to two distinct uses for spatial information. Thus, in his view, cerebral asymmetries arise in terms of the processing within the dorsal streams of the right and left hemispheres. Although he views those types of representations as qualitatively distinct, he does not make the stronger claim of exclusivity. Both hemispheres are capable of representing both categorical and coordinate. As in the DFF theory, the hemispheres differ in their relative efficiency for supporting such representations (Kosslyn et al., 1992).

In some respects Kosslyn's theory is narrower in scope than the DFF theory. Kosslyn's theory, at least as tested and developed in detail, focuses on asymmetries in the representation of spatial information. In the DFF theory we propose that the asymmetric representation of frequency information accounts for various laterality phenomena across different

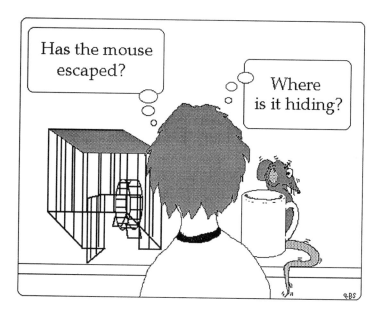

Figure 7.1 Two types of spatial relations. Categorical spatial relations are essential for determining the basic features of the scene. Has the mouse escaped? Is it inside or outside the cage? Coordinate spatial relations provide metrical information that is essential for action. To retrieve the mouse, it is essential to locate precisely where it is hiding.

modalities, and that it may also apply in the temporal domain. On the other hand, Kosslyn points out that the categorical/coordinate distinction could be a fundamental distinction, at least in human cognition. Categorization is one of the hallmarks of language at all levels, from the way articulatory gestures are linked to phonetic categories to the words we use to label perceptual and conceptual entities. Within those categories we are generally sensitive to idiosyncratic differences that could be considered to be coordinate information. Whereas many pieces of furniture can be called "chairs," for example, we are obviously sensitive to the differences among the thousands of varieties of dining room chairs. Thus, the categorical/coordinate distinction may well provide a general theory of hemispheric specialization.

Our main concern here, however, is to discuss similarities and differences between the DFF theory and Kosslyn's theory. We have already described in chapter 4 how both theories can account for the same set of experimental data. To review briefly, Kosslyn et al. (1989) compared two tasks, both of which involved the same stimuli. A lateralized stimulus composed of a bar and dot was presented in each trial. For the above versus below task, subjects judged whether the dot was above or below the bar (a categorical discrimination). For the near versus far task, subjects judged whether the dot was relatively close to or far from the bar (a metrical or coordinate discrimination). Subjects were faster at making coordinate judgments when the stimuli were in the left visual field and showed a trend favoring categorical judgments when the stimuli were in the right visual field. In our reanalysis of those tasks we proposed that the above versus below task would require processing of relatively higher spatial frequency information (see figure 3.22).

In the following section, we present a computer implementation of the DFF theory that produces this interaction. First, it is useful to consider related modeling of the bar-dot task. In a series of simulations of the task Kosslyn et al. (1992) employed a standard connectionist architecture composed of three layers corresponding to input, output, and so-called hidden layers (figure 7.2). Such networks are used to test how a set of inputs can be mapped onto a desired set of outputs (Rummelhart & McClelland, 1986). A stimulus is represented as a pattern of activation across the input units. The activation pattern is propagated through the hidden units to the output units; the level of activity in each unit is a function of both its input and the weighted connection between the sending and receiving unit. The resulting representation in the output units is compared with a desired output, and supervised learning algorithms use the difference between the two representations to generate an error signal. The error signal is then propagated backwards through the network (i.e., from output to input units) to modify the weights between the various units. Although backpropagation has been challenged as physiologically implausible, it nonetheless provides a tool by which a system can learn

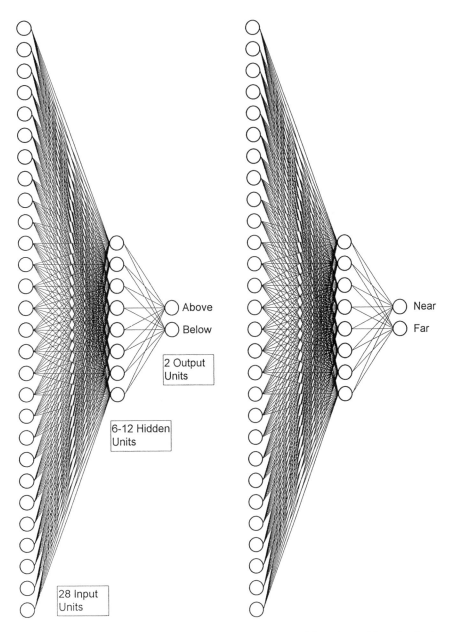

Figure 7.2 The standard connectionist architecture consists of three layers. The stimulus is represented across the input layer and the response of the network is represented by the output nodes. The hidden units allow the network to learn the mapping between the input and output layers. Kosslyn et al. (1992) used this architecture to explore hemispheric asymmetries in the representation of categorical and coordinate spatial relations. Although the architecture is similar for the two networks, the output units correspond to judgments for either the categorical task (left) or coordinate task (right). (Adapted from Kosslyn et al., 1992.)

A Computer Implementation of the DFF Theory

arbitrary mappings between input and output representations. Thus, simulations can be used to compare different types of network architectures or forms of representation.

In the simulations of Kosslyn et al. (1992) the input layer was used to represent the stimuli for the various conditions of the bar-dot task. Each of the 28 units in the input layer represented a particular location in a one-dimensional space. In each trial three of the input units were activated, two representing the position of the bar and one representing the position of the dot. Activation from the input units was transmitted to 10 hidden units that converged on two output units. In a network trained on the categorical task, the output units corresponded to judgments of "above" and "below." In a network trained on the coordinate task, the output units corresponded to judgments of "near" and "far." In their third study Kosslyn et al. assessed the size of the receptive fields of the hidden units within the two networks. That is, they measured the weights between the input and hidden units to determine the contiguous number of spatial positions that activated a given hidden unit. Intriguingly, they found that the hidden units in the categorical network developed receptive fields smaller than those in the coordinate network.

In the second part of the study Kosslyn et al. (1992) directly tested the hypothesis that receptive field differences can produce asymmetric performance on the two tasks. The input units were given their own fixed receptive fields, which operated on an earlier retinal array. Hence, an input unit did not represent a single point in space but instead integrated information over a contiguous region of space. The extent of the integration process depended on the size of the receptive field. The critical comparison was between the performance of two networks, one in which the input units had small receptive fields and the other in which the input units had large receptive fields. The network with small receptive fields was better at learning the categorical, above versus below, discrimination; the network with large receptive fields was better at learning the coordinate, near versus far, discrimination.

Those findings are interesting to consider from the perspective of the DFF theory. We have argued that the categorical task requires the use of relatively higher spatial frequency information than is required by the coordinate task. In accord with that analysis, Kosslyn et al. (1992) found that differences on the two tasks were related to receptive field size. Small receptive fields are generally most sensitive to high spatial frequencies whereas large receptive fields are optimally tuned to low spatial frequencies. Kosslyn et al. suggested that the right hemisphere may disproportionately receive input from lateral geniculate neurons that carry low spatial frequency information. However, that hypothesis would predict differences based on absolute frequency. As reviewed in this book, the evidence suggests that hemispheric asymmetries are best described in terms of relative frequency (Christman et al., 1991; but, see Kosslyn, Anderson, Hillger, & Hamilton, 1994).

Thus, whereas Kosslyn et al. motivate their modeling in terms of hemispheric specialization for task requirements, the simulations show that such differences may instead be an emergent property of asymmetric use of spatial frequency information. We now turn to an implementation of the DFF theory that takes an approach different from this divide-and-conquer strategy in which separate networks are specialized for deriving different types of spatial representations. In our theory we emphasize that each hemisphere is capable of performing all perceptual tasks and representing the full range of frequency information. Performance asymmetries emerge from differences in how each hemisphere transforms the sensory data.

IMPLEMENTATION OF THE DFF THEORY

We used a computer model to explore whether the DFF theory can provide a unified account of some prominent laterality effects in visual perception. Our overall goal was straightforward. Could one architecture prove sufficient to simulate laterality effects in three distinct tasks? The tasks we selected were grating identification, local/global form perception, and the two so-called categorical and coordinate discriminations with the bar-dot task.

Architecture of the Simulations

Figure 7.3 provides a sketch of the model architecture. There are five layers in the model. The middle three layers correspond to the standard connectionist architecture with input, hidden, and output units. Where our model differs is that the standard organization is repeated to form six independent modules, each composed of input units sensitive to a particular spatial frequency. In this manner, the structure captures the key assumption of the DFF theory: namely, that visual perception involves processing within a series of spatial frequency channels (De Valois & De Valois, 1990; Graham, 1989).

Located before those three-layer modules is a common stimulus array that provides a veridical representation of the stimulus, analogous to the image that falls on the retina. We used 192 units for the stimulus array. The stimulus array is transformed by spatial frequency filtering into activation along the 80 input units of each three-layer module. Those 80 units converge on eight hidden units, which in turn project to four output units per module. The final layer of the network corresponds to the ultimate decision of the network as a whole, and is represented by four decision units. In effect, the modules compete to impose their output patterns on the final decision layer. Thus, the decision layer reflects the integration of processing within the independent modules.

The input units were designed to reflect the receptive field properties of neurons in visual cortex. Thus, they capture two fundamental pieces

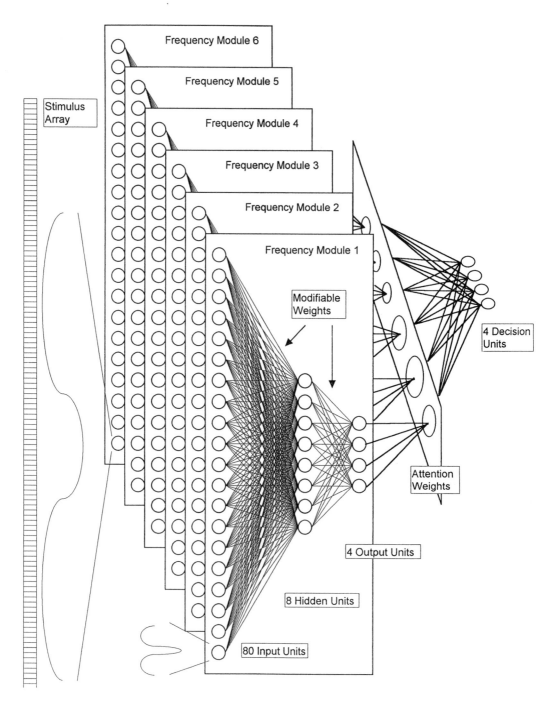

Figure 7.3 The architecture of our computer model of the DFF theory. The stimulus array provides a veridical representation of the stimulus. Activation from those units is fed into the input units for the six frequency modules. The activation in the input units is determined by the receptive field properties of each module. The receptive fields are largest for units in Module 6 (the wide center-surround function spanning most of the stimulus array). The receptive fields are smallest for units in Module 1 (the narrow center-surround function spanning just a few of the stimulus array units near the bottom of the figure). Within each

of information. First, they reflect the location of a stimulus. Within a module there is a complete representation of one-dimensional space, with each unit sensitive to a particular region of space. Second, the input units reflect the form of the stimulus through spatial frequency filtering. The modules differ in terms of the sizes of their receptive fields. In the module with the smallest receptive fields the input units are optimally tuned to changes in luminance at 5 cycles/degree. Input units in the module with the largest receptive fields are optimally tuned to changes in luminance at 0.20 cycles/degree. In essence, the input units provide a filtered representation of the stimulus array, integrating luminance information across the spatial dimension as a function of receptive field size (figure 7.4).

The hidden units do not have any receptive field properties built into them. Within a module each hidden unit is connected to all of the input units and projects to all of the output units. The activity of the hidden units is determined by standard connectionist rules, with the activation from each input unit weighted by a modifiable connection strength. Similarly, there are connections between all of the hidden and output units of each module, and those connections are also plastic. In all of the simulations the weights within a module are adjusted using the back propagation algorithm. The error is determined by comparing activation in the decision layer with the desired output. The weights between the stimulus array and input units, which produce the receptive field transformation, do not change with learning. Within the model, modules retain their spatial frequency sensitivity.

The weights between the module-specific output units and the decision units are modifiable, but in a manner designed to capture the initial selective filtering component of the DFF theory. As detailed in chapter 2, we assume that attention serves to focus processing on the stimulus information that is most relevant to the task at hand. Given frequency-based representations, that idea can be instantiated by varying the relative influence of the six modules. For example, consider two stimuli, one that spans a large portion of the stimulus array and a second that spans a small portion of the stimulus array. The critical information is carried at relatively lower frequencies in the former condition, and thus attention should favor processing within the module with larger receptive fields. To model such processing mechanisms the weights between module outputs and the decision layer were altered according to an assessment of the range of stimulus information. For example, the attentional weights were used to amplify the output from low-frequency channels when the

module the input units are connected to hidden units, which project to module-specific output units. The output units from the six modules project to the four decision units that represent the response of the network. The activation of the module-specific output units is modulated by the attentional weighting function.

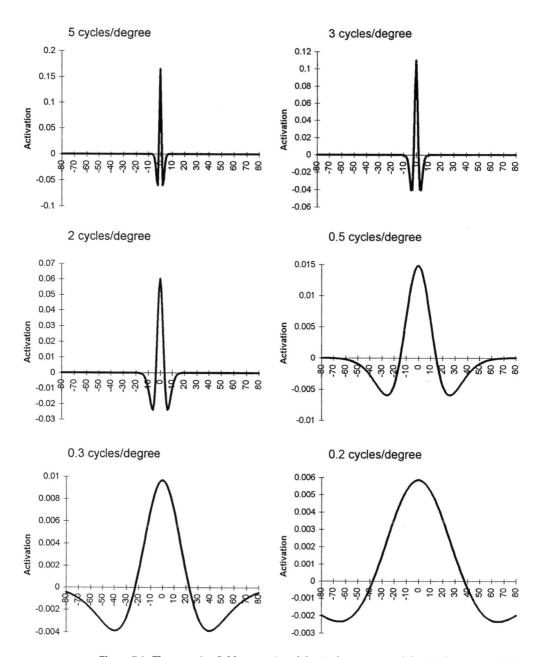

Figure 7.4 The receptive field properties of the six frequency modules. Each receptive field is a center-surround mechanism with an excitatory center region and symmetric, inhibitory flanking regions (calculated as the difference of two Gaussian functions). The modules differ in the size of their receptive fields.

stimulus was large. Note that in experiments such as the auditory studies of Ivry and Lebby (1993) attention is directed on the basis of task-relevant information rather than the overall range of frequency information. In the visual tasks we have modeled to date, the overall range of frequency information and task-relevant frequency information have covaried.

To this point, we have not addressed the most important issue, namely, hemispheric asymmetries in the representation of frequency information. The fundamental tenet of the DFF theory is that the right hemisphere is biased to represent information at relatively lower spatial frequencies than is the left hemisphere. To implement that asymmetry we used the attentional weights between the module outputs and the decision layer. Specifically, we varied the attentional weighting functions between two networks so that the attentional weights for the right hemisphere network emphasized lower frequency modules; in contrast, the attentional weights for the left hemisphere network emphasized higher frequency modules (figure 7.5).

Two critical features are captured in figure 7.5. First, the peak of each weighting function is centered over the same module for the two networks. This peak shifts, however, as a function of the focus of attention. In the top panel the focus is at Module 2; in the lower panel the focus is at Module 5. Second, the asymmetric weighting functions produce a consistent bias for the right hemisphere to emphasize relatively lower frequencies than those analyzed by the left hemisphere. In this manner the model reflects our hypothesis that the asymmetric use of information is based on relative frequencies rather than absolute frequencies. Importantly, the set of attentional weights is the same across the two networks, but the weights are differentially distributed. Although attentional weights are not altered by learning, they have significant consequences in terms of how processing within each network changes over the course of learning. Because the error signal starts at the decisional layer and is propagated back through the attentional weights, modules receiving greater emphasis have the potential for more dramatic changes during learning.

To summarize, the model architecture is consistent with the basic assumptions of the DFF theory. Each hemisphere has the capability to represent the full range of frequency information; indeed, the frequency modules are identical in the two hemispheric networks. Performance differences between the two networks, however, emerge from their asymmetric use of spectral information. Because of the way in which we implement selective attention, such differences should depend on relative frequencies. Thus, our model contrasts with the approach pursued by Kosslyn et al. (1992), which emphasized absolute frequency differences in the receptive field properties of the two hemispheres.

Our architecture also captures the idea that relative asymmetries in the use of frequency information result from two distinct filtering operations.

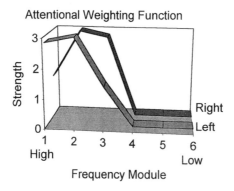

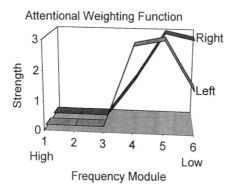

Figure 7.5 The attentional weighting functions used to modulate the connection strength between the output units and the decision units. The attentional weighting functions implement the two filtering stages of the DFF theory. First, both functions are centered over the frequency module that is expected to provide the most useful information for the task at hand. That position is over a higher frequency module (Module 2) in the top panel than it is in the lower panel (Module 5). Second, the shape of the weighting function is asymmetric. The right hemisphere function provides a low-pass filtering operation; the left hemisphere function provides a high-pass filtering operation. The shape of the hemispheric filters is invariant. The position of the filters is task-dependent but is the same for both hemispheres.

One mechanism determines the focus of attention and operates in an identical manner for each hemisphere (i.e., the peak of the attentional weighting function is centered over the same module). A second mechanism, the shape of the weighting functions, causes the two networks to emphasize different aspects of the internal representation of the stimulus.

Finally, our architecture treats the two hemispheres as essentially autonomous structures. There are no connections between the two hemispheres. Indeed, in all of the simulations reported in the next sections, we contrast performance of the right and left hemisphere networks when tested separately on the same problem. Of course, this is not possible in research with humans, not even with those with severed corpus callosi, for whom interactions can still occur via subcortical mechanisms. Future work should examine different forms of hemispheric interaction (e.g., convergence directly from hemispheric modules onto a single set of decision units); we currently focus on demonstrating how a common architecture that exploits the asymmetric representation of frequency information may underlie laterality effects across a diverse set of tasks.

Identification of Spatial Frequency Gratings

For our initial test of the model we modified the grating identification task of Kitterle et al. (1990). As described in chapters 2 and 3 a sinusoidal grating of either 1 or 9 cycles/degree was presented to either the left or right visual fields of healthy, young subjects. The low-frequency grating was identified faster when presented in the left visual field, while the high-frequency grating was identified faster when presented in the right visual field. Christman et al. (1991) showed that the effect was one of relative frequency. When they used stimuli composed of multiple sinusoids the inclusion of a 2 cycle/degree component produced opposite laterality effects depending on whether it was the relatively lowest or highest frequency in the stimulus.

In Simulation 1 the stimuli in our identification task were single gratings. The network was trained to determine whether the pattern along the stimulus array varied at either a low or high frequency. The activation levels for each of the 192 units in the stimulus array were determined by the sine function, which was normalized so that the values varied from −1 to +1. The frequency was set to either 1 or 3 cycles/degree. Note that the difference between the frequencies was less than that used by Kitterle et al. (1990). Our network was not sensitive to frequencies above 5 cycles/degree, due to constraints of network size and the requirements of later simulations (figure 7.6).

The network was trained to classify a set of 80 stimuli, which included 20 versions of each sinusoid, each differing in phase. The phase variations prevented the network from relying on a limited set of units to learn the discrimination. The remaining 40 stimuli were "catch trials," with activation levels set to zero for all of the stimulus array units. Without the catch trials the network would have been able to learn by detecting the absence of activity within certain modules. By including the catch trials, inactivity within a module no longer provided sufficient information.

In each trial a stimulus was randomly selected and the output from the decision units was compared to a target output pattern. Target output patterns of 1000 and 0100 corresponded to the low- and high-frequency patterns, and 0010 corresponded to the catch trials. Thus, although there were four decision units, only three were used in the first simulation. Activity in the decision units was an integration of the output units of the six frequency modules. Learning occurred after each trial, and the difference between the activation of the decision units and the target

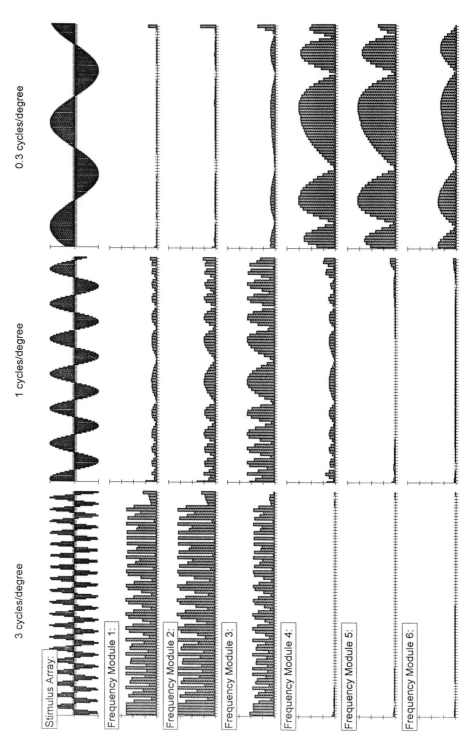

Figure 7.6 The activation across the stimulus array and across the input units for each of the six modules for the stimuli in Simulations 1 and 2. (Left column) 3 cycles/degree stimulus. (Middle column) 1 cycle/degree stimulus. (Right column) 0.3 cycle/degree stimulus. Note how the locus of activity shifts for the three stimuli. Whereas the low-frequency modules are insensitive to the high-frequency stimulus, activity is restricted to those modules with the lowest frequency stimulus.

pattern was used as an error signal. For each trial the difference between each decision unit and its corresponding target unit was squared, and the sum of those four values constituted our error measure. With this method, the maximum error score would be 4 if all four decision units had values opposite to those in their corresponding target units. By chance, however, the error score should be 1, assuming activation values of 0.5 in the decision units (squared sum difference between 0.5 and the target values). The error score was calculated across the full set of 80 stimuli.

Separate simulations were run for a left hemisphere and a right hemisphere network. As described previously, the only difference between the two networks was in the profile of the attentional weighting function. For both networks that function was centered over the second-highest frequency module, a position that was based on assessment of the distribution of activity across the module inputs.

Each network was trained on 10 runs, with the initial weights randomized between runs. A run consisted of 20 blocks with the 80 stimuli, and a performance probe was made after every two blocks. Both the right and left hemisphere networks had little trouble learning the discrimination (figure 7.7); indeed, by the tenth block (fifth probe), the error was quite small, averaging less than 0.2 per stimulus. The error value was reduced to approximately 0.1 per stimulus by the end of the twentieth block, at which point performance was near asymptote. The results were consistent across the 10 runs; all reported effects are statistically reliable.

As predicted, there was a hemisphere-by-frequency interaction. At all 10 probes, the right hemisphere network was more accurate than the left hemisphere network in classifying the 1 cycle/degree stimuli. Similarly, the left hemisphere network was always more accurate in classifying the 3 cycles/degree stimuli. The difference was present even though the higher frequency stimulus was easier to learn overall.

Simulation 2 was designed to demonstrate that the laterality effect was based on relative frequency. The same networks were trained to discriminate between sinusoidal gratings of either 0.3 or 1.0 cycle/degree. The target output patterns for the 1.0 cycle/degree and catch trials were as before; for the new 0.3 cycle/degree stimulus the fourth decision unit was used, with a target output pattern of 0001. The position of the attentional weighting function was again determined by the distribution of activity in the module inputs. Reflecting the fact that the stimuli spanned a lower range of frequencies, the weighting function also shifted to a center over the third-highest module.

The laterality effect was essentially identical to that obtained in the first simulation (figure 7.7). Of particular interest in the second simulation was how the hemispheric networks performed when presented with the 1.0 cycle/degree stimuli. When those stimuli constituted the lower frequency members of the training set, the right hemisphere network performed

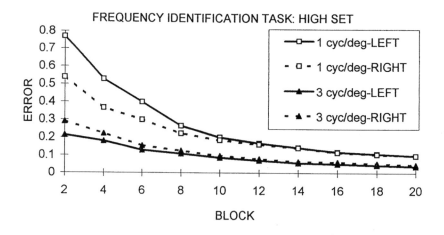

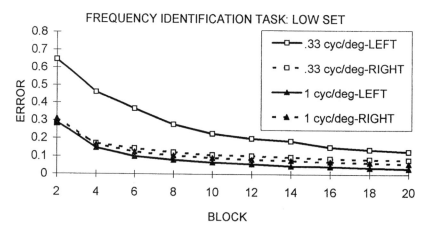

Figure 7.7 Learning functions for each stimulus within the right hemisphere and left hemisphere networks. The mean error rate is calculated per stimulus. (Top panel) Simulation 1 results. (Bottom panel) Simulation 2 results. The relative frequency effect is most apparent in the results with the 1 cycle/degree stimulus. The right hemisphere network is better than the left hemisphere network in classifying the 1 cycle/degree stimulus when it is paired with the 3 cycle/degree stimulus. In contrast, the left hemisphere shows an advantage when the 1 cycle/degree stimulus is paired with the 0.3 cycle/degree stimulus.

better than the left hemisphere network. However, when the exact same patterns constituted the higher frequency members, the advantage reverted to the left hemisphere network. Together, the first two simulations demonstrate that the combination of two filtering stages—the attentional weighting function and the hemispheric filters—produces representational differences in terms of relative frequency rather than absolute frequency.

Two additional results from Simulation 2 are noteworthy. First, as in Simulation 1, the average error was lower for the higher frequency member of the pair, even though its absolute frequency changed. Second, the overall error rates were comparable in the two simulations. In combination with the reversed laterality effect for the 1 cycle/degree stimulus, the results make it difficult to attribute the interactions to synergies between receptive field properties and particular frequencies. Rather, the interactions must be ascribed to differential weighting of activity within the frequency-sensitive modules. Shifting the position of the weighting function allows attention to be focused on task-relevant information while maintaining the asymmetric use of that information by the two hemispheres. Those two processes embody the central tenets of the DFF theory.

Same Stimuli, Different Tasks

The results of these initial simulations are encouraging, but they are not very surprising. The weighting function amplified lower frequency information in the right hemisphere network compared to the left hemisphere network. The effect should be expected to be one of relative frequency, since the center of the weighting function shifted between the two sets of stimuli. A more impressive demonstration would be to show that laterality effects are contingent on task demands even when the stimuli remain unchanged. In the first two simulations the laterality effect was independent of particular stimuli: the task remained the same but the stimuli changed across the simulations. In the next set of simulations the stimuli were constant and the task was varied. If emergent laterality effects are task dependent, then different regions of the frequency spectrum must contain the critical information for the particular tasks. By constructing the simulation in this way, we ensure that the laterality effects are not attributed to generic properties of the stimuli.

For our simulation, we chose to emulate the study of Kitterle et al. (1992). In their study subjects performed two tasks with the same set of stimuli. The stimuli were varied on two dimensions: fundamental frequency (1 or 3 cycles/degree) and component structure (sinusoids or square waves). For one task subjects had to base their responses on the fundamental, judging whether the stripes were wide or narrow. For the second task subjects had to consider the component structure of the stimuli, judging whether the edges of the stripes were fuzzy or sharp (see figure 2.8). The wide versus narrow discrimination was performed faster when the stimuli were presented in the left visual field, whereas the fuzzy versus sharp discrimination was performed faster when the stimuli were presented in the right visual field.

For Simulation 3 we created 80 patterns, 20 for each combination of fundamental frequency and component structure. Given the constraints of our simulations, we opted to use fundamentals of 0.3 and 1.0 cycle/degree. Square wave stimulus patterns were created from the sinusoidal patterns by setting all positive activation values to 1.0 and all negative activation values to –1.0. As before, the only difference within a set of 20 stimuli was in the phase. The target patterns over the four decision units corresponded to the four response categories: 1000 = wide; 0100 = narrow; 0010 = fuzzy; 0001 = sharp. Separate networks were trained on the two tasks, and for each task there were right hemisphere and left hemisphere networks. The attentional weighting function was centered over the third-highest module in all of the simulations, the same position that was used in Simulation 2. As in the first two simulations, the networks were trained over 20 blocks, and performance was evaluated after every other block.

Figure 7.8 presents the learning functions for each of the two hemispheric networks on the two tasks. The data points correspond to the mean error, averaged over all 80 patterns. In accord with the results of Kitterle et al. (1992) there was a hemisphere-by-task interaction. Specifically, at all of the performance probes the right hemisphere network outperformed the left hemisphere network on the wide versus narrow task; the reverse was true for the fuzzy versus sharp task.

Simulation 3 differs in a fundamental way from the preceding two simulations. In Simulations 1 and 2 the hemispheric networks differed in how they classified particular stimuli, with the right hemisphere network more adept at identifying the relatively lower frequency stimulus. In Simulation 3 the laterality effects were obtained in comparisons across the same stimulus sets. That finding is consistent with the hypothesis that task requirements force the networks to exploit different sources of information.

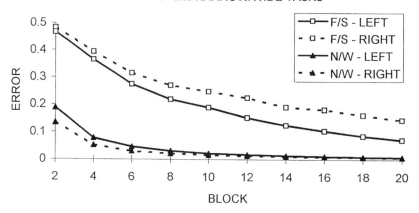

Figure 7.8 Learning functions in Simulation 3. In accord with the findings of Kitterle et al. (1992), the laterality effect was highly task-dependent, and it reversed when the classification rule changed. The mean error rate was lower in the right hemisphere network for the narrow versus wide task, which is a discrimination that should require the analysis of the fundamental frequency. The advantage shifted to the left hemisphere network for the fuzzy versus sharp task, which is a discrimination that requires the analysis of the harmonic structure of the stimuli.

The results of Simulation 3 reinforce an important feature of the DFF theory. The theory assumes that hemispheres are not specialized for particular tasks. Rather, each hemisphere is in principle capable of representing the information required for all perceptual tasks. However, task differences may emerge because the representations are asymmetric. The asymmetry leads to an advantage for one hemisphere because it amplifies the critical information for a given task. Thus, in Simulation 3, each hemisphere could independently learn to correctly classify the stimuli according to either scheme. Nonetheless, there were consistent differences between the left and right hemisphere networks on the tasks, presumably because the tasks required analysis of different spectral regions. The fundamental frequency was critical for the wide versus narrow task, and thus performance was better on that task for the right hemisphere network, since it amplified the lower frequency information. When the same stimuli were classified in the fuzzy versus sharp task, the networks had to rely on higher frequency information, and the left hemisphere network proved more adept.

Identification of Hierarchical Patterns

To this point, the simulations of the DFF theory have all involved tasks that classify spatial frequency gratings. We now turn to a broader application of the model: How does the model perform when the stimuli are less tailored to the frequency-sensitive modular structure of our implementation? Specifically, can the same architecture used in the previous simulations mimic the robust laterality effects reported in identification tasks with hierarchical stimuli? As reviewed extensively in this book, evidence reveals that identification of local elements in such patterns is favored within the left hemisphere, whereas identification of global elements is favored within the right hemisphere.

Our fourth simulation addresses a central assumption in the hierarchical pattern perception literature. Global patterns by definition have power at relatively lower spatial frequencies than do local elements. Nonetheless, the lower frequencies are not essential, as evidenced by the fact that people can identify the global shape of high-pass filtered stimuli (Hughes et al., 1990). Given that high-frequency information is sufficient, it remains possible that a laterality model based on frequency analysis will not produce the observed behavioral interaction.

Simulation 4 was developed to explore those questions. We devised stimuli that could be accommodated by our network architecture, which required modification of the traditional two-dimensional hierarchical patterns so that the structure could be represented in a single dimension. The essence of hierarchical patterns is that a global shape is formed by the composition of a repeated local element. In divided-attention tasks a target letter can either occur globally or locally, with a distractor letter

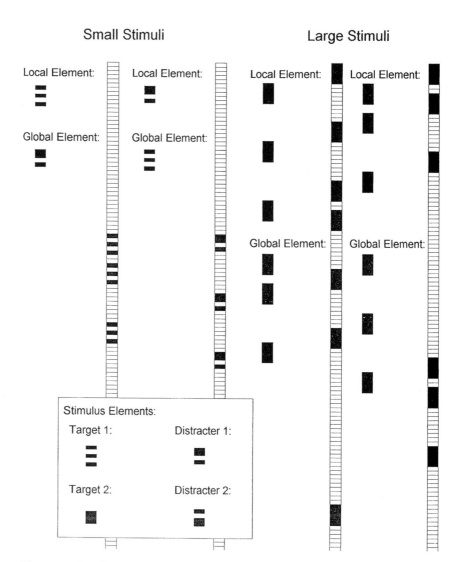

Figure 7.9 One-dimensional versions of hierarchical patterns. The patterns for the two targets and two distractors are shown in the inset. They are created by activating three elements in a five-element array (e.g., in Target 1, the first, third, and fifth elements are active; in Target 2, the second, third, and fourth elements are active). As shown on the left of each stimulus, the patterns occur at either the local or global level; one level is used for the target and the other is used for the distractor. In the small stimuli, the local pattern is created across five contiguous units and the global pattern is created across groups of five units. In the large stimuli, the small pattern is created across groups of five units and the global pattern is created across groups of 25 units. The small and large stimuli were tested in separate simulations.

appearing at the other level. We sought to maintain this logic in our one-dimensional stimulus arrays.

Examples of our stimuli are depicted in figure 7.9. Within each stimulus the local element is defined by the pattern across five contiguous units. In the stimulus shown in the left column of figure 7.9 the pattern consists of an alternation between active and inactive units. Similarly, in the other local elements, three units are active and two are inactive, but the sequence of active and inactive units differs. The global shapes are created by using the same four sequences, but with the repetition occurring over local elements of five units. To match the typical hierarchical letter stimuli, we include a space of two units between each local element.

There were a total of eight basic stimuli, formed by the combination of two targets and two distractors, with the target appearing at either the local or global level. The total stimulus set consisted of 160 patterns and included 20 versions of each stimulus with the exact placement varied within the 192-unit stimulus array. The variation over the 20 displacements spanned approximately 1 degree of visual angle. The procedure was identical to that used to vary phase in the grating simulations. As described previously, by using various displacements, the network is not able to learn the classification based on activity in a limited set of input units.

The frequency modules were the same as in the previous simulations. Activation across the stimulus array was converted into an input pattern through the receptive field properties of the input units, and from there was propagated through the hidden units to the module outputs. The module outputs converged on four decision units. The attentional weighting function was centered over the second-highest frequency module, based on an assessment of the activity across the input arrays. In the current simulation the decision units represented the two targets, with each target separately represented at the local and global level. An error signal was generated by comparing the activation in the decision units with four target patterns: 1000 = target 1, local; 0100 = target 2, local; 0010 = target 1, global; 0001 = target 2, global.

The right hemisphere and left hemisphere networks were each trained on 10 runs. Over the first 20 blocks the results showed the predicted interaction (figure 7.10). When the target was at the local level the mean error was lower in the left hemisphere network than in the right hemisphere network. Conversely, the mean error was lower in the right hemisphere network when the target was at the global level. The model provides converging support for the assumption that local and global processing are preferentially dependent on relatively higher and lower spatial frequency information, respectively.

The network produced considerably more error after 20 blocks on the local/global task in comparison to the grating identification tasks. That effect confirms our intuition that classification of those complex patterns

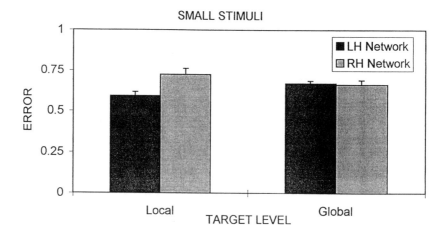

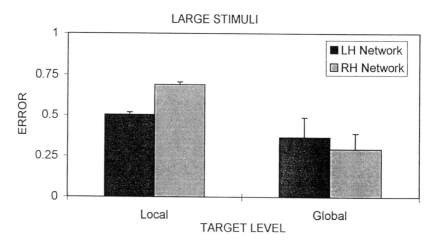

Figure 7.10 Mean error by each network in classifying the hierarchical stimuli at the end of the twentieth training block. (Top panel) There is a hemisphere-by-level interaction; the left hemisphere network produces an advantage when the target is at the local level for the small stimuli. (Bottom panel) The interaction is even more pronounced with the large stimuli.

is a more difficult task than is the identification of simple gratings. We proceeded to train each network for an additional 80 blocks, with performance reaching an asymptotic level after about 60 blocks. The hemisphere-by-level interaction was not consistently obtained in the additional blocks. At probes between the thirtieth and sixtieth blocks, performance was generally better in the left hemisphere network for both local and global targets, although the advantage was more pronounced for the local targets. In the final probes, performance was either equal in the two hemispheric networks or there was a right hemisphere advantage for both types of targets. Although we are unaware of any studies with hierarchical patterns that report changes in laterality effects over practice, researchers using other visual tasks have reported an attenuation of laterality effects with practice (e.g., Kosslyn et al., 1989).

Local and global relations are by definition relative. As discussed in chapter 3, hemispheric asymmetries in classification of hierarchical patterns are maintained across a range of absolute stimulus sizes. We ran a second simulation with our one-dimensional local global patterns in which we increased the size of the stimuli by a factor of five. In the large stimuli the local elements were defined by the pattern across five contiguous units, grouped into five clusters of five units each. Across the five clusters the elements formed the same sequences as with the small stimuli. The global shapes were again created by using those sequences, but with the repetition occurring over clusters of 25 units. The position of the attentional weighting function was centered over the second-lowest frequency module, reflecting the increased activity in the lower frequency modules.

The hemisphere-by-level interaction was even more pronounced with the larger stimuli (figure 7.10). The interaction persisted across all 100 blocks, although the left hemisphere network eventually became better at identifying both local and global targets. Interestingly, with the larger stimuli a general advantage was observed for the global figures, a result that may correspond to global precedence (Navon, 1977).

The results of these four simulations show that our computer model of the DFF theory produces a range of laterality effects similar to those that have been reported in the visual perception literature. The results with hierarchical stimuli show that the effects are not dependent on stimuli that are explicitly manipulated along the frequency dimension. The model transforms the stimulus into a frequency-based representation and, through its learning mechanism, exploits the task-relevant frequency information. Hemispheric advantages emerge because the right hemisphere and left hemisphere networks provide an asymmetric representation of the information.

Modeling a Frequency-Based Interpretation of the Distinction Between Categorical and Coordinate Tasks

In the final simulation we turn to the claim that the two hemispheres are biased to extract qualitatively different types of spatial representations. As reviewed previously, Kosslyn et al. (1989; see, also, Hellige & Michimata, 1989) postulate that the left hemisphere is more adept at representing categorical relations and that the right hemisphere is more adept at representing coordinate relations. In contrast, we hypothesize that predictions derived from a categorical/coordinate interpretation are identical to those yielded by the DFF theory when consideration is given to the spectrally based discriminations required by such tasks. Thus, our theory provides a more parsimonious account. One might argue that narrow versus wide judgments involve a coordinate discrimination and that sharp versus fuzzy distinctions are categorical. However, it is difficult to see how the categorical/coordinate distinction could apply to asymmetries in local/global processing.

The fifth simulation was quite similar to the study reported in Kosslyn et al. (1992). We used stimuli consisting of a bar and a dot (figure 7.11). In separate runs the network had to determine whether the dot was above or below the bar (categorical task) or whether the dot was near to or far from the bar (coordinate task). Kosslyn et al. (1992) showed that learning was better on the coordinate task in a network with large receptive fields, whereas learning was better on the categorical task in a network with smaller receptive fields. Replicating that result with our model is important for two reasons. First, our input units operate as band-pass filters, using on-center/off-surround receptive fields. Kosslyn et al. used on-only receptive field properties, and their results therefore do not reflect spatial frequency analyzers. Second, we wanted to examine that task with the same architecture used in the previous simulations. In particular, in our network there are six simultaneously active spatial frequency modules. The studies of Kosslyn et al. (1992) focused on a comparison between single-channel networks.

In Simulation 5 we followed the stimulus parameters reported in Hellige and Michimata (1989) in constructing our stimuli. Again, we made some modifications in translating their two-dimensional displays into a one-dimensional stimulus array. There were a total of 12 stimuli (figure 7.11). For each stimulus four units were active in the stimulus array, three for the dot and one for the bar. Since we could not capture the horizontal extent of the bar, we set the activation for that unit at twice that for the three units representing the dot. The only difference between the 12 stimuli was the distance between the dot and the bar. The distances were 7, 15, 23, 39, 47, and 55 units above or below the bar in the stimulus array. Thus, those distances formed four clusters of three stimuli each: two clusters near the bar (≤ 23 units) and two clusters far from the bar (≥ 39 units), with the two near and far clusters differing on whether they were above or below the bar.

Twenty versions of each of the 12 stimuli were made, with the exact position within the 192-unit stimulus array varying across the versions. Processing within the frequency modules was the same as in all of the other simulations, and attention was always centered at the second-lowest frequency module. The four decision units in this simulation corresponded to the four possible stimulus categories. Activation across the decision units was compared to target patterns of 1000 (above), 0100 (below), 0010 (near), and 0001 (far). The two tasks were simulated separately, and so perfect performance would require only two of the decision units to be active within a run. Separate left and right hemisphere networks were trained on each of the two tasks.

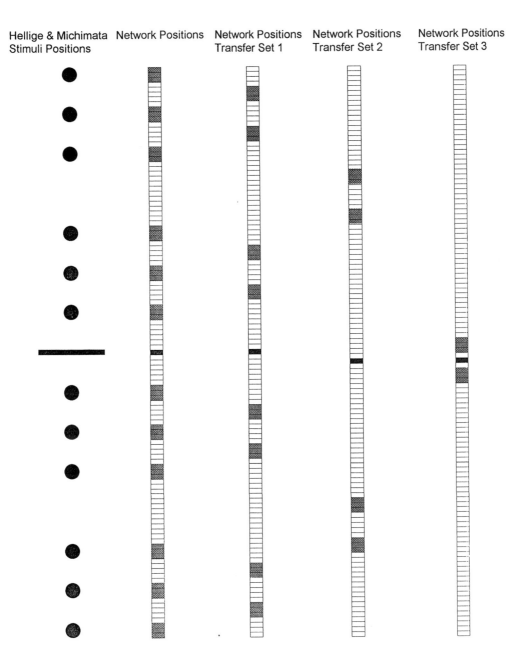

Figure 7.11 The stimuli used in Simulation 5 of the bar-dot task. The left column shows the 12 possible positions of the dot in the experiment of Hellige and Michimata (1989). Our primary simulation of the task used the positions in the second column from the left. The dot was represented by activation across three units and the bar was represented by activation across a single unit. The intensity of the bar unit was set to twice the level of the dot units. The last three columns show the position of the stimuli used in the transfer studies.

A Computer Implementation of the DFF Theory

In accord with the results of Kosslyn et al. (1992), the mean error rate on the above versus below task was lower in the left hemisphere network than in the right hemisphere network (figure 7.12). The reverse was true for the near versus far task. The interaction was observed at every performance probe up to 50 blocks. Thus, we can now add those two tasks to the list of laterality effects that are produced by our implementation of the DFF theory. Although we can describe the tasks in terms of categorical or coordinate spatial relations, the simulation demonstrates that it is not necessary to assume that qualitatively different forms of spatial representation underlie the laterality effects reported in the behavioral studies. The DFF theory provides a unified framework for a range of laterality results, including those that would not be predicted on the basis of the categorical/coordinate distinction.

It is important to consider similarities and differences between the fifth simulation and the other four simulations. First, as in Simulation 4, responses on the above versus below and near versus far tasks do not explicitly require the analysis of spatial frequency information. Second, as in Simulation 3, the same set of stimuli are used in two tasks that differ in how the stimuli are mapped onto response categories. Thus, the hemispheric interaction cannot arise because the left hemisphere and right hemisphere networks confer advantages in processing particular stimuli; rather, the interaction must be due to the fact that different components of information are essential for the two tasks.

In the first four simulations the tasks can be best described as identification tests; in each case there are only two levels along the task-relevant dimension. In the bar-dot task, however, the task is one of discrimination (or categorization). There are six levels within each

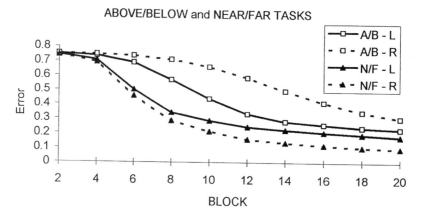

Figure 7.12 Learning functions for each network on the two tasks with the stimulus set that corresponded to the sets used by Hellige and Michimata (1989). For all probes the left hemisphere network was more accurate on the categorical above versus below task, and the right hemisphere network was more accurate on the coordinate near versus far task.

category, and the network (or person) must learn the similarities among the stimuli assigned to a common response. This again suggests that the networks do not learn to respond to idiosyncratic features of the stimulus set, but rather to more general spatial properties.

To further explore that hypothesis we used a transfer paradigm to see how the networks generalized. In the transfer tests right hemisphere and left hemisphere networks were trained either on the above versus below or near versus far task for 50 blocks. At that point error rates were fairly low. Transfer was tested by examining how well the networks classified novel stimuli. During the transfer tests no error feedback was given; thus, the performance of the networks was based solely on what had been learned during training with the original stimulus set.

Three sets of transfer stimuli were used. There were eight stimuli in the first set (figure 7.11), spaced at distances within the clusters (bar-dot distances of 11, 19, 43, and 51). Again, there were 20 versions of each stimulus. Despite the fact that the network had never before been exposed to the transfer stimuli, the mean error rate per stimulus was even less than had been obtained during the final training block of the original simulation (figure 7.13). Moreover, the hemisphere-by-task interaction was unaffected. The transfer of the laterality effect was expected, since the novel stimuli did not significantly alter the correspondence between spatial frequency information and the response categories.

The second and third transfer tests manipulated that correspondence. Four stimuli were used in the second test (figure 7.11). The dot was located at intermediate positions between the near and far clusters

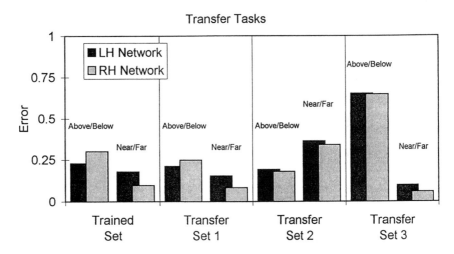

Figure 7.13 Mean error on the bar-dot tasks. The left panel shows the hemisphere-by-task interaction with the training set after 20 training blocks. For the three transfer sets, the weights were fixed after 20 blocks and the networks were probed with the transfer stimuli. In each case, the results were in accord with predictions derived by considering the frequency information contained in the transfer sets.

(bar-dot distances of 27 and 35). Consideration of figure 7.11 suggests that transfer should be differentially affected for the two tasks. With the transfer stimuli the above versus below task should become easier since the minimum distance between the bar and dot was increased. In contrast, the near versus far task should become more difficult with the transfer set since the gap between the near and far stimuli was reduced from 16 to 8 units.

Those predictions were confirmed. Mean error was lower with the novel stimuli on the above versus below task than it had been at the end of training with the original set. For the near versus far task the error rate was much higher during transfer. Furthermore, the laterality effect also changed in this transfer test. On the above versus below task the right hemisphere network produced less error than did the left hemisphere network. This suggests that with the transfer stimuli the most useful information for making the above versus below judgments was carried in lower frequency modules, which were the ones amplified by the right hemisphere attentional weighting function. Those modules were better able to discriminate between the positions closest to the bar as the minimum distance was increased. Although a similar reversal was not obtained for the near versus far task, the right hemisphere advantage was greatly attenuated. The relative contribution of higher frequency information likely increased as the distance between the two response categories was reduced.

The final transfer set consisted of only two stimuli, positioned either 1 pixel above or below the bar (figure 7.11). Both the left and right hemisphere networks were severely taxed by those stimuli on the above versus below task. With such close spacings and with the attentional weighting function positioned over the lower channels, the modules were unable to make the subtle above versus below discrimination. However, with those distances the networks were easily able to generalize for the near versus far response.

The transfer tests provided a convincing demonstration that the performance of the networks in our simulations was determined by the spatial frequency information provided by the stimuli. In all of the tests the weights of the network were fixed after the initial training period with the standard set of patterns. Thus, the networks could not learn to classify the transfer stimuli. Rather, the transfer stimuli provided a test of how well performance would generalize when the networks were given novel stimuli. Not only could the networks classify the new stimuli (with the exception of the third set on the above versus below task), but in some cases performance was actually superior to that obtained with the training set. If the networks had learned an arbitrary classification scheme, good transfer would not be expected because there was no overlap in the representation of the dot in the input array between the training and transfer sets (see Cook, Fruh, & Landis, 1995).

In all cases, the results were in accord with expectations based on an analysis of the frequency content of the transfer stimuli. When cruder spatial discriminations were sufficient to classify the stimuli, performance improved for the right hemisphere network. When the classifications required finer spatial distinctions, right hemisphere advantages were attenuated. The performance of the networks was a function of not just the task, but also of the stimuli.

The simulations challenge the idea that categorical and coordinate representations provide two qualitatively different ways to capture spatial relations (Kosslyn, 1987). The results indicate that that distinction may be an epiphenomenon, dependent on differences in the spatial frequency properties of the stimuli.

The critical test of our claim, of course, requires experiments with human subjects. We would predict that the pattern of laterality effects on the bar-dot task would also depend on the exact set of stimuli. For example, akin to the transfer simulations, we would expect that the categorical coordinate asymmetry could be reversed. If the stimuli were repositioned so that distinctions at higher frequencies were required for the near versus far coordinate task, for example, then a right hemisphere advantage should disappear. To date, our empirical efforts provide only minimal support. In one preliminary study we presented a circle and dot on each trial, similar to what had been done by Kosslyn et al. (1989, Experiment 1). In the categorical task the subjects judged whether the dot was on or off the circle. In the coordinate task the subjects judged whether the dot was near to or far from the circle. Two stimulus sets were compared. In one, the dot was either 0, 1, or 10 cm from the circle. In the other, the dot was either 0, 8, or 10 cm from the circle. By Kosslyn's theory we predicted that for both sets categorical judgments would be better when the stimuli were shown in the right visual field and that coordinate judgments would show a left visual field advantage. However, by the DFF theory we predicted a reversal of the laterality effects for the two stimulus sets. For the 0, 1, 10 cm set, the spatial discrimination is finest for the categorical task because the 0 and 1 cm stimuli are assigned to different categories. For the 0, 8, 10 set, the finest discrimination is on the coordinate task because the 8 and 10 cm stimuli are assigned to different categories.

The results were in accord with the predictions of the DFF theory. A 16 ms right visual field advantage on the categorical task with the 0, 1, 10 cm set reversed to a 23 ms left visual field advantage with the 0, 8, 10 cm set. Similarly, a 5 ms left visual field advantage on the coordinate task with the 0, 1, 10 cm set reversed to a 15 ms right visual field advantage with the 0, 8, 10 cm set. However, this interaction was only present when the analysis was restricted to the first block of trials. No laterality effects were obtained in subsequent blocks (see, also, Kosslyn et al., 1989, Experiment 3; Rybash & Hoyer, 1992).

Moreover, we have failed in a series of studies to obtain a similar reversal with the bar-dot task. Our problem in those studies was that we were unable to replicate the basic asymmetry using parameters similar to those of Kosslyn et al. (1989) and Hellige and Michimata (1989), even when the analysis was restricted to the initial test blocks. The reasons for our failures remain unclear but underscore the frustration of laterality research with healthy people. Asymmetries in visual perception are subtle and likely reflect the general similarity in how the two hemispheres process information.

SUMMARY

This chapter reviewed the computer simulations we used to demonstrate that the DFF theory can provide a unified account of how the asymmetric representation of frequency information may underlie laterality effects in a diverse set of tasks. An architecture was implemented that incorporates the basic ideas of the theory. First, for all of the tasks the stimuli were processed in parallel by a set of modules, each of which was tuned to represent information at different spatial scales. Second, an asymmetric weighting function differentially amplified the output from the modules for the two networks, with the right hemisphere network biased to represent lower frequency information compared to the left hemisphere network. Third, the weighting function was constrained by the attentional requirements of the different tasks.

To this point our modeling work has been primarily geared toward providing a sufficiency demonstration of the DFF theory as a general account of hemispheric asymmetries in visual perception. Our modeling work clearly contains limitations. Future studies are required to test the robustness of the model. Our choice of parameters, both for the tuning of the frequency modules and the attention weighting function, was relatively arbitrary. To keep the size of the networks reasonable we limited the model to six modules per network, using a range of receptive field sizes that would allow the networks to solve each of the tasks. It is important to test the model with parameters that resemble the spatial frequency channels that have been described for human vision (Graham, 1989). We also used a fairly crude method to implement attention; namely, we used an assessment of the spatial extent of the stimuli, an algorithm reminiscent of behavioral evidence suggesting that early visual processes either perform grouping operations (Driver, Baylis, & Rafal, 1992) or assess the overall mass of a stimulus (Grabowecky et al., 1993). In future work we will test alternative methods for allocating attention. For example, the sequential effects reported by Robertson (1996) may require that the position of the attention function be influenced by how the networks respond on previous trials.

We can envision two other extensions of the modeling work. First, the model could easily be modified to examine laterality effects in audition. Of course, the input would have to be altered to represent sound frequencies so that the modules would have distinctive tuning functions in that dimensional space. But the asymmetric representation of sound frequency information, coupled with a flexible attention function, would likely produce many of the laterality effects that were reported in chapters 5 and 6.

Second, the architecture could be converted into a more process-oriented model. In our implementation we tested the right and left hemisphere networks in separate simulations, focusing on a comparison of learning rates. In a process-oriented model both networks could have access to a common input, and comparisons would focus on the time course of activation in the decision units. A process-oriented model would more closely mimic normal perception, in which both hemispheres are simultaneously active. Whether that simultaneous activity reflects the operation of relatively independent processors or two interactive subsystems remains a subject of debate, a topic we turn to in chapter 9. But performance is unified. The linking of our networks is a prerequisite for making explicit whether the DFF theory can account for how action is guided by the asymmetric representation of frequency information.

8 The DFF Theory at Work

This book has so far focused on developing an account of perceptual and attentional factors that contribute to important aspects of hemispheric specialization. We have emphasized the study of neurological patients with focal brain lesions in order to support the basic tenets of the theory and to link cognitive dysfunction with specific brain regions. The DFF theory proposes a model of how different computations associated with different brain areas contribute to humans' ability to perceive and apprehend a complex world. Our work has thus far been very much in the mainstream of cognitive neuroscience, but the theory also provides a framework for exploration of other more clinically relevant questions.

The current emphasis in cognitive neuroscience is on an interdisciplinary approach to understanding the relationship between mind and brain. The focus is on questions that can be addressed by basic research: What are the component operations of a complex process like spatial attention? How are those operations realized in the normal brain? What computational processes are required for normal interactions between those component operations? The goal of cognitive neuroscience is to understand how the normal brain subserves normal cognition. However, any theory of normal cognition is strengthened if it can account for cognitive dysfunction as well.

Cognitive neuroscience has spawned new efforts to account for the neural pathology that underlies a wide range of disorders, even those that are not easily linked to particular brain structures. In such clinically oriented studies, the methodologies of cognitive psychology have provided a fine-grained analysis of the cognitive sequelae of diseases that may include a multifarious set of symptoms. Those studies have also provided new techniques for testing hypotheses about how different brain regions may be affected by degenerative diseases and by other diseases that have diffuse effects on neural structures.

In this chapter we provide a few examples of how the basic ideas of the DFF theory may be applied. Those examples are accompanied by a discussion of how the procedures developed to test the theory may be used to facilitate understanding of some behavioral problems seen in patients with diffuse disorders. The review focuses on the syndromes of chronic alcoholism, schizophrenia, and dementia and is meant to be exemplary and not exhaustive.

People with these disorders typically demonstrate a host of cognitive abnormalities. Indeed, their behavior tends to be more indicative of a breakdown in general brain function than of lesions restricted to specific brain regions. They may have difficulty comprehending language, or they may produce slurred or inarticulate speech. They may be unable to solve the kinds of problems that characterize fluent human cognition. Motor performance may become uncoordinated.

Although it is unlikely that simple hypotheses can sufficiently account for the full complexity of those disorders, it is still important to identify those functions that are disproportionately affected by these disorders. In keeping with the theme of this book, we focus on deficits in perception and attention, with a particular eye on how those disorders may disrupt normal functioning in the two cerebral hemispheres.

Our discussion of applied research is selective. For the most part we describe studies analyzing patients' performance on tasks using the hierarchical patterns that were extensively discussed in chapter 3 and 4. Our focus is twofold: how might the different components of the DFF theory help explain the patterns of deficits that have been observed in different patient populations, and might it prove useful in developing new hypotheses about cognitive deficits associated with a disease? The research reviewed here is in its infancy, but the hierarchical patterns nonetheless provide a model task for studying hemispheric asymmetry in visual perception. There is even a standard test that has been developed and used within clinical neuropsychology for that purpose (Delis, 1989). Future work will need to examine how well the results of such tests generalize to audition as well as to more natural tasks of visual perception and other perceptual domains.

ALCOHOLICS AND ALCOHOL INTOXICATION

It has long been known that alcohol abuse affects performance on visual tasks more than on verbal tasks (Ellenberg, Rosenbaum, Goldman, & Whitman 1980; Fabian & Parsons, 1983; Jones, 1971; Miglioli, Buchtel, Campanini, & DeRisio, 1979; Parsons & Leber, 1981). Alcohol has also been closely linked to deficits in selective attention (Chandler & Parsons, 1975; Miller & Orr, 1980; Smith & Oscar-Berman, 1991). Some of those deficits have often been observed under conditions of acute alcohol intoxication, but they have also been found when all traces of alcohol were absent from the blood. Sober alcoholics have demonstrated lingering attentional and perceptual problems even after a sobriety period of three weeks or more.

Sober alcoholics often draw the Rey-Osterrieth pattern (see figure 1.6) by starting with the local parts to construct the whole. Such performance

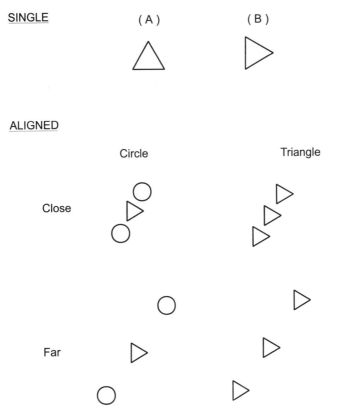

Figure 8.1 Example of a single equilateral triangle (top). Triangle A can be seen to point in the direction of 12, 4, or 8 o'clock; triangle B can be seen to point in the direction of 3, 7, or 11 o'clock. The examples of aligned elements (bottom) show stimulus conditions in which the global alignment is created by flanking circles or triangles that are either similar or dissimilar and either close to or far from the target triangle. (Adapted from Palmer, 1980.)

is similar to that of patients with right hemisphere damage. As would be expected, the drawing abnormalities in alcoholics tend to be less dramatic than in patients who have recently suffered a right hemisphere stroke. However, their local bias is hard to ignore. That bias, coupled with the fact that alcoholics perform more poorly on visual tests than on verbal tests, has led to the proposal that right hemisphere function may be disproportionately affected by long-term alcohol abuse.

More systematic experimental studies using hierarchically arranged patterns have further explored the possibility of a right hemisphere deficit that is disproportional to left hemisphere deficit in sober chronic alcoholics. When judging the orientation of a central triangle (figure 8.1), a group of alcoholics was less likely to be influenced by the global alignment created by surrounding circles or triangles (Robertson, Stillman, & Delis, 1985). The data are presented in figure 8.2. Similarly, in reaction-time studies with hierarchical letter stimuli, alcoholics showed

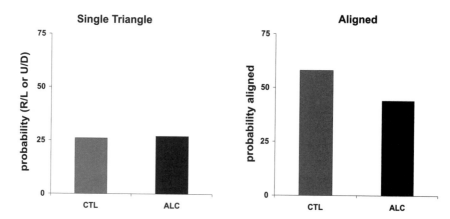

Figure 8.2 Performance of control subjects (CTL) and sober alcoholics (ALC) on single and aligned triangle trials (compare to patient data in figure 3.12). (Adapted from Robertson, Stillman, & Delis, 1985.)

an increased bias to respond to the local level compared to appropriately matched control subjects. The magnitude of alcoholics' local bias has been shown to correlate with performance on more typical neuropsychological tests like the Block Design test (Kramer et al., 1989).

In the Block Design test patients are given between four and nine cubes with white and red on each cube. Subjects are shown a standard pattern (e.g., a red V shape on a white background) that can be replicated when the red and white portions of the cubes are arranged in a particular way. It is the patients' task to arrange the cubes appropriately (see figure 3.8). Patients with right hemisphere damage tend to arrange the individual blocks into something that might resemble a line or angle of the V. The cubes are not neatly arranged next to each other as they should be, but instead appear inappropriately placed. In contrast, patients with left hemisphere damage tend to cluster the cubes correctly but are more likely to make a local error such as rotating one cube.

The hypothesis that this is related to the global and local asymmetry discussed throughout this book is supported by a study of alcoholics showing that their errors on the Block Design test were more like those of patients with right hemisphere damage than like those with left hemisphere damage. In other words, the alcoholic subjects' errors—like the right hemisphere patients'—were mostly of a configural nature. More importantly, the number of configural errors on the Block Design test positively correlated with the magnitude of a local bias for hierarchically arranged stimuli; that effect is also similar to the effects obtained in studies of patients with right hemisphere damage (Kramer et al., 1989).

Interestingly, those effects may be a direct consequence of the subjects' exposure to alcohol and may not be related to a secondary mechanism resulting from their chronic condition. Young, intoxicated nonalcoholic subjects showed a pattern similar to the sober alcoholics' when responding to hierarchical stimuli (Lamb & Robertson, 1987). They were slower than control subjects to identify global shapes in studies measuring reaction time using hierarchical letter patterns as stimuli. In those studies, young volunteers were given a liquid drink that included a measure of alcohol calculated by each subject's weight to approximate a desired blood alcohol level. One group received a placebo that contained no alcohol. The drink mix masked whether or not alcohol was included in the drink. Subjects were then tested after their breath alcohol levels reached a predetermined level. Another two groups were given enough alcohol before participation to become either moderately or heavily intoxicated. The blood alcohol level of the moderately intoxicated group was below 0.05%, and the level of the heavily intoxicated group was closer to 0.1%. Alcohol disproportionately increased response time to global targets compared to the response times for the placebo group, and the magnitude of the increase was greater for the group with blood alcohol levels closer to 0.1%. As blood alcohol level increased, its effect on global identification increased as well. Being drunk had surprisingly little effect on local target identification time.

At present, it is not clear how those effects can be best accounted for within the framework of the DFF theory. However, the theory may be used as a guide for exploring different hypotheses. One hypothesis is that right hemisphere damage disrupts the asymmetrically skewed filters that amplify lower spatial frequency information. Alternatively, alcohol may disrupt the ability to switch attention from the local target level to the global target level. Alcoholics may fail to redirect attention to lower frequency information, even when that information can facilitate performance. The DFF theory does not predict which of those two hypotheses is most likely, but the evidence from patients and imaging studies suggests that the left hemisphere is more involved than the right hemisphere in switching attention between objects at different levels (Robertson et al., 1988; Schneider, 1993). A third hypothesis is that alcohol disrupts a spatial attentional mechanism that determines the size of the "spotlight" over which attention is spread.

Some evidence favors the attentional spotlight hypothesis. A study by Post et al. (1996) demonstrated that healthy intoxicated subjects were actually better at detecting a foveally presented target than were control subjects who were given a placebo. However, when the task required responses to more peripheral targets, the placebo group outperformed the intoxicated group. It was as if attentional resources had been focused on foveal information at the expense of peripheral information. Although such findings could account for previous findings with alcoholics, it would not predict the correlation between performance on Block Design and global identification; two tasks that have been associated with right hemisphere dysfunction (Kramer et al., 1989). Of course, it is always possible that both the spotlight of attention and the ability to recognize a global form are both affected by alcohol.

It is obvious that a great deal of further study is required to come to any firm conclusions. It also will be necessary to determine whether intoxicated nonalcoholics have difficulty detecting peripheral targets for the same reason that sober alcoholics have difficulty seeing global information. It is possible that acute consumption of alcohol has a disproportionate effect on peripheral vision in comparison to foveal vision, although such a disproportionate effect does not explain the performance advantage in foveal vision for intoxicated subjects over placebo control subjects in Post's experiment.

Given the complex behavioral syndrome associated with alcoholism, chronic exposure is likely to damage several neural mechanisms related to perception and attention. However, the evidence indicates that alcohol may have more pronounced effects on mechanisms that are linked to posterior regions of the right hemisphere than it has on those of the left.

SCHIZOPHRENIA

Schizophrenia is a complicated and severely disabling psychiatric condition. Patients with schizophrenia seem detached from the world, lost in the cacophony of their idiosyncratic obsessions and internal confusion. Their language and actions suggest a loss of connection to the reality of the surrounding environment.

While the disorder clearly reflects a widespread breakdown of cognitive function, it nonetheless seems critical to establish how people with schizophrenia represent the external world and which neural systems are affected by the disease or by its variations. Are their percepts normal, and do their problems reflect an inability to attach appropriate meaning to the representations? Or are they working with internal representations that have distorted perceptual reality?

Many theorists have proposed that a fundamental problem in many forms of schizophrenia involves a selective attention deficit. An innocuous event may turn into a threatening monster; an insignificant stimulus may become the focus of their world. Studies of spatial attention using hierarchical patterns or spatial-cuing methods have revealed some of the ways in which these patients represent visual-spatial information and how their abnormal representations may influence attentional processes.

The most important finding for the current discussion is that schizophrenia appears to affect the left hemisphere to a greater extent than the right hemisphere. Both imaging and behavioral data have supported that hypothesis (Early, Posner, Reiman & Raichle, 1989; Nordahl, Robertson, Carter, Chaderjian, & O'Shora-Celaya, 1994). Although many imaging studies have emphasized abnormalities of the frontal lobe (Berman, Illowsky, & Weinberger, 1988; Weinberger, Berman, & Zec, 1986), recent findings have implicated more ventral regions in the area of the left superior temporal plane and temporal lobes.

Behavioral data are consistent with the hypothesis that many symptoms of schizophrenia are primarily associated with left hemisphere dysfunction. For example, patients with schizophrenia are typically slower to detect visual targets presented in the right visual field when the targets are preceded by a cue in the left visual field than vice versa (Posner et al., 1988; see, also, Carter, Robertson, Chaderjian, Celaya, & Nordahl, 1992). That problem in disengaging attention from an invalidly cued location is similar to that observed in patients with posterior damage (Posner et al., 1984). For neurological patients the problem is more pronounced to the contralateral side of the lesion. Left parietal damage makes it difficult to shift attention from a cue in the left visual field to a target in the right visual field, and right parietal damage makes it difficult to shift attention 'from a cue in the right visual field to a target in the left. By inference, the deficits in shifting attention in patients with schizophrenia are more consistent with disruption of visual attention processes of the left hemisphere.

Other behavioral evidence using hierarchical patterns also supports the hypothesis that schizophrenia affects left hemisphere function more than right hemisphere function. Schizophrenia patients had more difficulty than healthy subjects in identifying the relatively local targets in hierarchical patterns (Carter, Robertson, & Nordahl, 1996). However, the patients did not show an inability to selectively attend to the global or local pattern as the probability of a pattern appearing at one level or the other changed (Robertson, Lamb & Knight, 1988). Together, those results indicate a deficit in the left hemisphere filtering operation that favors local identification. Effects that have been associated with the left parietal lobe were not present in this group of schizophrenia patients, whereas those associated with the left temporal lobe were.

Research with schizophrenia patients participating in clinical drug trials provide further opportunity to explore hemispheric dysfunction associated with this disease. Clinical trials are part of the last stage of drug development: Food and Drug Administration regulations require that efficacy in humans be demonstrated before final approval. Volunteers in clinical trials are required to undergo a "wash-out period" to control for lingering effects of their old medications or for unexpected interactions between old and new medication. This transition period presents a special opportunity to test schizophrenia patients in an unmedicated state (see Salo, Robertson, & Nordahl, 1996). Such research is important, given that the drugs used to treat schizophrenia produce direct effects on cognitive processes. For example, if a patient experiencing auditory hallucinations finds relief through antipsychotics, the drug has effectively altered the neural mechanisms that sustain such hallucinations.

Carter et al. (1996) tested a group of unmedicated schizophrenia patients using hierarchical patterns. As might be expected, patients with schizophrenia who can tolerate three weeks of washout from their usual medication are not the most severely impaired. In the Carter et al. study (1996) patients were high-functioning individuals compared to many schizophrenic patients. They were shown hierarchical patterns and asked to indicate which of two targets was present. A target could appear at either the global or local level in every trial, and the probability that the target would be at one level or the other was varied across blocks. In one block of trials global targets were more probable and in another block of trials local targets were more probable. The subjects were verbally informed by the experimenter of the probability schedules.

Two critical results were obtained in that experiment. First, the patients' performance was worse than that of matched control subjects when the targets appeared at the local level. Second, the patients were influenced by the probability schedules to the same extent as were the control subjects. That is, reaction times were faster for targets appearing at the more probable level and slower for targets appearing at the less probable level. The magnitude of the trade-off did not differ significantly between the patient and control groups. Thus, the patients were able to selectively attend to one level or another appropriately, but had an overall problem in identifying local targets.

In other words, patients with schizophrenia produced a pattern of performance that was very similar to that seen in patients with focal lesions of the left temporal-parietal cortex. Because their trade-offs were normal over probability schedules, the patients' left parietal lobe may be functioning normally in spatial frequency selection. According to the DFF theory, the problem is at the second filtering stage with the process that amplifies relatively higher frequency information. The selective attention mechanism may be appropriately shifted to amplify the region of frequency space that contains the relevant frequency information for target identification. However, the relatively higher frequency information necessary for identifying the local targets is not appropriately amplified by the left temporal-parietal filter in schizophrenia patients.

The placement of this problem in the second filtering stage, based on the DFF theory, may at first seem at odds with the cuing data, which requires simple detection. However, the cuing data may reflect a very early problem in space-based selection. Selection within hierarchical patterns does not require the same type of spatial information. Instead, selection occurs through a series of spatial filters that we have argued are linked to spatial frequency information. The time course of the two processes may be quite different. Despite these differences, both methods have implicated a greater role of the left posterior areas than the right in schizophrenia.

More direct evidence that schizophrenia involves abnormal function of the left hemisphere temporal-parietal region comes from a recent PET study. A subset of the patients in the Carter et al. experiment were injected with a radioactively labeled tracer, 2-fluoro-2D-deoxyglucose (FDG). Because it has a relatively long half-life of approximately 40 minutes, FDG is difficult to use in studies of on-line processing where events take place on the order of milliseconds. However, it is very powerful when comparing basal metabolic activity, across groups of subjects. Unlike oxygen tracers that dissipate in a few minutes and measure areas of increased bloodflow, FDG directly measures the metabolic activity in neurons.

Overall, the schizophrenia patients as a group showed notable hypometabolism in the posterior middle temporal region of the left hemisphere (Nordahl et al., 1994). The center of the abnormality was inferior and somewhat anterior to the region of maximal overlap in the Robertson et al. (1988) group of patients with focal lesions. Nonetheless, it is striking that the two methodologies implicate neighboring regions in ventral areas. A correlation analysis between the behavioral and anatomical data revealed a significant effect in the schizophrenia group. Due to technical limitations, whole-brain images were not obtained. Excluded regions included early visual areas of extrastriate cortex and most of the frontal and parietal lobes. However, the cingulate was included, and decreased activity in that area was also evident.

DEMENTIA

Alzheimer's disease is a degenerative neurological condition that becomes more debilitating as the disease progresses. The onset of symptoms is insidious, perhaps beginning with a continual failure to find words to describe things or with a tendency to forget to turn off the stove after using it. As the disease progresses friends and relatives may become difficult to recognize, which is one of the many memory failures that become commonplace over time. These memory problems are typical in Alzheimer's disease, but it has become increasingly evident that selective attention is also affected.

Nearly all tasks—including those involving language and perception—become more difficult as the disease takes its ugly toll. With so many systems involved, it can be difficult to determine when there is a direct breakdown in language or perception or when such problems can be attributed to more generalized memory problems. When the concern is to establish a plan for daily care, mild problems in visual-spatial or attentional functions tend to be ignored. There are far more pressing concerns from the perspective of both the clinician and the major caregivers.

The neuropathology associated with Alzheimer's disease is diffuse, and patients form a heterogeneous population. Studies of their ability to perceive spatial structure reflect this heterogeneity. For example, some patients may show a local bias, whereas others may show a global bias.

Of course, we might expect such a distribution in a normal population of subjects as well; in any given set of trials, some subjects will be faster in responding to one level compared to the other. However, in Alzheimer's disease, such differences may reflect individual pathology.

PET studies reveal that some patients show relatively more right hemisphere hypometabolism, whereas others show more left hemisphere hypometabolism. This is the type of pattern that would be expected if there were no preferential side to the disease. The pattern is important, however, for purposes of understanding what a patient's difficulties might be. The fact that some individuals show signs of more right hemisphere involvement and others show signs of more left hemisphere involvement means that planned care for the different types of patients and predictions about the course of the disease may be quite different.

The qualitative difference in observed deficits that can result from damage to the right or left hemisphere after stroke can also be seen in Alzheimer's patients with either more right or more left hemisphere involvement. The importance of the distinction has received support from correlational studies that suggest that Alzheimer patients do in fact cluster into different profiles that seem to reflect the chance occurrence of more right or more left hemisphere involvement (Delis et al., 1992). Patients who score poorly on verbal subtests of standard neuropsychological batteries are more likely to show a global bias. These results would suggest relatively greater involvement of the left hemisphere in the disease process. In contrast, poor performance on visual subtests is correlated with a local bias. This outcome would indicate that the right hemisphere is more affected than the left hemisphere.

One curious result has emerged in the performance of Alzheimer's patients when tested with hierarchical stimuli. Filoteo, Delis, Masserman et al. (1992) used the standard divided-attention task in which the target could appear at either the local or global level. Recall that normal subjects showed a sequential priming effect with this task. (Robertson Egly et al. 1993; Robertson, 1996). Responses were faster when the target appeared at the same level in successive trials compared to trials in which the target level changed. That effect was independent of whether or not the identity of the target (i.e., the shape) changed or remained the same. Thus, the effect can be attributed to repetition priming related to the attended level on the previous trial.

Filoteo, Delis, Masserman et al. analyzed sequential priming effects in Alzheimer's patients. As with normal subjects, response times were faster when the target was at the same level in successive trials than when the target level changed. However, the priming effect was even greater in the patient group. It was as if patients found it more difficult to switch attention from one level to the other than did other control groups. The greater priming effect may be partly due to the normal aging process. Healthy elderly subjects also show more substantial sequential priming than do younger subjects. Nonetheless, the enhancement is even more pronounced with Alzheimer's patients.

Consider the mechanisms that are purported to underlie sequential priming effects. We have argued that these effects reflect a form of attentional memory, or what Robertson (1996) has called an attentional print. We assume that attention shifts towards the level that contains a target. After the target is identified, people appear to attend to that level better in the next trial. Either attention remains at the level that had been informative on the preceding trial, or else attention is attracted to the same level through common features and mechanisms that are reactivated when a new stimulus appears. The evidence reported by Robertson (1996) supports the latter view. Whatever the details of the priming mechanism, attention acts as if it remains at a given level until required to shift to another level.

Based on their observations, Filoteo, Delis, Masserman et al. concluded that patients with Alzheimer's disease have difficulty disengaging attention to shift between the levels of hierarchical stimuli. The evidence that level-specific priming may be related to the spatial frequency value of the previous target (Kim, Ivry, & Robertson, submitted; Robertson, 1996) suggests that Alzheimer's disease reduces the ability of patients to switch attention from one frequency range to another. Note that this result is opposite to what is observed in patients with left parietal lobe damage. For those patients, switching was reduced, indicating that the attentional print was deactivated or faded over the time between trials. The patients in the study of Filoteo et al. were not divided into groups based on neuropsychological evidence of more left or right involvement (see Delis et al., 1992). Thus, the data cannot be easily analyzed in terms of the DFF theory. However, this would be a fruitful area for future investigation into hypotheses generated by the theory.

SUMMARY

As the foregoing sections demonstrate, the research on visual and attentional function using paradigms initially developed in cognitive psychology have been broadly applied. To date, these broad applications have been most productive in articulating component processes associated with different areas of the human brain. However, the knowledge we have gained from this endeavor has begun to have a strong influence on the study of cognitive dysfunction produced either by traumatic brain injury or by other diseases that diffusely affect cerebral functioning. We have discussed a few examples in this chapter, and there are more examples that we have not discussed (e.g., Martin et al., 1995).

Research using common tasks with various populations has uncovered potential answers to some long-asked questions, but such research has also opened new doors for hypothesis testing. The DFF theory is but a beginning attempt to articulate the way in which spatial information at different spatial scales contributes to hemispheric differences and how areas within each hemisphere contribute different computations to spatial attention and object perception. The fact that so many different neurological problems affect some aspect of processing forms in hierarchically arranged stimuli is intriguing, but it also should be expected. Hierarchical spatial organization is seen in the external world almost every waking minute of every day. We perceive the world of objects to be organized in spatial hierarchies. Each object appears to be a part of a larger object or visual scene. This is the structure of the world in which animals evolved. Thus, it should not be surprising to find that rather large areas of the brain contribute to perception of hierarchical structures. For the same reasons, it is also not surprising that perception of hierarchically organized information breaks down with many different diseases that affect the cortex in different ways.

The clinical results described in this chapter demonstrate that the dissociations we have discussed throughout this book can also be observed by comparisons of different profiles between patients with schizophrenia, patients with progressive dementia, and long-term alcoholics. Again, we see that one component process of the DFF theory can be affected without affecting others to the same extent. The evidence implicates more right than left hemisphere dysfunction in alcoholics, more left than right hemisphere dysfunction in patients with schizophrenia, and problems in attentional selection associated with parietal lobes in patients with Alzheimer's disease.

Perhaps more importantly, we also see that scientific results can contribute to understanding problems in a cross section of patient populations with cognitive deficits. The DFF theory provides hypotheses about which cognitive processes may be most affected by diseases that cause such deficits. The theory may also be used as a guide to explore more specific component processes that may underlie perceptual dysfunction in groups as a whole and in individuals.

9 The Two Sides of Perception

The human brain is a most impressive processing machine. We perceive and act in the world with remarkable efficiency. We recognize the familiar sights, sounds, and smells of the city as we walk down a street at rush hour, smoothly navigating a baby stroller and avoiding the turning cars at a crowded intersection. The ease with which we perform and integrate complex cognitive operations remains a mystery. Even our most advanced artificial intelligence systems pale in comparison when we consider the relatively limited domains within which they operate.

And yet, the human brain is a severely limited information processing system. When chatting with some friends at a sidewalk cafe, we fail to notice the street magician trying to entice us with her bag of tricks. We are amazingly facile in recognizing the familiar faces of our friends, even when we meet someone who has been out of town for a few years. But our memories are also quite fallible. Within a few seconds the name of a new acquaintance can slip from memory. Our limitations are even more pronounced in the action domain. As impressive as is the dexterity with which we use our hands or produce fluent speech, such gestures are tightly constrained. When we greet a friend with a handshake and pat on the back, the two relatively unrelated gestures are as tightly coupled as the childhood act of rubbing one's stomach while patting the head.

The word "limitation" is misleading. It is not unreasonable to assume that, if it were to our evolutionary benefit, such constraints would be minimal. Those limitations, however, are an essential part of our cognitive competence. Being limited in the amount of information that can be attended to at any point in time provides a useful mechanism for highlighting the particular information that is most relevant to current goals. Memory retrieval should also be selective, lest we be overwhelmed by trivial associations. And actions can only be purposeful if the motor system is able to coordinate them across a large number of muscle groups, ensuring that the right hand and the left hand are both working toward a common goal.

The integration and control of our cognitive machinery remains one of the preeminent problems of psychology and neuroscience. What underlies the constraints in information processing capabilities? How are the processes associated with perception, memory, and action linked together? How is it that the activity of billions of relatively simple processing elements is efficiently integrated to produce coherent behavior? City planners must devise elaborate control schemes to segregate pedestrian and vehicular traffic, restrict the flow of movement at intersections, and enforce violations of these schemes. Does the brain use analogous control processes? Are there specialized systems that regulate and direct the flow of information processing and others that sort through the incoming information to determine the most appropriate action?

In this concluding chapter we do not attempt to answer these thorny questions. Rather, we raise those issues here because they highlight some of the primary motivations for the DFF theory. At the heart of the theory is the notion that the brain is composed of a series of highly specialized, distributed processors. That idea is central to cognitive neuroscience. Theories of visual perception have focused on the idea that the brain adopts a divide-and-conquer strategy. In visual perception we understand that the complex array of information impinging on the retina is quickly channeled into a set of processing streams, each with its particular specialization for representing elementary features such as color, shape, and motion. In audition the localization of sound entails separable mechanisms for detecting the minute differences in the time and amplitude with which the ears respond to changes in sound pressure level. Of course, we do not perceive amorphous patches of color or floating elements of shape. The outputs from these specialized modules are eventually integrated, allowing us to form percepts of coherent objects occupying specific locations in space. Computational specialization allows us to extract the relevant cues in an efficient manner.

HEMISPHERIC SPECIALIZATION AS AN EMERGENT PROPERTY OF THE ASYMMETRIC REPRESENTATION OF FREQUENCY INFORMATION

In a similar vein, we have argued that a divide-and-conquer approach offers the proper computational framework for understanding hemispheric specialization. This idea is certainly not unique to the DFF theory. Indeed, it has been the hallmark of laterality research throughout the century. Early theories of hemispheric specialization advocated perhaps the most extreme form of the divide-and-conquer strategy, linking specific task domains to either the left or right hemisphere. In such theories the hemispheres tended to be viewed each as the sole province for processing certain types of material. For example, the left hemisphere was thought to be uniquely suited for comprehending language, implying that speech signals within the right hemisphere either dissolved into oblivion or were shuttled across the corpus callosum.

With the advent of more sophisticated methods of analysis it has become clear that the division of labor is not so extreme. Differences between the two hemispheres appear to be more a matter of degree rather than kind. Testimony to that fact has come from a variety of sources. Patients with large lesions in posterior regions of the left hemisphere may initially show a severe Wernicke's aphasia, but in most cases the comprehension problems become attenuated over time. Although such attenuation could reflect reorganization within intact areas of the damaged hemisphere, PET evidence suggests that homologous regions in the right hemisphere become functionally more relevant (Weiller et al., 1995). Research with callosotomy patients is also revealing, in that those patients can generally follow verbal instructions when responding to perceptual inputs restricted to either hemisphere. It is difficult to make inferences about normal processing from such cases, given the startling new insights we have gained about cortical plasticity. However, even with healthy individuals, current models emphasize a difference in the degree to which each hemisphere represents semantic information (e.g., Beeman, Friedman, Grafman, Perez, et al., 1994).

At the heart of the DFF theory is the idea that each hemisphere comes equipped with a similar set of processing mechanisms. This does not mean that processing within each hemisphere yields identical representations. Rather, the asymmetric filtering properties of the hemispheres provide a mechanism for highlighting different information. Such a model does not entail complex control structures devoted to determining whether a particular task requires information to be shuttled to one hemisphere or the other. Rather, the asymmetric contributions of the two hemispheres for particular task domains is an emergent property of their asymmetric representations. When a task requires the analysis of the constituent elements that form a complex pattern the left hemisphere representation will be most efficient, since it amplifies the relatively higher frequency signals that carry information about local elements. Conversely, the right hemisphere representation will prove most efficient for tasks that require the analysis of lower frequency information, such as identification of the global shape of a pattern. Assuming that both hemispheres have access to the same sensory input, either through central presentation or through interhemispheric transfer, processing within each hemisphere progresses in parallel. But parallelism here does not mean equality. Each hemisphere has some degree of competence for performing all types of perceptual analysis, but their representational asymmetries confer an advantage for one hemisphere over the other depending on the spectral content of the critical information for a given task.

The asymmetric processing of frequency information can be seen as another manifestation of a divide-and-conquer strategy. Analogous to the way in which visual inputs are partitioned into channels specialized to represent features such as color and motion, the two hemispheres appear to have evolved such that they produce different perceptual representations of the world. In essence, rather than providing a redundant representation of the world, asymmetric filtering offers a means for extracting nonidentical representations. By recognizing the limited-capacity nature of human information processing, we can see the advantages of nonidentical representations. Processing within the two hemispheres yields two sides of perception. Higher-level processes, reflecting both our experience and current goals, will help determine which of the two sides of perception is most useful for solving the task at hand. The overall computational competence of a limited-capacity system is enhanced by specialized representations, each of which is uniquely suited for highlighting different sources of information.

We have argued that the asymmetric representation of frequency information provides an important cross-modal characterization of hemispheric specialization. The evidence is most compelling for vision. As shown through our implementation of the DFF theory, a number of seemingly unrelated tasks can be related by considering how the tasks all demand the analysis of either low or high spatial frequency information. Thus, at a minimum, the DFF theory represents a parsimonious account for hemispheric specialization in visual perception. Our extension of the model to audition is admittedly more speculative, primarily motivated by consideration of laterality effects in music and speech perception that only indirectly involve the manipulation of lower and higher frequency information. This is obviously an area of research that will require future study, both to assess the validity of our cross-modal generalization and to determine the causal basis for the similarity. As briefly reviewed in chapter 2, there are some provocative correlations between spectral cues in the two modalities. On the other hand, the similarity may not extend beyond the fact that in both modalities the utility of asymmetric representations reflects a general principle of brain function.

COMPUTATIONAL SPECIFICITY OF THE DFF THEORY

The goals of cognitive neuroscience extend beyond simply providing general descriptions of brain function. To develop a true biology of the mind we need to delineate the mental computations required for performing a particular task, determine the neural structures associated with those computations, and specify how those neural structures implement their specialized computations. The study of hemispheric lateralization is only in its infancy in terms of this level of specification. Indeed, the study of hemispheric specialization has earned the scorn of many researchers because the work frequently appears to offer little beyond general descriptions of the differences between the two hemispheres.

In some respects, we are guilty of perpetuating that tradition. At the most basic level the DFF theory offers a simple description of a fundamental asymmetry between the two hemispheres. Earlier theories focused on dichotomies such as verbal versus spatial, serial versus parallel, and detail versus whole (Bradshaw & Nettleton, 1981). Superficially, one could argue that the DFF theory simply provides a new dichotomy, in which the left hemisphere is seen as amplifying the relatively higher frequency information in a stimulus, and the right hemisphere as amplifying relatively lower frequency information.

However, we believe the theory provides a significant advance over its predecessors. Consider the problems associated with a dichotomy based on local and global processing. How do we define what is local and global, especially when we want our description to be independent of the phenomena we are trying to explain? The DFF theory, by its computational nature, does not face this circular dilemma. We have specified a set of processing mechanisms that are closely linked to more general theories of perception. A frequency-based analysis is fundamental to all theories of auditory perception. Similarly, visual perception includes an analysis of spatial frequency information, although the appropriate characterization of that analysis remains controversial. In both modalities information is carried at different scales, and the processing mechanisms inherent in the DFF theory are designed to exploit that difference. As such, the DFF theory provides a rigorous means for specifying what is meant by the terms "local" and "global."

We have also proposed that the hemispheric representations are essentially flexible, an idea that is captured by the attentional filtering stage of the theory. The study of perceptual systems is currently undergoing a revolution of sorts, with many studies showing that we cannot view perceptual mechanisms simply as passive processors of sensory signals (see Desimone & Duncan, 1995). Rather, signal processing at almost all levels of cortical processing is modulated by the current task demands. We have provided a computationally reasonable scheme to incorporate that idea into the DFF theory. The attentional selection mechanism indicates that the asymmetric representations must be viewed as differences in relative frequency rather than absolute frequency. The two hemispheres provide an asymmetric representation of the world, but the representations are tailored to maximize information relevant to current processing goals.

We can already see the benefits offered by postulating computational mechanisms underlying hemispheric specialization in perception. First, as shown by the computer simulations in chapter 7, we can develop existence proofs to demonstrate the plausibility of the theory. Although there is a clear need to incorporate stricter biological constraints into the model, the simulations show how the asymmetric representation of frequency information can account for a diverse set of tasks that produce laterality effects in visual perception. Moreover, the model offers an explicit account of the two filtering stages that form the basis of the theory. It is likely that mechanisms similar to those encompassed by the

DFF theory would be needed to implement more descriptive dichotomies like local versus global processing.

Second, the computational mechanisms of the DFF theory offer a principled way to evaluate the contributions of different brain structures within each hemisphere. Our understanding of the specializations of those structures is greatly facilitated by detailed processing models. As reviewed in chapters 3 and 4, the evidence suggests that the two filtering stages of the DFF theory are linked with separable neural systems. Neuropsychological studies have implicated regions in the temporal-parietal junction as critical for asymmetric filtering of spatial frequency information. Although spatial resolution information is limited in lesion studies with humans, more recent neuroimaging studies point to a critical focus within the superior aspects of the temporal lobe. In contrast, the attentional filtering mechanism appears to depend on parietal mechanisms. Thus, we can begin to see how computational theories offer the opportunity to go beyond simple dichotomous descriptions of hemispheric specialization. Not only can we develop a catalog of how the two hemispheres make asymmetric contributions in different processing domains, but we are in a position to link particular component operations to specific neural systems.

HEMISPHERIC INTERACTIONS: COOPERATION OR COMPETITION?

The asymmetric operation of the two hemispheres is striking. Nonetheless, it remains clear that overt behavior is not fractionated. Although the hemispheres may afford two sides of perception, our actions emerge as an integration of complex processing that occurs both within and between the two hemispheres. At this point the DFF theory does not offer an account of hemispheric interactions or integration. In considering how this integration occurs, we can consider two extreme positions in terms of how processing is coordinated between the two hemispheres.

At one extreme is the hypothesis that the two hemispheres operate in a completely integrated fashion. The corpus callosum contains more than 200 million fibers, providing interhemispheric connections at just about all stages of processing. In combination with subcortical pathways, the callosum would seem to be an ideal system for allowing the two hemispheres to operate in an integrated, cooperative manner (for a thorough review, see Hellige, 1993).

Interhemispheric coordination is an essential component of task-based models of hemispheric specialization. Without transfer, it would not be possible to perform a task unless the information was directed to the appropriate hemisphere. For example, in dichotic-listening tasks, people are able to report some of the words presented to the left ear. If the left hemisphere is assumed to be solely responsible for speech comprehension, then it is necessary to assume that left-ear stimuli are either projected directly to the left hemisphere, or that the information is from the right hemisphere across the corpus callosum. Similarly, some theorists have posited models of perception in which each hemisphere is essential for separable stages of stimulus elaboration. For example, Warrington (1985) has proposed a right hemisphere specialization for perceptual categorization, or for processes required for maintaining object constancy, and a left hemisphere specialization for semantic categorization, or for the linking of perceptual information to semantic knowledge. In her model object constancy precedes semantic categorization. Thus, interhemispheric transfer provides the means for routing information through those specialized modules.

Even in less restrictive models, transcallosal communication may be viewed as a cooperative process. As perceptual representations are embellished, interhemispheric processing may allow the two hemispheres to converge on common long-term representations in memory. In that view each hemisphere provides the other with a record of its current representational state, and perceptual coherence arises through those interactions. Thus, whereas the right hemisphere may only have a weak representation of the higher frequency local elements in a hierarchical pattern, that representation may be facilitated by signals from the left hemisphere. Lesion studies have shown how interhemispheric signals can allow access to associations stored in either hemisphere (Ungerleider & Mishkin, 1982).

At the other extreme, the two hemispheres may be viewed as competitors, at least in terms of their perceptual functions (Reuter-Lorenz et al., 1990). Cook (1984) has proposed that homotopic callosal connections are primarily inhibitory. As activation accrues in one region within a hemisphere, processing within the homologous region in the other hemisphere is diminished or attenuated. Ringo, Doty, Demeter, and Simard (1994) provide one argument for why cooperation may not be the appropriate metaphor for interhemispheric communication. Unlike the lightening speed with which computers operate, neural communication is a relatively slow process determined by the size of axonal fibers and the distance to be traveled. Ringo et al. (1994) estimate that the average conduction delay for callosal fibers would be on the order of 30 ms. Such delays could seriously handicap a pattern recognition system since the intra- and interhemisphere inputs would be desynchronized. Indeed, based on a series of computer simulations, Ringo et al. (1994) conclude that slow interhemispheric conduction delays result in a system in which the two hemispheres operate with relative independence.

That view is consistent with cognitive models that assume capacity limitations are primarily manifest at later stages of processing (e.g., Allport, 1980). According to such theories, different perceptual channels perform their specialized operations on the sensory input with little interference or cross talk, producing outputs that compete for access to response systems. Integration occurs at relatively late stages when the perceptual information is used to guide action. A late bottleneck imposes little restriction on upstream processes but ensures that the final action is the coherent result of a winner-take-all competitive process.

In the extreme, we might suppose that each hemisphere independently performs its specialized perceptual analysis, with the outputs from that analysis providing votes that eventually result in the selection of a single response. We can create situations in which this process is truly competitive; for instance, with hierarchical letter stimuli the hemispheres may end up promoting different responses. But in most situations the asymmetric representations converge on the same response, at least when coupled with task-specific goals. For example, when viewing a global S composed of local Ts, the right hemisphere will produce a strong representation of the S and a weak representation of the T. The reverse will characterize the left hemisphere. However, if the response set is limited to either S or H, then the output from each hemisphere will converge on S. If the stimuli are lateralized we will observe a left visual field advantage, but not because stimuli in the right visual field need to be shuttled across the callosum to the right hemisphere for global analysis. Rather, the laterality effect will emerge because the representation of the global S is less salient in the left hemisphere. Similarly, the patient with a lesion encompassing the temporal-parietal junction of the right hemisphere will be slow to identify S because her representation of the global structure is handicapped in the high-pass filtered image provided by the intact left hemisphere.

In our current development of the DFF theory we have emphasized how processing within each of the hemispheres considered in isolation can account for laterality effects in a variety of task domains. Our current lack of consideration of interhemispheric communication is an obvious weakness of the theory but is also a consequence of the fact that the nature of callosal function remains mysterious. Although transcortical communication is surely an essential component of our integrated behavior, asymmetric processing within each of the two hemispheres may still yield two sides of perception.

CONCLUSIONS

In this concluding chapter we have attempted to highlight some of the strengths of the DFF theory as well as point to some of the important, unresolved issues. As noted throughout this monograph the theory is limited to an account of hemispheric asymmetries in perception. Within this limited domain the theory offers a novel slant on hemispheric specialization both in terms of the computational mechanisms involved and by providing a parsimonious account of laterality effects across a wide range of task domains.

New scientific theories are rarely in direct conflict with older theories. Rather, they offer new insights into the analysis of long-standing problems. Hemispheric specialization remains one of the most important aspects of human cognition, inspiring many theoretical attempts to capture the functional asymmetries. There are obvious links between the DFF theory and its predecessors. For example, the analytic versus holistic dichotomy easily maps onto the current hypothesis that the left hemisphere is biased to amplify high-frequency information and the right hemisphere is biased to amplify low-frequency information. Where we hope to make our most significant contributions is by providing an explicit computational account for how those asymmetries arise. In this way we seek to retain the parsimony offered in earlier descriptive accounts, while offering specific, testable hypotheses.

References

Abramson, A. S. (1975). The tones of central Thai: Some perceptual experiments. In J. G. Harris and J. R. Chamberlain (Eds.), *Studies in Thai linguistics in honor of William J. Gedney* (pp. 1–6). Bangkok: Central Institute of English Language, Office of State Universities.

Akelaitis, A. J. (1941). Studies on the corpus callosum. *Archives of Neurology and Psychiatry, 45,* 788–796.

Alivisatos, B. & Wilding, J. (1982). Hemispheric differences in matching Stroop-type letter stimuli. *Cortex, 18,* 5–22.

Allport, D. A. (1980). Attention and performance. In G. Claxton (Ed.), *Cognitive psychology: New directions* (pp. 112–153). London: Routledge and Kegan Paul.

Amirkhiabani, G. & Lovegrove, W. J. (1966). Role of eccentricity and size in the global precedence effect. *Journal of Experimental Psychology: Human Perception and Performance, 22,* 1434–1447.

Andersen, R. A. (1987). Inferior parietal lobule function in spatial perception and visuomotor integration. In V. B. Mountcastle, F. Plum & S. R. Geiger (Eds.), *Handbook of physiology.* (Vol. 5, pp. 483–518). Baltimore: American Physiological Society.

Arrigoni, G. & De Renzi, E. (1964). Constructional apraxia and hemispheric locus of lesion. *Cortex, 1,* 180–197.

Badal, J. (1888). Contribution a l'etude des cecites psychiques. Alexie, agraphie, hemianopsie inferieure, trouble du sens d'l'espace. *Archives d'Ophtalmologie et Revue Generale d'Ophtalmologie, 140,* 97–117. (In De Renzi, 1982).

Balint, R. (1909). Seelenlahmung des "Schauens," optische Ataxie, raumliche Storung der Aufmerksamkeit. *Monatsschrift fuer Psychiatrie und Neurologie,* 51–81. (Translated in *Cognitive Neuropsychology, 12,* 265–281).

Bartholomeus, B. (1974). Effects of task requirements on ear superiority for sung speech. *Cortex, 10,* 215–223.

Barton, M. I., Goodglass, H., & Shai, A. (1965). Differential recognition of tachistoscopically presented English and Hebrew words in right and left visual fields. *Perceptual and Motor Skills, 21,* 431–437.

Basso, A., Casati, G., & Vignolo, A. (1977). Phonemic identification defect in aphasia. *Cortex, 13,* 84–95.

Baylis, G. C. & Driver, J. (1992). Visual parsing and response competition: The effect of grouping factors. *Perception and Psychophysics, 51,* 145–162.

Baylis, G. C., Driver, J., Baylis, L., & Rafal, R. D. (1994). Reading of letters and words in a patient with Balint's syndrome. *Neuropsychologia, 32,* 1273–1286.

Beaumont, J. G. (Ed.) (1982). Divided visual field studies of cerebral organization. New York: Academic Press.

Beeman, M., Friedman, R. B., Grafman, J., Perez, E., et al. (1994). Summation priming and coarse semantic coding in the right hemisphere. *Journal of Cognitive Neuroscience, 6*, 26–45.

Behrmann, M. & Moscovitch, M. (1996). Object-centered neglect in patients with unilateral neglect: Effects of left-right coordinates of objects. *Journal of Cognitive Neuroscience, 6*, 1–16.

Behrmann, M., Moscovitch, M., & Winocur, G. (1994). Intact visual imagery and impaired visual perception in a patient with visual agnosia. *Journal of Experimental Psychology: Human Perception and Performance, 20*, 1068–1087.

Benton, A. L. (1973). Visuoconstructive disability in patients with cerebral disease: Its relationship to side of lesion and aphasic disorder. *Documenta Ophthalmology, 34*, 67–76.

Benton, A. L. & Fogel, M. L. (1962). Three-dimensional constructional praxis. *Archives of Neurology, 7*, 347–354.

Benton, A. L. & Van Allen, M. W. (1968). Impairment in facial recognition in patients with cerebral disease. *Cortex, 4*, 344–358.

Berman, K. F., Illowsky, B. P., & Weinberger, D. R. (1988). Physiological dysfunction of dorsolateral prefrontal cortex in schizophrenia: Further evidence for regional and behavioral specificity. *Archives of General Psychiatry, 43*, 126–135.

Bever, T. G. & Chiarello, R. J. (1974). Cerebral dominance in musicians and nonmusicians. *Science, 185*, 537–539.

Black, F. W. & Strub, R. L. (1976). Constructional apraxia in patients with discrete missile wounds of the brain. *Cortex, 12*, 212–220.

Blakemore, C. & Campbell, F. W. (1969). On the existence of neurones in the human visual system selectively sensitive to the orientation and size of retinal images. *Journal of Physiology (London), 203*, 237–260.

Blonder, L. X., Bowers, D., & Heilman, K. M. (1991). The role of the right hemisphere in emotional communication. *Brain, 114*, 1115–1127.

Blumstein, S. E., Baker, E., & Goodglass, H. (1977). Phonological factors in auditory comprehension in aphasia. *Neuropsychologia, 15*, 19–30.

Blumstein, S. E. & Cooper, W. E. (1974). Hemispheric processing of intonation contours. *Cortex, 10*, 146–158.

Blumstein, S. E., Cooper, W. E., Zurif, E. B., & Caramazza, A. (1977). The perception and production of voice-onset time in aphasia. *Neuropsychologia, 15*, 371–383.

Bogen, J. E. & Gazzaniga, M. S. (1965). Cerebral commissurotomy in man: Minor hemisphere dominance for certain visuospatial functions. *Journal of Neurosurgery, 23*, 394–399.

Boles, D. B. (1984). Global versus local processing: Is there a hemispheric dichotomy? *Neuropsychologia, 22*, 445–455.

Boring, E. G. (1965). *A source book in the history of psychology*. Cambridge, Mass.: Harvard University Press.

Bradshaw, J. (1986). *Basic experiments in neuropsychology*. Amsterdam: Elsevier Science Publications.

Bradshaw, J. L. & Nettleton, N. C. (1981). The nature of hemispheric specialization in man. *Behavior and Brain Sciences, 4*, 51–63.

Broadbent, D. E. (1954). The role of auditory localization in attention and memory span. *Journal of Experimental Psychology, 47,* 191–196.

Broadbent, D. E. (1958). *Perception and communication.* New York: Pergamon.

Broadbent, D. E. (1977). The hidden preattentive process. *American Psychologist, 32,* 109–118.

Broca, P. (1861). Remarques sur le siege de la aculte du langage articule suivie d'une observation d'aphemie. *Bulletin of the Society of Anatomy, 6,* 330. Trans. J. Kann (1950), *Journal of Speech and Hearing Disorders, 15,* 16–20.

Brodal, A. (1981). (3rd ed.). *Neurological anatomy in relation to clinical medicine.* New York: Oxford University Press.

Brown, H. D. & Kosslyn, S. M. (1995). Hemispheric differences in visual object processing: Structural versus allocation theories. In R. J. Davidson & K. Hugdahl (Eds.), *Brain asymmetry.* Cambridge, Mass.: MIT Press.

Brown, M. W. (1947). *Read to me storybook.* New York: Thomas Crowell Co.

Bruce, V. & Green, P. R. (1990). *Visual perception: Physiology, psychology and ecology.* Hillsdale, N.J.: Lawrence Erlbaum & Associates.

Bruce, V. & Humphreys, G. W. (1994). *Object and face recognition.* Hillsdale, N.J.: Lawrence Erlbaum & Associates.

Brugge, J. F. & Merzenich, M. M. (1973). Response of neurons in auditory cortex of the macaque monkey to monaural and binaural stimulation. *Journal of Neurophysiology, 36,* 1138–1158.

Bryden, M. P. (1982). *Laterality: Functional asymmetry in the intact brain.* New York: Academic Press.

Burton, A., Morton, N., & Abbess, S. (1989). Mode of processing and hemisphere divergences in the judgment of musical stimuli. *British Journal of Psychology, 80,* 169–180.

Calvanio, R., Petrone, P. M., & Levine, D. N. (1987). Left visual spatial neglect is both environmental-centered and body-centered. *Neurology, 37,* 1179–1183.

Campbell, F. W., Cooper, G. F., & Enroth-Cugell, C. (1969). The spatial selectivity of the visual cells of the cat. *Journal of Physiology, 203,* 223–235.

Campbell, F. W. & Robson, J. G. (1968). Application of Fourier analysis to the visibility of gratings. *Journal of Physiology, 197,* 551–566.

Carter, C. S., Robertson, L. C., Chaderjian, M. R., Celaya, L. J., & Nordahl, T. E. (1992). Attentional asymmetry in schizophrenia: Controlled and automatic processes. *Biological Psychiatry, 31,* 909–918.

Carter, C. S., Robertson, L. C., Chaderjian, M. R., O'Sora-Celaya, L., & Nordahl, T. (1994). Attentional asymmetry in schizophrenia: The role of illness subtype and symptomatology. *Progress in Neuro-Psychopharmacology, 18,* 661–683.

Carter, C. S., Robertson, L. C., Nordahl, T. E., Chaderjian, M., & Oshora-Celaya, L. (1996). Perceptual and attentional asymmetries in schizophrenia: Further evidence for a left hemisphere deficit. *Psychiatry Research, 62,* 111–119.

Catlin, J. & Neville, H. (1976). The laterality effect in reaction time to speech stimuli. *Neuropsychologia, 14,* 141–143.

Celesia, G. G. (1976). Organization of auditory cortical areas in man. *Brain, 99,* 403–414.

Chandler, B. C. & Parsons, O. A. (1975). Visual search on the ascending and descending limbs of the blood alcohol curve. *Alcohol Technical Reports, 4,* 23–27.

Cheney, D. L. & Seyfarth, R. M. (1990). *How monkeys see the world: Inside the mind of another species*. Chicago: University of Chicago Press.

Chi, J. G., Dooling, E. C., & Gilles, F. H. (1977). Left-right asymmetries of the temporal speech areas of the human fetus. *Archives of Neurology, 34,* 346–348.

Chiarello, C., Senehi, J., & Soulier, M. (1986). Viewing conditions and hemispheric asymmetry for lexical decision. *Neuropsychologia, 24,* 521–530.

Christman, S., Kitterle, F. L., & Hellige, J. (1991). Hemispheric aysmmetry in the processing of absolute versus relative spatial frequency. *Brain and Cognition, 16,* 62–73.

Chung, D. Y., Mason, K., Gannon, P. R., & Wilson, G. N. (1983). The ear effect as a function of age and hearing loss. *Journal of the Acoustical Society of America, 73,* 1277–1282.

Coltheart, M. (1985). Cognitive neuropsychology and the study of reading. In M. I. Posner & O. S. M. Marin (Eds.), *Attention and performance XI* (pp. 3–37). Cambridge, Mass.: Lawrence Erlbaum & Associates.

Cook, N. D. (1984). Homotopic callosal inhibition. *Brain and Language, 23,* 116–125.

Cook, N. D., Fruh, H., & Landis, T. (1995). The cerebral hemispheres and neural network simulations: Design considerations. *Journal of Experimental Psychology: Human Perception and Performance, 21,* 410–422.

Corballis, M. C. (1991). *The lopsided ape: Evolution of the generative mind*. Oxford: Oxford University Press.

Corbetta, M., Miezin, F. M., Shulman, G. L., & Petersen, S. E. (1993). Shifts of visuo-spatial attention: A PET study. *Journal of Neuroscience, 13,* 1202–1226.

Corbetta, M., Shulman, G. L., Miezin, F. M., & Petersen, S. E. (1995). Superior parietal cortex activation during spatial attention shifts and visual feature conjunction. *Science, 270,* 802–805.

Coslett, H. B. & Saffran, E. M. (1991). Simultanagnosia: To see but not to see. *Brain, 113,* 1523–1545.

Costa, L. D. & Vaughan, H. G. (1962). Performance of patients with lateralized cerebral lesions. *Journal of Nervous and Mental Disorders, 134,* 162–168.

Cowin, E. L. & Hellige, J. B. (1994). Categorical versus coordinate spatial processing: Effects of blurring on hemispheric asymmetry for processing spatial information. *Journal of Cognitive Neuroscience, 6,* 156–164.

Cutting, J. (1974). Two left-hemisphere mechanisms in speech perception. *Perception and Psychophysics, 16,* 601–612.

Damasio, A. R. (1990). Category-related recognition defects as a clue to the neural substrates of knowledge. *Trends in Neurosciences, 13,* 95–98.

Damasio, A. R. & Damasio, H. (1986). In R. Bruyer (Ed.), *The neuropsychology of face perception and facial expression*. Hillsdale, N.J.: Lawrence Erlbaum & Associates.

Damasio, H., Grabowski, T. J., Tranel, D., Hichwa, R. D., & Damasio, A. D. (1996). A neural basis for lexical retrieval. *Nature, 380,* 499–505.

Damasio, A. R. & Tranel, D. (1993). Nouns and verbs are retrieved with differently distributed neural systems. *Proceedings of the National Academy of Sciences of the United States of America, 90,* 4957–4960.

Davidson, R. J. & Hughdahl, K. (Eds.) (1995). *Brain asymmetry*. Cambridge, Mass.: MIT Press.

Davis, E. T. (1981). Allocation of attention: Uncertainty effects when monitoring one or two visual gratings of noncontiguous spatial frequencies. *Perception and Psychophysics, 29,* 618–622.

Davis, E. T. & Graham, N. (1981). Spatial frequency uncertainty effects in the detection of sinusoidal gratings. *Vision Research, 21,* 705–712.

DeArmond, S. J., Fusco, M. M., & Dewey, M. M. (1989). *Structure of the human brain.* New York: Oxford University Press.

Delis, D. C. (1989). Neuropsychological assessment of learning and memory. In F. Boller & J. Grafman (Eds.), *Handbook of neuropsychology* (Vol. 3). Amsterdam: Elsevier Science Publications.

Delis, D. C., Kramer, J. H., & Kiefner, M. G. (1988). Visuospatial functioning before and after commissurotomy: Disconnection in hierarchical processing. *Archives of Neurology, 45,* 462–465.

Delis, D. C., Massman, P. J., Butters, N., Salmon, D. P., Shear, P. K., Demadura, T., & Filoteo, J. V. (1992). Spatial cognition in Alzheimer's disease: Subtypes of global-local impairment. *Journal of Clinical and Experimental Psychology, 14,* 463–477.

Delis, D. C., Robertson, L. C., & Efron, R. (1986). Hemispheric specialization of memory for visual hierarchical stimuli. *Neuropsychologia, 24,* 205–214.

Denes, G., Semenza, C., Stoppa, E., & Lis, A. (1982). Unilateral spatial neglect and recovery from hemiplegia. A follow-up study. *Brain, 105,* 543–552.

De Renzi, E. (1966). Balints-Holmes syndrome. In C. Code, C. W. Wallesch, Y. Joanette, & A. R. Lecours (Eds.), *Classic cases in neuropsychology.* Hove, UK: Erlbaum, Taylor & Francis.

De Renzi, E. (1982). *Disorders of space exploration and cognition.* Chichester: John Wiley & Sons.

De Renzi, E. & Spinnler, H. (1966). Facial recognition in brain-damaged patients: An experimental approach. *Cortex, 16,* 634–642.

de Schonen, S. & Mathivet, E. (1989). First come, first served: A scenario about the development of hemispheric specialization in face recognition during infancy. *European Bulletin of Cognitive Psychology, 9,* 3–44.

Desimone, R. & Duncan, J. (1995). Neural mechanisms of selective visual attention. *Annual Review of Neuroscience, 18,* 193–222.

Desimone, R., Schein, S. J., & Albright, T. D. (1985). Form, color and motion analysis in prestriate cortex of the macaque. In C. Chagas, R. Gattass, & C. Gross (Eds.), *Pattern recognition mechanisms.* Berlin: Springer.

Desimone, R., Stanley, J. S., Moran, J., & Ungerleider, L. G. (1985). Contour, color and shape analysis beyond the striate cortex. *Vision Research, 25,* 441–452.

Deutsch, D. (1974). An auditory illusion. *Nature, 251,* 307–309.

Deutsch, D. (1975). Musical illusions. *Scientific American, 233,* 92–104.

Deutsch, D. (1985). Dichotic listening to melodic patterns and its relationship to hemispheric specialization of function. *Music Perception, 3,* 127–154.

Deutsch, D. & Roll, P. L. (1976). Separate "what" and "where" decision mechanisms in processing a dichotic tonal sequence. *Journal of Experimental Psychology, 2,* 23–29.

De Valois, R. L., Albrecht, D. G., & Thorell, L. G. (1982). Spatial frequency selectivity of cells in macaque visual cortex. *Vision Research, 22,* 545–559.

De Valois, R. L. & De Valois, K. K. (1990). *Spatial vision.* New York: Oxford University Press.

De Valois, R. L., Morgan, H., & Snodderly, D. M. (1974). Psychophysical studies of monkey vision III. Spatial luminance contrast sensitivity tests of macaque and human observers. *Vision Research, 14,* 75–81.

Di Stefano, M., Morelli, M., Marzi, C. A., & Berlucchi, G. (1980). Hemispheric control of unilateral and bilateral movements of proximal and distal parts of the arm as inferred from simple reaction time to lateralized light stimuli in man. *Experimental Brain Research, 38,* 197–204.

Doyon, J. & Milner, B. (1991). Right temporal-lobe contributions to global visual processing. *Neuropsychologia, 19,* 343–360.

Driver, J., Baylis, G., & Rafal, R. (1992). Preserved figure-ground segmentation and symmetry perception in a patient with visual neglect. *Nature, 360,* 73–75.

Driver, J. & Halligan, P. W. (1991). Can visual neglect operate in object-centered coordinates? An affirmative single case study. *Cognitive Neuropsychology, 8,* 475–496.

Duncan, J. (1984). Selective attention and the organization of visual information. *Journal of Experimental Psychology: General, 113,* 501–517.

Early, T. S., Posner, M. I., Reiman, E., & Raichle, M. E. Left striato-pallidal hyperactivity in schizophrenia. Part II: Phenomenology and thought disorder. *Psychiatric Developments, 2,* 109–121.

Edmondson, J. A., Chan, J. L., Seibert, G. B., & Ross, E. D. (1987). The effect of right-brain damage on acoustical measures of affective prosody in Taiwanese patients. *Journal of Phonetics, 15,* 219–233.

Efron, R. (1990). *The decline and fall of hemispheric specialization.* Hillsdale, N.J.: Lawrence Erlbaum & Associates.

Eglin, M. (February 1992). Modes of visual attention. Symposium paper presented at the International Neuropsychological Society: San Diego, CA.

Eglin, M., Robertson, L. C., & Knight, R. T. (1989). Visual search performance in the neglect syndrome. *Journal of Cognitive Neuroscience, 4,* 372–381.

Eglin, M., Robertson, L. C., Knight, R. T., & Brugger, P. (1994). Search deficits in neglect patients are dependent on size of the visual scene. *Neuropsychology, 4,* 451–463.

Egly, R., Driver, J., & Rafal, R. D. (1994). Shifting visual attention between objects and locations: Evidence from normal and parietal lesion subjects. *Journal of Experimental Psychology: General, 123,* 161–177.

Egly, R. & Homa, D. (1984). Sensitization in the visual field. *Journal of Experimental Psychology, 10,* 778–793.

Egly, R., Rafal, R. D., Driver, J., & Starreveld, Y. (1995). Hemispheric specialization for object-based attention in a split-brain patient. *Psychological Science, 5,* 380–383.

Egly, R., Rafal, R., & Henik, A. (October 1993). Reflexive and voluntary covert orienting in detection and discrimination tasks. Paper presented at the 34th Annual Meeting of the Psychonomic Society, Washington, D.C.

Ellenberg, L., Rosenbaum, G., Goldman, M. S., & Whitman, R. D. (1980). Recoverability of psychological functioning following alcohol abuse: Lateralization effects. *Journal of Consulting and Clinical Psychology, 48,* 502–510.

Ellis, A. W. (1986). Processes underlying face recognition. In R. Bruyer (Ed.), *The neuropsychology of face perception and facial expression.* Hillsdale, N.J.: Lawrence Erlbaum & Associates.

Ellis, A. W. & Young, A. W. (1988). *Human cognitive neuropsychology*. Hillsdale, N.J.: Lawrence Erlbaum & Associates.

Elmo, T. (1987). Hemispheric asymmetry of auditory evoked potentials to comparisons within and across phonetic categories. *Scandinavian Journal of Psychology, 28*, 251–266.

Enns, J. T. & Kingstone, A. (1995). Access to global and local properties in visual search for compound stimuli. *Psychological Science, 6*, 283–291.

Eriksen, C. W. & St. James, J. D. (1986). Visual attention within and around the field of focal attention: A zoom lens model. *Perception and Psychophysics, 40*, 225–240.

Eriksen, C. W. & Yeh, Y. (1985). Allocation of attention in the visual field. *Journal of Experimental Psychology: Human Perception and Performance, 11*, 583–597.

Fabian, M. S. & Parsons, O. A. (1983). Differential improvement of cognitive functions in recovering alcoholic women. *Journal of Abnormal Psychology, 92*, 87–95.

Farah, M. J. (1990). *Visual agnosia*. Cambridge, Mass.: MIT Press.

Farah, M. J., Brunn, J. L., Wong, A. B., Wallace, M. A., & Carpenter, P. A. (1990). Frames of reference for allocating attention to space: Evidence from the neglect syndrome. *Neuropsychologia, 28*, 335–347.

Farmer, M. E. & Klein, R. M. (1995). The evidence for a temporal processing deficit linked to dyslexia. *Psychonomic Bulletin and Review, 2*, 460–493.

Fendrich, R. & Gazzaniga, M. (1990). Hemispheric processing of spatial frequencies in two commissurotomy patients. *Neuropsychologia, 28*, 657–664.

Fiez, J. A., Raichle, M. E., Balota, D. A., Tallal, P., & Petersen, S. E. (1996). PET activation of posterior temporal regions during auditory word presentation and verb generation. *Cerebral Cortex, 6*, 1–10.

Fiez, J. A., Raichle, M. E., Miezin, F. M., Petersen, S. E., Tallal, P., & Katz, W. F. (1995). PET studies of auditory and phonological processing: Effects of stimulus characteristics and task demands. *Journal of Cognitive Neuroscience, 7*, 357–375.

Fiez, J., Raife, E., Balota, D., Schwartz, J., & Raichle, M. (1996). A positron emission tomography study of the short-term maintenance of verbal information. *Journal of Neuroscience, 16*, 808–822.

Filoteo, J. V., Delis, D. C., Demadura, T., Salmon, D. P., Roman, M. J., & Shults, C. W. (1992). Abnormally rapid disengagement of covert attention to global and local stimulus levels may underlie the visuoperceptual impairment in Parkinson's patients. *Neuropsychology, 8*, 210–217.

Filoteo, J. V., Delis, D. C., Massman, P. J., Demadura, T., Butters, N., & Salmon, D. P. (1992). Directed and divided attention in Alzheimer's disease: Impairments in shifting of attention to global and local stimuli. *Journal of Clinical and Experimental Neuropsychology, 14*, 871–883.

Finger, S. (1994). *Origins of neuroscience*. New York: Oxford University Press.

Fink, G., Halligan, P., Marshall, J., Frith, C., Frackowiak, R., & Dolan, R. (1996). Where in the brain does visual attention select the forest and the trees? *Nature, 15*, 626–628.

Fiorentini, A., Maffei, L., & Sandini, G. (1983). The role of high spatial frequencies in face perception. *Perception, 12*, 195–201.

Foss, D. J. & Hakes, D. T. *Psycholinguistics: An introduction to the psychology of language*. Englewood Cliffs, N.J.: Prentice-Hall.

Freyd, J. (1987). Dynamic mental representations. *Psychological Review, 94*, 427–438.

Friedman-Hill, S. R., Robertson, L. C., & Treisman, A. (1995). Parietal contributions to visual feature binding: Evidence from a patient with bilateral lesions. *Science, 269,* 853–855.

Gaede, S. E., Parsons, O. A., & Bertera, J. H. (1978). Hemispheric differences in music perception: Aptitude versus experience. *Neuropsychologia, 16,* 369–373.

Gainotti, G. & Tiacci, C. (1972). Patterns of drawing disability in right and left hemispheric patients. *Neuropsychologia, 8,* 379–384.

Galaburda, A. & Livingstone, M. (1993). Evidence for a magnocellular defect in developmental dyslexia. *Annals of the New York Academy of Sciences, 682,* 70–82.

Galaburda, A. M., Menard, M. T., & Rosen, R. D. (1994). Evidence for aberrant auditory anatomy in developmental dyslexia. *Proceedings of the National Academy of Sciences of the United States of America, 91,* 8010–8013.

Gandour, J. & Dardarananda, R. (1983). Identification of tonal contrasts in Thai aphasic patients. *Brain and Language, 18,* 98–114.

Garay, M. R. & Johnson, D. S. (1979). *Computers and intractability.* New York: W. H. Freeman.

Gates, A. & Bradshaw, J. L. (1977). The role of the cerebral hemispheres in music. *Brain and Language, 4,* 403–431.

Gattass, R., Sousa, A. P. B., & Covey, E. (1985). Cortical visual areas of the macaque: Possible substrates for pattern recognition mechanisms. In C. Chagas, R. Gattass, & C. Gross (Eds.), *Pattern recognition mechanisms.* Berlin: Springer.

Gazzaniga, M. S. (1967). The split brain in man. *Scientific American, 217,* 24–29. San Francisco: W. H. Freeman.

Gazzaniga, M. S. (1970). *The bisected brain.* New York: Appleton-Century-Crofts.

Gazzaniga, M. S. (Ed.). (1995). *The cognitive neurosciences.* Cambridge, Mass.: MIT Press.

Gazzaniga, M. S. & Alan, K. (1995). Subcortical transfer of higher order information: More illusory than real? *Neuropsychology, 9,* 321–328.

Gazzaniga, M. S., Bogen, J. E., & Sperry, R. W. (1962). Some functional effects of sectioning the cerebral commissures in man. *Proceedings of the National Academy of Science, 48,* 1765–1769.

Gazzaniga, M. S., Bogen, J. E., & Sperry, R. W. (1965). Observations on visual perception after disconnexion of the cerebral hemispheres in man. *Brain, 88,* 221–236.

Gazzaniga, M. S. & Hillyard, S. A. (1971). Language and speech capacity of the right hemisphere. *Neuropsychologia, 9,* 273–280.

Gazzaniga, M. S. & Ladavas, E. (1987). Disturbances in spatial attention following lesion or disconnection of the right parietal lobe. In M. Jeannerod (Ed.), *Neurophysiological and neuropsychological aspects of spatial neglect.* Amsterdam: Elsevier Science Publishers.

Gazzaniga, M. S. and Smylie, C. S. (1984). Dissociation of language and cognition: A psychological profile of two disconnected right hemispheres. *Brain, 107,* 145–153.

Gazzaniga, M. S. & Sperry, R. W. (1967). Language after section of the cerebral commissures. *Brain, 90,* 131–148.

Geschwind, N. & Galaburda, A. M. (1987). *Cerebral lateralization: Biological mechanisms, associations, and pathology.* Cambridge, Mass.: MIT Press.

Gialanella, B. & Mattioli, F. (1992). Anosognosia and extrapersonal neglect as predictors of functional recovery following right hemisphere stroke. *Neuropsychological Rehabilitation, 2,* 169–178.

Ginsburg, A. (1978). Visual information processing based on spatial filters constrained by biological data. Doctoral dissertation. Cambridge University, England.

Goldman, M. S. (1983). Cognitive impairment in chronic alcoholics: Some cause for optimism. *American Psychologist, 10,* 1045–1054.

Goldman-Rakic, P. S. (1992). Working memory and the mind. *Scientific American, 267,* 111–117.

Goldmeier, E. (1972). Similarity in visually perceived forms. *Psychological monographs, 8,* (Whole no. 29). (Originally published 1936).

Goldstein, K. (1995). *The Organism.* New York: Zone Books. Originally published 1934.

Goodglass, H. & Calderon, M. (1977). Parallel processing of verbal and musical stimuli in right and left hemispheres. *Neuropsychologia, 15,* 397–407.

Gordon, H. W. (1974). Auditory specialization of the right and left hemispheres. In M. Kinsbourne & W. L. Smith (Eds.), *Hemispheric disconnection and cerebral function* (pp. 126–136). Springfield, Ill: Charles C. Thomas.

Gordon, H. W. (1980). Degree of ear asymmetries for perception of dichotic chords and for illusory chord localization in musicians of different levels of competence. *Journal of Experimental Psychology: Human Perception and Performance, 6,* 516–527.

Gould, S. J. & Vrba, E. S. (1982). Exaptation—a missing term in the science of form. *Paleobiology, 8,* 4–15.

Grabowecky, M., Robertson, L. C., & Treisman, A. (1993). Preattentive processes guide visual search: Evidence from patients with unilateral visual neglect. *Journal of Cognitive Neuroscience, 5,* 288–302.

Grafton, S. T., Hazeltine, E., & Ivry, R. (1995). Functional mapping of sequence learning in normal humans. *Journal of Cognitive Neuroscience, 7,* 497–510.

Graham, N. V. S. (1989). *Visual pattern analyzers.* New York: Oxford University Press.

Graham, N., Kramer, P., & Haber, N. (1985). Attending to the spatial frequency and spatial position of near-threshold visual patterns. In M. I. Posner & O. S. M. Marin (Eds.), *Attention and performance XI.* Hillsdale, N.J.: Lawrence Erlbaum & Associates.

Graziano, M. & Gross, C. G. (1995). Multiple pathways for processing visual space. In T. Inui & J. McClelland (Eds.), *Attention and performance XVI.* Cambridge, Mass.: MIT Press.

Green, D. M. (1976). *An introduction to hearing.* Hillsdale, N.J.: Erlbaum & Associates.

Grossman, M., Shapiro, B. E., & Gardner, H. (1981). Dissociable musical processing strategies after localized brain damage. *Neuropsychologia, 19,* 425–433.

Guiard, Y. (1987). Asymmetric division of labor in human skilled bimanual action: The kinematic chain as a model. *Journal of Motor Behavior, 19,* 486–517.

Halligan, P. W. & Marshall, J. C. (1993). Homing in on neglect: A case study of visual search. *Cortex, 29,* 167–174.

Halligan, P. W. & Marshall, J. C. (1994). Toward a principled explanation of unilateral neglect. *Cognitive Neuropsychology, 11,* 167–206.

Hardyck, C. (1991). Shadow and substance: Attentional irrelevancies and perceptual constraints in hemispheric processing of language stimuli. In F. L. Kitterle (Ed.), *Cerebral laterality: Theory and research.*

Harmon, L. D. (1973). The recognition of faces. *Scientific American, 229,* 71–82.

Harrington, A. (1995). Unfinished business: Models of laterality in the nineteenth century. In R. J. Davidson and K. Hugdahl (Eds.), *Brain asymmetry.* Cambridge, MA: MIT Press.

Hart, J., Berndt, R. S., & Caramazza, A. (1985). Category-specific naming deficit following cerebral infarction. *Nature, 316,* 439–440.

Hecaen, H. & Angelergues, R. (1962). Agnosia for faces (prosopagnosia). *Archive of Neurology, 7,* 92–100.

Heilman, K. M. & Valenstein, E. (Eds.). (1985). *Clinical neuropsychology.* New York: Oxford University Press.

Heilman, K. M., Watson, R. R., & Valenstein, E. (1985). Neglect and related disorders. In K. M. Heilman & E. Valenstein (Eds.), *Clinical neuropsychology* (pp. 243–293). New York: Oxford University Press.

Heilman, K. M. & Van Den Abell, T. (1980). Right hemisphere dominance for attention: The mechanism underlying hemispheric asymmetries of inattention (neglect). *Neurology, 30,* 327–330.

Heinze, H. J., Johannes, S., Munte, T. F., & Mangun, G. R. (1994). The order of global- and local-level information processing: Electrophysiological evidence for parallel perceptual processes. In H. J. Heinze, T. F. Munte, & G. R. Mangun (Eds.), *Cognitive electrophysiology.* Cambridge, Mass.: Birkhauser Boston.

Heinze, H. J., Mangun, G. R., Burchert, W., Hinrichs, H., Munte, M., Scholz, A., Johannes, M., Scherg, H., Hundeshagen, H., Gazzaniga, M. S., & Hillyard, S. A. (1994). Combined spatial and temporal imaging of brain activity during visual selective attention in humans. *Nature, 372,* 543–546.

Heinze, H. J. & Munte, T. F. (1993). Electrophysiological correlates of hierarchical stimulus processing: Dissociation between onset and later stages of global and local target processing. *Neuropsychologia, 31,* 841–852.

Hellige, J. B. (1980). Effects of perceptual quality and visual field of probe stimulus presentation on memory search for letters. *Journal of Experimental Psychology: Human Perception and Preformance, 6,* 639–651.

Hellige, J. B. (1983). Feature similarity and laterality effects in visual masking. *Neuropsychologia, 21,* 633–639.

Hellige, J. B. (1993). *Hemispheric asymmetry.* Cambridge, Mass.: Harvard University Press.

Hellige, J. B. & Michimata, C. (1989). Categorization versus distance: Hemispheric differences for processing spatial information. *Memory and Cognition, 17,* 770–776.

Hillyard, S. A., Mangun, G. R., Woldorff, M. G., & Luck, S. J. (1995). Neural systems mediating selective attention. In M. Gazzaniga (Ed.), *The cognitive neurosciences* (pp. 665–681). Cambridge, Mass.: MIT Press.

Holmes, G. (1918). Disturbances of visual orientation. *British Journal of Ophthalmology, 2,* 449–468.

Holmes, G. & Horrax, G. (1919). Disturbances of spatial orientation and visual attention with loss of stereoscopic vision. *Archives of Neurology and Psychiatry, 1,* 385–407.

Houtsma, A. J. M. & Goldstein, J. L. (1972). The central origin of the pitch of complex tones: Evidence from musical interval recognition. *Journal of the Acoustical Society of America, 51,* 520–529.

Hubel, D. H. & Wiesel, T. N. (1977). The Ferrier lecture: Functional architecture of macaque monkey visual cortex. *Proceedings of the Royal Academy of London, Series B, 198,* 1–59.

Hugdahl, K. & Webster, K. (1992). Dichotic listening studies of hemispheric asymmetry in brain damaged patients. *International Journal of Neuroscience, 63,* 17–29.

Hughes, H. C., Fendrich, R., & Reuter-Lorenz, P. A. (1990). Global versus local processing in the absence of low spatial frequencies. *Journal of Cognitive Neuroscience, 2,* 272–282.

Hummel, J. & Biederman, I. (1992). Dynamic binding in a neural network for shape recognition. *Psychological Review, 99,* 480–517.

Humphreys, G. W. & Riddoch, M. J. (1993). Interactions between object and space systems revealed through neuropsychology. In D. E. Meyer & S. Kornblum (Eds.), *Attention and performance XIV* (pp. 183–218). Cambridge, Mass.: MIT Press.

Ivry, R. (1993). Cerebellar involvement in the explicit representation of temporal information. *Annals of the New York Academy of Sciences, 682,* 214–230.

Ivry, R. (1996). The representation of temporal information in perception and motor control. *Current Opinion in Neurobiology, 6,* 851–857.

Ivry, R. & Gopal, H. (1992). Speech perception and production in patients with cerebellar lesions. In D. E. Meyer and S. Kornblum (Eds.), *Attention and performance XIV: Synergies in experimental psychology, artificial intelligence, and cognitive neuroscience* (pp. 771–802). Cambridge, Mass.: MIT Press.

Ivry, R. & Lebby, P. (1993). Hemispheric differences in auditory perception are similar to those found in visual perception. *Psychological Science, 4,* 41–45.

Ivry, R. & Lebby, P. (in press). The neurology of consonant perception: Specialized module or distributed processors? In M. Beeman and C. Chiarello (Eds.), *Right hemisphere language comprehension: Perspectives from cognitive neuroscience.* Hillsdale, N.J.: Erlbaum & Associates.

James, W. (1890). *The principles of psychology.* New York: Dover Publications.

Jenkins, W. M. & Masterson, R. B. (1982). Sound localization: Effects of unilateral lesions in central auditory system. *Journal of Neurophysiology, 47,* 987–1016.

Jenkins, W. M. & Merzenich, M. M. (1984). Role of cat primary auditory cortex for sound-localization behavior. *Journal of Neurophysiology, 52,* 819–847.

Jerrison, H. J. (1980). The evolution of intelligence. *Separata, 5,* 273–280.

Johnson, D. M. & Hafter, E. R. (1980). Uncertain-frequency detection: Cueing and condition of observation. *Perception and Psychophysics, 28,* 143–149.

Jones, B. M. (1971). Verbal and spatial intelligence in short and long term alcoholics. *Journal of Nervous and Mental Disease, 153,* 292–297.

Jonsson, J. E. & Hellige, J. B. (1986). Lateralized effects of blurring: A test of the visual spatial frequency model of cerebral hemisphere asymmetry. *Neuropsychologia, 24,* 361–362.

Jouandet, M. L., Tramo, M. J., Herron, D. M., Herman, A., Loftus, W. C., Bazell, J., & Gazzaniga, M. (1989). Brainprints: Computer-generated two-dimensional maps of the cerebral cortex in vivo. *Journal of Cognitive Neuroscience, 1,* 88–117.

Kannan, P. M. & Lipscomb, D. M. (1974). Bilateral hearing asymmetry in a large population. *Journal of the Acoustical Society of America, 55,* 1092–1094.

Kaplan, E. (August 1976). The role of the noncompromised hemisphere in focal organic disease. Paper presented at the American Psychological Association meeting, Washington, D.C.

Kaplan, E. (1983). Process and achievement revisited. In S. Wagner & B. Kaplan (Eds.), *Toward a holistic developmental psychology.* Hillsdale, N.J.: Lawrence Erlbaum & Associates.

Kelly, J. P. (1981). Auditory system. In Kandel, E. R. and Schwartz, J. H. (Eds.), *Principles of Neuroscience* (pp. 258–268). New York: Elsevier North Holland.

Kiang, N. Y. S. (1965). *Discharge patterns of single fibers in the cat's auditory nerve.* Cambridge, Mass.: MIT Press.

Kim, N., Ivry, R. B., & Robertson, L. C. Sequential priming in hierarchical figures. Submitted manuscript.

Kimchi, R. & Palmer, S. (1982). Form and texture in hierarchically constructed patterns. *Journal of Experimental Psychology: Human Perception and Performance, 8,* 521–535.

Kimura, D. (1961a). Cerebral dominance and the perception of verbal stimuli. *Canadian Journal of Psychology, 15,* 166–171.

Kimura, D. (1961b). Some effects of temporal lobe damage on auditory perception. *Canadian Journal of Psychology, 15,* 156–165.

Kimura, D. (1964). Left-right differences in the perception of melodies. *Quarterly Journal of Experimental Psychology, 16,* 355–358.

Kimura, D. (1969). Spatial localization in left and right visual fields. *Canadian Journal of Psychology, 23,* 445–458.

Kimura, D. (1973). The asymmetry of the human brain. *Scientific American, 228,* 70–78.

Kinchla, R. A. (1974). Detecting target elements in multielement arrays: A confusability model. *Perception and Psychophysics, 15,* 149–158.

Kinchla, R. A., Solis-Macias, V., & Hoffman, J. (1983). Attending to different levels of structure in a visual image. *Perception and Psychophysics, 33,* 1–10.

Kinchla, R. A. & Wolfe, J. (1979). The order of visual processing: "Top-down," "bottom-up," or "middle-out." *Perception and Psychphysics, 33,* 1–10.

King, L. F. & Kimura, D. (1972). Left-ear superiority in dichotic perception of vocal nonverbal sounds. *Canadian Journal of Psychology, 26,* 111–116.

Kinsbourne, M. (1975). The mechanism of hemispheric control of the lateral gradient of attention. In P. M. A. Rabbit & S. Dornic (Eds.), *Attention and performance V.* New York: Academic Press.

Kinsbourne, M. (1987). Mechanisms of unilateral neglect. In M. Jeannerod (Ed.) *Neurophysiological and neuropsychological aspects of spatial neglect* (pp. 69–86). Amsterdam: Elsevier Science Publishers.

Kinsbourne, M. & Cook, J. (1971). Generalized and lateralized effects of concurrent verbalization on a unimanual skill. *Quarterly Journal of Experimental Psychology, 23,* 341–345.

Kitterle, F. & Christman, S. (1991). Symmetries and asymmetries in the processing of sinusoidal gratings. In F. Kitterle (Ed.), *Cerebral laterality: Theory and research. The Toledo symposium.* Hillsdale, N.J.: Lawrence Erlbaum & Associates.

Kitterle, F., Christman, S., & Hellige, J. (1990). Hemispheric differences are found in the identification, but not the detection, of low versus high spatial frequencies. *Perception and Psychophysics, 48,* 297–306.

Kitterle, F. L., Hellige, J. B., & Christman, S. (1992). Visual hemispheric asymmetries depend on which spatial frequencies are task relevant. *Brain and Cognition, 20,* 308–314.

Kitterle, F. & Kay, R. (1985). Hemispheric symmetry in contrast and orientation sensitivity. *Perception and Psychophysics, 37,* 391–396.

Kitterle, F. L. & Selig, L. M. (1991). Visual field effects in the discrimination of sine-wave gratings. *Perception and Psychophysics, 50,* 15–18.

Kleist, K. (1934). Kriegsverletzungen des Gehirns in ihrer Bedeutung fur die Hirnlikalisation und Hirnpathologie. Leipzig: Barth. (In De Renzi, 1982).

Knight, R. T. (1997). Distributed cortical network for visual attention. *Journal of Cognitive Neuroscience, 1,* 75–91.

Koffka, K. (1935). *Principles of Gestalt psychology.* New York: Harcourt Brace.

Konishi, M. (1993). Listening with two ears. *Scientific American, 268,* 66–73.

Kosslyn, S. M. (1986). Toward a computational neuropsychology of high level vision. In T. J. Knapp & L. C. Robertson (Eds.), *Approaches to cognition: Contrasts and controversies.* Hillsdale, N.J.: Lawrence Erlbaum & Associates.

Kosslyn, S. M. (1987). Seeing and imaging in the cerebral hemispheres: A computational approach. *Psychological Review, 94,* 148–175.

Kosslyn, S. M. (1988). Aspects of cognitive neuroscience of mental imagery. *Science, 240,* 1621–1626.

Kosslyn, S. M., Anderson, A. K., Hillger, L. A., Hamilton, S. E. (1994). Hemispheric differences in sizes of receptive fields or attentional biases? *Neuropsychology, 8,* 139–147.

Kosslyn, S. M., Chabris, C. F., Marsolek, C. J., Koenig, O. (1992). Categorical versus coordinate spatial relations: Computational analyses and computer simulations. *Journal of Experimental Psychology: Human Perception and Performance, 18,* 562–577.

Kosslyn, S. M., Flynn, R. A., Amsterdam, J. B., & Wang, G. (1990). Components of high-level vision: A cognitive neuroscience analysis and accounts of neurological syndromes. *Cognition, 34,* 203–277.

Kosslyn, S. M., Holtzman, J., Farah, M. J., & Gazzaniga, M. A. (1985). A computational analysis of mental image generation: Evidence from functional dissociations in split-brain patients. *Journal of Experimental Psychology: General, 114,* 311–341.

Kosslyn, S. M. & Koenig, O. (1992). *Wet mind: The new cognitive neuroscience.* New York: Free Press.

Kosslyn, S. M., Koenig, O., Barret, A., Cave, C. B., Tang, J., & Gabrieli, J. D. E. (1989). Evidence for two types of spatial representations: Hemispheric specialization for categorical and coordinate relations. *Journal of Experimental Psychology, 15,* 723–735.

Kramer, A. F. & Jacobson, A. (1991). Perceptual organization and focused attention: The role of objects and proximity in visual processing. *Perception and Psychophysics, 50,* 267–284.

Kramer, J. H., Blusewicz, M. J., Robertson, L. C., & Preston, K. (1989). The effects of chronic alcoholism on perception of hierarchical visual stimuli. *Alcoholism: Clinical and Experimental Research, 13,* 240–245.

Krech, D. & Calvin, A. (1953). Levels of perceptual organization and cognition. *Journal of Abnormal and Social Psychology, 48,* 394–400.

Krechevsky, I. (1938). An experimental investigation of the principle of proximity in the visual perception of the rat. *Journal of Experimental Psychology, 22,* 497–523.

Krieman, J. & Van Lancker, D. (1988). Hemispheric specialization for voice recognition: Evidence from dichotic listening. *Brain and Language, 34,* 246–252.

LaBerge, D. & Brown, V. (1989). Theory of attentional operations in shape identification. *Psychological Review, 96,* 101–124.

LaBerge, D. & Buchsbaum, M. S. (1990). Positron emission tomographic measurements of pulvinar activity during an attention task. *Journal of Neuroscience, 10,* 613–619.

Ladavas, E. (1987). Is the hemispatial deficit produced by right parietal lobe damage associated with retinal or gravitational coordinates? *Brain, 110,* 167–180.

Laeng, B. (1994). Lateralization of categorical and coordinate spatial functions: A study of unilateral stroke patients. *Journal of Cognitive Neuroscience, 6,* 189–203.

LaGasse, L. L. (1993). Effects of good form and spatial frequency on global percedence. *Perception and Psychophysics, 53,* 89–105.

Lamb, M. R. & Robertson, L. C. (1987). The effect of acute alcohol on attention and the processing of hierarchical patterns. *Alcoholism: Clinical and Experimental Research, 11,* 243–248.

Lamb, M. R., & Robertson, L. C. (1988). The processing of hierarchical stimuli: Effects of retinal locus, locational uncertainty and stimulus identity. *Perception and Psychophysics, 44,* 172–181.

Lamb, M. R. & Robertson, L. C. (1989). Do response time advantage and interference reflect the order of processing of global and local level information? *Perception and Psychophysics, 46,* 254–258.

Lamb, M. R. & Robertson, L. C. (1990). The effects of visual angle on global and local reaction times depends on the set of visual angles presented. *Perception and Psychophysics, 47,* 489–496.

Lamb, M. R., Robertson, L. C., & Knight, R. T. (1989). Attention and interference in the processing of global and local information: Effects of unilateral temporal-parietal junction lesions. *Neuropsychologia, 4,* 471–483.

Lamb, M. R. & Robertson, L. C., & Knight, R. T. (1990). Component mechanisms underlying the processing of hierarchically organized patterns: Inferences from patients with unilateral cortical lesions. *Journal of Experimental Psychology: Learning, Memory and Cognition, 16,* 471–483.

Lamb, M. R. & Yund, E. W. (1993). The role of spatial frequency in the processing of hierarchically organized stimuli. *Perception and Psychophysics, 54,* 773–784.

Lamb, M. R. & Yund, E. W. (1996). Spatial frequency and attention: Effects of level-, target-, and location-repetition on the processing of global and local forms. *Perception and Psychophysics, 58,* 363–373.

Lauter, J. L., Herscovitch, P., Formby, C., & Raichle, M. E. (1985). Tonotopic organization in the human auditory cortex revealed by positron emission tomography. *Hearing Research, 20,* 199–205.

LeDoux, J. E., Wilson, D. H., & Gazzaniga, M. S. (1977). Manipulospatial aspects of cerebral lateralization: Clues to the origin of lateralization. *Neuropsychologia, 15,* 743–750.

Lehiste, I. (1970). *Suprasegmentals.* Cambridge, Mass.: MIT Press.

Levy, J., Trevarthen, C., & Sperry, R. (1972). Perception of bilateral chimeric figures following hemisphere disconnection. *Brain, 5,* 61–68.

Ley, R. G. & Bryden, M. P. (1982). A dissociation of right and left hemisphere effects for recognizing emotional tone and verbal content. *Brain and Cognition, 1*, 3–9.

Liberman, A. M., Cooper, F. S., Shankweiler, D. P., & Studdert-Kennedy, M. (1967). Perception of the speech code. *Psychological Review, 74*, 431–461.

Liberman, A. M., Delattre, P. C., & Cooper, F. S. (1958). Some cues for the distinction between voiced and voiceless stops in initial position. *Language and Speech, 1*, 153–167.

Liberman, A. M. & Mattingly, I. G. (1989). A specialization for speech perception. *Science, 243*, 489–494.

Lieberman, P. (1991). *Uniquely human: The evolution of speech, thought, and selfless behavior.* Cambridge, Mass.: Harvard University Press.

Lisker, L. (1975). Is it VOT of a first-formant transition detector? *Journal of the Acoustical Society of America, 56*, 1547–1551.

Lisker, L. & Abramson, A. (1964). A cross-language study of voicing in initial stops: Acoustical measurements. *Word, 20*, 384–422.

Livingstone, M. S., Rosen, G. D., Drislane, F. W., & Galaburda, A. M. (1991). Physiological and anatomical evidence for a magnocellular defect in developmental dyslexia. *Proceedings of the National Academy of Science U.S.A., 88*, 7943–7947.

Logan, G. D. (1995). Linguistic and conceptual control of visual spatial attention. *Cognitive Psychology, 28*, 103–174.

Lovegrove, W. (1993). Weakness in the transient visual system: A causal factor in dyslexia? *Annals of the New York Academy of Sciences, 682*, 57–69.

Luck, S. J., Hillyard, S. A., Mangun, G. R., & Gazzaniga, M. S. (1994). Independent attentional scanning in the separated hemispheres of split-brain patients. *Journal of Cognitive Neuroscience, 6*, 84–91.

Luria, A. R., Tsvetkova, L. S., & Futer, J. C. (1965). Aphasia in a composer. *Journal of Neurological Science, 2*, 288–292.

Maglioli, B. S., Buchtel, H. A., Campanini, T., & DeRisio, C. (1979). Cerebral hemispheric lateralization of cognitive deficits due to alcoholism. *Journal of Nervous and Mental Disease, 167*, 212–217.

Majkowski, J., Bochenek, Z., Bochenek, W., Knapik-Fijalkowska, D., & Kopec, J. (1971). Latency of averaged evoked potentials to contralateral and ipsilateral auditory stimulation in normal subjects. *Brain Research, 25*, 416–419.

Makela, J. P., Ahonen, A., Hamalainen, M., Hari, R., Ilmoniemi, R., Kajola, M., Knuutila, J., et al. (1993). Functional differences between auditory cortices of the two hemispheres revealed by whole-head neuromagnetic recordings. *Human Brain Mapping, 1*, 48–56.

Mandelbrot, B. (1977). *Fractals—Form, Chance and Dimension.* San Francisco: W. H. Freeman.

Mangun, G. R. & Heinze, H. J. (1995). Combining electrophysiology with neuroimaging in the study of human cognition. In H. Mueller-Gartner (Ed.), *Supercomputers in brain research from tomography to neural networks* (pp. 61–74). N.J.: World Scientific Publications.

Mangun, G. R., Woldorff, M. G., & Luck, S. J. (1995). Neural systems mediating selective attention. In M. Gazzaniga (Ed.), *The cognitive neurosciences* (pp. 665–682). Cambridge, Mass.: MIT Press.

Marr, D. (1982). *Vision.* San Francisco: W. H. Freeman.

Martin, M. (1979a). Local and global processing: The role of sparsity. *Memory and Cognition, 7*, 476–484.

Martin, M. (1979b). Hemispheric specialization for local and global processing. *Neuropsychologia, 17*, 33–40.

Martin, E. M., Pitrak, D. L., Robertson, L. C., Novak, R. M., Mullane, D. M., & Pursell, K. J. (1995). Divided attention in HIV-1 infection. *Neuropsychology, 9*, 102–109.

Martinez, A., Moses, P., Frank, L., Blaettler, D., Stiles, J., Wong, E., & Buxton, R. (June 1996). Lateralized differences in spatial processing: Evidence from RT and fMRI. Paper presented at the Second International Conference on Functional Mapping of the Human Brain, Boston.

Mazziotta, J. C., Phelps, M. E., Carson, R. E., & Kuhl, D. E. (1982). Tomographic mapping of human cerebral metabolism: Auditory stimulation. *Neurology, 32*, 921–937.

McFie, J., Piercy, M. F., & Zangwill, O. L. (1950). Visual-spatial agnosia associated with lesions of the right cerebral hemisphere. *Brain, 73*, 167–190.

McFie, J. & Zangwill, O. L. (1960). Visual-constructive disabilities associated with lesions of the left cerebral hemisphere. *Brain, 83*, 243–260.

Merzenich, M. M., Jenkins, W. M., Johnston, P., Schreiner, C., Miller, S. L., & Tallal, P. (1996). Temporal processing deficits of language-learning impaired children ameliorated by training. *Science, 271*, 77–81.

Michel, F. & Henaff, M. A. (March 1996). Two types of visual agnosia: Occipital-temporal versus occipito-parietal. Paper presented at meeting of the Cognitive Neurosciences Society, San Francisco.

Michimata, C. & Hellige, J. B. (1987). Effects of blurring and stimulus size on the lateralized processing of nonverbal stimuli. *Neuropsychologia, 25*, 397–407.

Miglioli, H., Buchtel, H. A., Campanini, T., & DeRisio, C. (1979). Cerebral hemispheric lateralization of cognitive deficits due to alcoholism. *Journal of Nervous Disorders, 167*, 212–217.

Miller, S. L., Delaney, T. V., & Tallal, P. (1995). Speech and other central auditory processes: Insights from cognitive neuroscience. *Current Opinion in Neurobiology, 5*, 198–204.

Miller, W. R. & Orr, J. (1980). Nature and sequence of neuropsychological deficits in alcoholics. *Journal of Studies in Alcohol, 41*, 325–337.

Milner, B. (1962). Laterality effects in audition. In V. B. Mountcastle (Ed.), *Interhemispheric relations and cerebral dominance* (pp. 177–195). Baltimore: Johns Hopkins University Press.

Milner, B. (1968). Visual recognition and recall after right temporal lobe excision in man. *Neuropsychologia, 6*, 191–209.

Milner, B., Taylor, L., & Sperry, R. W. (1968). Lateralized suppression of dichotically presented digits after commissural section in man. *Science, 161*, 184–185.

Mishkin, M. & Forgays, D. G. (1952). Word recognition as a function of retinal locus. *Journal of Experimental Psychology, 43*, 43–48.

Mody, M., Studdert-Kennedy, M., & Brady, S. (in press). Speech perception deficits in poor readers: Auditory processing or phonological coding? *Journal of Experimental Child Psychology.*

Molfese, D. L. (1978a). Left and right hemisphere involvement in speech perception: Electrophysiological correlates. *Perception and Psychophysics, 23*, 237–243.

Molfese, D. L. (1978b). Neuroelectrical correlates of categorical speech perception in adults. *Brain and Language, 5*, 25–35.

Molfese, D. L. (1980). Hemispheric specialization for temporal information: Implications for the perception of voicing cues during speech perception. *Brain and Language, 11,* 285–299.

Molfese, D. L. & Hess, T. (1978). Hemispheric specialization for VOT perception in preschool children. *Journal of Experimental Child Psychology, 26,* 71–84.

Monrad-Krohn. (1947). Dysprosody or altered "melody of language." *Brain, 70,* 405–415.

Moon, C., Cooper, R. P., and Fifer, W. P. (1993). Two-day-olds prefer their native language. *Infant Behavior and Development, 16,* 495–500.

Morais, J. & Bertelson, P. (1975). Spatial position versus ear of entry as determinant of the auditory laterality effects: A stereophonic test. *Journal of Experimental Psychology: Human Perception and Performance, 1,* 253–262.

Moran, J. & Desimone, R. (1985). Selective attention gates visual processing in the extrastriate cortex. *Science, 229,* 782–784.

Morrow, L. & Ratcliffe, G. (1988). The disengagement of covert attention and the neglect syndrome. *Psychobiology, 16,* 261–269.

Mountcastle, V. B. (1978). Brain mechanisms for directed attention. *Journal of the Royal Society of Medicine, 71,* 14–28.

Navon, D. (1977). Forest before the trees: The precedence of global features in visual perception. *Cognitive Psychology, 9,* 353–393.

Nebes, R. D. (1972). Dominance of the minor hemisphere in commissurotomized man on a test of figural unification. *Brain, 95,* 633–638.

Nebes, R. D. (1973). Perception of spatial relationships by the right and left hemispheres in commissurotomized man. *Neuropsychologia, 11,* 285–289.

Newcombe, F. (1969). *Missile wounds of the brain: A study of psychological deficits.* Oxford: Oxford University Press.

Newcombe, F., De Haan, E. H. F., Ross, J., & Young, A. W. (1989). Face processing, laterality and contrast sensitivity. *Neuropsychologia, 27,* 523–538.

Newcombe, F. & Russell, W. R. (1969). Dissociated visual perceptual and spatial deficits in focal lesions of the right hemisphere. *Journal of Neurology, Neurosurgery, and Psychiatry, 32,* 73–81.

Nordahl, T. E., Kusubov, N., Carter, C., Salamat, S., Cummings, A. M., O'Shora-Celaya, L., Eberling, J., Robertson, L. C., Huesman, R. H, Jagust, W., & Budinger, T. F. (1996). Temporal lobe glucose metabolic differences in medication-free out-patients with schizophrenia via the PET-600. *Neuropsychopharmacology, 15,* 542–554.

Nordahl, T. E., Robertson, L. C., Carter, C., Chaderjian, M., & O'Shora-Celaya, L. (1994). Left midtemporal metabolic activity correlates with a global/local task parameter in unmedicated patients with schizophrenia. Paper presented at the West Coast Society for Biological Psychiatry, Lake Tahoe, Calif.

O'Boyle, M. W. & Hellige, J. B. (1982). Hemispheric asymmetry, early visual processes and serial memory comparison. *Brain and Language, 1,* 224–243.

Ogden, J. A. (1987). The "neglected" left hemisphere and its contribution to visuospatial neglect. In M. Jeannerod (Ed.), *Neurophysiological and neuropsychological aspects of spatial neglect.* Amsterdam: Elsevier Science Publications.

Palmer, S. E. (1980). What makes triangles point: Local and global effects in configurations of ambiguous triangles. *Cognitive Psychology, 12,* 285–305.

Palmer, S. E. (1982). Symmetry, transformation, and the structure of perceptual systems. In J. Beck (Ed.), *Organization and representation in perception*. Hillsdale, N.J.: Lawrence Erlbaum & Associates.

Palmer, S. E. & Kimchi, R. (1986). The information processing approach to cognition. In T. J. Knapp & L. C. Robertson (Eds.), *Approaches to cognition: Contrasts and controversies*. Hillsdale, N.J.: Lawrence Erlbaum & Associates.

Pantev, C., Hoke, M., Lutkenhoner, B., & Lehnertz, K. (1989). Tonotopic organization of the auditory cortex: Pitch versus frequency representation. *Science, 246,* 486–488.

Paquette, C., Bourassa, M., & Peretz, I. (1996). Left ear advantage in pitch perception of complex tones without energy at the fundamental frequency. *Neuropsychologia, 34,* 153–157.

Parsons, O. A. & Farr, S. P. (1981). The neuropsychology of alcohol and drug use. In S. Filskov & T. Boll (Ed.), *Handbook of clinical psychology*. New York: John Wiley & Sons.

Parsons, O. A. & Leber, W. R. (1981). The relationship between cognitive dysfunction and brain damage in alcoholics: Causal, interactive or epiphenomenal? *Alcoholism, 5,* 326–343.

Patterson, K., Vargha-Khadem, F., & Polkey, C. E. (1989). Reading with one hemisphere. *Brain, 112,* 39–63.

Penfield, W. & Perot, P. (1963). The brain's record of auditory and visual experience. *Brain, 86,* 595–697.

Peretz, I. (1990). Processing of local and global musical information by unilateral brain-damaged patients. *Brain, 113,* 1185–1205.

Peretz, I. & Babai, M. (1992). The role of contour and intervals in the recognition of melody parts: Evidence from cerebral asymmetries in musicians. *Neuropsychologia, 30,* 277–292.

Peretz, I. & Morais, J. (1980). Modes of processing melodies and ear asymmetry in non-musicians. *Neuropsychologia, 18,* 477–489.

Peretz, I. & Morais, J. (1987). Analytic processing in the classification of melodies as same or different. *Neuropsychologia, 25,* 645–652.

Peretz, I. & Morais, J. (1993). Specificity for music. In F. Boller & J. Grafman (Eds.), *Handbook of neuropsychology* (pp. 373–389). New York: Elsevier Science Publishers.

Petersen, S. E., Fox, P. T., Posner, M. I., Mintun, M., & Raichle, R. E. (1988). Positron emission tomographic studies of the cortical anatomy of single-word processing. *Nature, 331,* 585–589.

Peterzell, D. H. (1991). On the nonrelation between spatial frequency and cerebral hemispheric competence. *Brain and Cognition, 15,* 62–68.

Peterzell, D. H., Harvey, L. O. J., & Hardyck, C. D. (1989). Spatial frequencies and the cerebral hemispheres: Contrast sensitivity, visible persistence, and letter classification. *Perception and Psychophysics, 46,* 443–445.

Phillips, C., Marantz, A., Poeppel, D., Pesetsky, D., Wexler, K., & Yellin, E. (June 1995). Categorical perception in auditory cortex: Continuous and categorical representations of VOT. Paper presented at the First Annual Human Brain Mapping Conference, Paris.

Phillips, D. P. & Gates, G. R. (1982). Representation of the two ears in the auditory cortex: A re-examination. *International Journal of Neuroscience, 16,* 41–46.

Phillips, D. P. & Irvine, D. R. F. (1981). Responses of single neurons in physiologically-defined area A1 of cat cerebral cortex: Sensitivity to interaural intensity differences. *Hearing Research, 4,* 299–307.

Piercy, M., Hacaen, H., & de Ajuriaguerra, J. (1960). Constructional apraxia associated with unilateral cerebral lesions: Left and right sided cases compared. *Brain, 83,* 225–242.

Piercy, M. & Smyth, V. O. G. (1962). Right hemisphere dominance for certain nonverbal intellectual skills. *Brain, 85,* 775–790.

Pisoni, D. B. & Martin, C. S. (1989). Effects of alcohol on the acoustic-phonetic properties of speech: Perceptual and acoustic analyses. *Alcoholism: Clinical and Experimental Research, 13,* 577–587.

Pomerantz, J. R. (1983). Global and local precedence: Selective attention in form and motion perception. *Journal of Experimental Psychology: General, 112,* 516–540.

Poppelreuter, W. (1917). Die psychiscen Schaedigungen durch Kopfschuss im Kriege, 1914–1916. Band 1. Die Storungen der niederen und hoheren Seheleistungen durch Verletzungen des Okzipitalhirns. Leipzig: L. Voss. (In De Renzi, 1982).

Posner, M. I. (1978). *Chronometric explorations of mind.* Hillsdale, N.J.: Erlbaum Associates.

Posner, M. I. (1980). Orienting of attention. *Quarterly Journal of Experimental Psychology, 32,* 3–25

Posner, M. I. & Raichle, M. E. (1994). *Images of Mind.* New York: W. H. Freeman.

Posner, M. I., Early, R. S., Reiman, E., Pardo, P. J., & Dhawan, M. (1988). Asymmetries in hemispheric control of attention in schizophrenia. *Archives of General Psychiatry, 45,* 814–821.

Posner, M. I., Inhoff, A. W., Friedrich, F. J., & Cohen, A. (1987). Isolating attentional systems: A cognitive-anatomical analysis. *Psychobiology, 15,* 107–121.

Posner, M. I. & Petersen, S. E. (1990). The attention system of the human brain. *Annual Review of Neuroscience, 13,* 25–42.

Posner, M. I., Walker, J. A., Friedrich, F. J., & Rafal, R. D. (1984). Effects of parietal injury on covert orienting of attention. *Journal of Neuroscience, 4,* 1863–1874.

Post, R. B., Lott, L. A., Maddock, R. J., & Beede, J. I. (1996). An effect of alcohol on the distribution of spatial attention. *Journal of Studies on Alcohol, 57,* 260–266.

Previc, F. H. (1991). A general theory concerning the prenatal origins of cerebral lateralization in humans. *Psychological Review, 98,* 299–334.

Rafal, R. (1996). Balint's syndrome. In T. W. Feinberg & M. J. Farah (Eds.), *Behavioral neurology and neuropsychology.* New York: McGraw-Hill.

Rafal, R. & Henik, A. (1994). The neurology of inhibition: Integrating controlled and automatic processes. In D. Dagenbach & T. H. Carr (Eds.), *Inhibitory processes and attention, memory, and language.* San Diego: Academic Press.

Rafal, R. & Robertson, L. (1995). The neurology of visual attention. In M. S. Gazzaniga (Ed.), *The cognitive neurosciences.* Cambridge, Mass.: MIT Press.

Rao, S. M., Rourke, D., & Whitman, R. D. (1981). Spatio-temporal discrimination of frequency in the right and left visual fields: A preliminary report. *Perceptual and Motor Skills, 53,* 311–316.

Rasmussen, T. & Milner, B. (1977). The role of early left-brain injury in determining lateralization of cerebral speech functions. In S. J. Dimond & D. A. Blizard (Eds.), (pp. 355–369). New York Academy of Sciences.

Rebai, M., Mecacci, L., Bagot, J. D., & Bonnet, C. (1989). Influence of spatial frequency and handedness on hemispheric asymmetry in visually steady-state evoked potentials. *Neuropsychologia, 27,* 315–324.

Reuter-Lorenz, P. A., Kinsbourne, M., & Moscovitch, M. (1990). Hemispheric control of spatial attention. *Brain and Cognition, 12,* 240–266.

Rhodes, D. L. & Robertson, L. C. (1996, April). Scene-based processing in spatial attention. Paper presented at the annual meeting of Cognitive Neuroscience Society, San Francisco.

Ringo, J. L., Doty, R. W., Demeter, S., & Simard, P. Y. (1994). Time is of the essence: A conjecture that hemispheric specialization arises from interhemispheric conduction delay. *Cerebral Cortex, 4,* 331–43.

Robertson, I. H. & Marshall, J. C. (Eds.) (1993). *Unilateral neglect: Clinical and experimental studies.* Hove, UK: Lawrence Erlbaum.

Robertson, L. C. (1986). From gestalt to neo-gestalt. In T. J. Knapp and L. C. Robertson (Eds.), *Approaches to cognition: Contrasts and controversies.* Hillsdale, N.J.: Lawrence Erlbaum & Associates.

Robertson, L. C. (1994). Hemisphere specialization and cooperation in processing complex visual patterns. In F. L. Kitterle (Ed.), *Hemispheric communication: Mechanisms and models.* Hillsdale, N.J.: Lawrence Erlbaum & Associates.

Robertson, L. C. (1995a). Covert orienting biases in scene-based reference frames: Orientation priming and visual field differences. *Journal of Experimental Psychology: Human Perception and Performance, 21,* 707–718.

Robertson, L. C. (1995b). Perceptual disturbances in focal neurological diseases. In B. S. Fogel, R. B. Shiffer, & S. M. Rao (Eds.), *Neuropsychiatry: A comprehensive textbook* (pp. 345–364). Baltimore: Williams & Wilkins.

Robertson, L. C. (1996). Attentional persistence for features of hierarchical patterns. *Journal of Experimental Psychology: General, 125,* 227–249.

Robertson, L. C. & Delis, D. C. (1986). "Part-whole" processing in unilateral brain damaged patients: Dysfunction of hierarchical organization. *Neuropsychologia, 24,* 363–370.

Robertson, L. C. & Eglin, M. (1993). Attention search in unilateral visual neglect. In I. Robertson & J. Marshall (Eds.), *Unilateral neglect: Clinical and experimental studies* (pp. 169–191). London: Taylor and Francis.

Robertson, L. C., Egly, R., Lamb, M. R., & Kerth, L. (1993). Spatial attention and cuing to global and local levels of hierarchical structure. *Journal of Experimental Psychology: Human Perception and Performance, 19,* 471–487.

Robertson, L. C. & Lamb, M. R. (1988). The role of perceptual reference frames in visual field asymmetries. *Neuropsychologia, 26,* 145–152.

Robertson, L. C. & Lamb, M. R. (1989). Judging the reflection of misoriented patterns in the right and left visual fields. *Neuropsychologia, 27,* 1081–1089.

Robertson, L. C. & Lamb, M. R. (1991). Neuropsychological contributions to theories of part/whole organization. *Cognitive Psychology, 23,* 299–330.

Robertson, L. C., Lamb, M. R., & Knight, R. T. (1988). Effects of lesions of temporal-parietal junction on perceptual and attentional processing in humans. *Journal of Neuroscience, 8,* 3757–3769.

Robertson, L. C., Lamb, M. R., & Knight, R. T. (1991). Normal global-local analysis in patients with dorsolateral frontal lobe lesions. *Neuropsychologia, 29,* 959–967.

Robertson, L. C., Lamb, M. R., & Zaidel, E. (1993). Interhemispheric relations in processing hierarchical patterns: Evidence from normal and commissurotomized subjects. *Neuropsychology, 7,* 325–342.

Robertson, L. C., Palmer, S. E., & Gomez, L. M. (1987). Reference frames in mental rotation. *Journal of Experimental Psychology: Learning, Memory and Cognition, 13,* 368–379.

Robertson, L. C., Stillman, R., & Delis, D. C. (1985). The effect of alcohol on establishing perceptual references frames. *Neuropsychologia, 23,* 69–76.

Robertson, L. C., Knight, R. T., Rafal, R., & Shimamura, A. P. (1993). Cognitive neuropsychology is more than single-case studies. *Journal of Experimental Psychology: Learning, Memory, & Cognition, 19,* 710–717.

Robertson, L. C., Triesman, A., Friedman-Hill, S., & Grabowecky, M. (1997). The interaction of spatial and object pathways: Evidence from Balint's syndrome. *Journal of Cognitive Neuroscience, 9,* 295–317.

Robin, D. A., Tranel, D., & Damasio, H. (1990). Auditory perception of temporal and spectral events in patients with focal left and right cerebral lesions. *Brain and Language, 39,* 539–555.

Robinson, G. M. & Solomon, D. J. (1974). Rhythm is processed by the speech hemisphere. *Journal of Experimental Psychology, 102,* 508–511.

Robson, J. G. (1966). Spatial and contrast sensitivity functions of the visual system. *Journal of the Optical Society of America, 56,* 1141–1142.

Rose, D. (1983). An investigation into hemisphere differences in adaptation to contrast. *Perception and Psychophysics, 34,* 89–95.

Rosenzweig, M. R. (1951). Representation of the two ears at the auditory cortex. *American Journal of Physiology, 167,* 147–158.

Ross, E. D. (1981). The aprosodias: Functional-anatomic organization of the affective components of language in the right hemisphere. *Archives of Neurology, 38,* 561–567.

Ross, E. D., Edmondson, J. A., & Seibert, G. B. (1986). The effect of affect on various acoustic measures of prosody in tone and non-tone languages: A comparison based on computer analysis of voice. *Journal of Phonetics, 14,* 283–302.

Ross, E. D., Edmondson, J. A., Seibert, G. B., & Homan, R. W. (1988). Acoustic analysis of affective prosody during right-sided Wada test: A within-subjects verification of the right hemisphere's role in language. *Brain and Language, 33,* 128–145.

Ross, E. D. & Mesulam, M. M. (1979). Dominant language functions of the right hemisphere? Prosody and emotional gesturing. *Archives of Neurology, 36,* 144–148.

Rovamo, J., Virsu, V., & Nasanen, R. (1978). Cortical magnification factor predicts the photopic contrast sensitivity of peripheral vision. *Nature, 271,* 54–56.

Rozin, P. (1976). The evolution of intelligence and access to the cognitive unconscious. *Progress in psychobiology and physiological psychology* (Vol. 6). New York: Academic Press.

Rummelhart, D. E. & McClelland, J. L. (1986). *Parallel distributed processing: Explorations in the microstructure of cognition.* Cambridge, Mass.: MIT Press.

Rybash, J. M. & Hoyer, W. J. (1992). Hemispheric specialization for categorical and coordinate spatial representations: A reappraisal. *Memory and Cognition, 20,* 271–276.

Salo, R., Robertson, L., & Nordahl, T. (1996). Normal sustained effects of selective attention are absent in unmedicated patients with schizophrenia. *Psychology Research, 62,* 121–130.

Scharf, B., Quigley, S., Aoki, C., Peachey, N., & Reeves, A. (1987). Focused auditory attention and frequency selectivity. *Perception and Psychophysics, 42,* 215–223.

Schlauch, R. S. & Hafter, E. R. (1991). Listening bandwidths and frequency uncertainty in pure-tone signal detection. *Journal of the Acoustical Society of America, 90,* 1332–1339.

Schneider, W. (October 1993). Functional MRI: Mapping the visual system with mm resolution. Paper presented at the 34th Annual Meeting of the Psychonomic Society, Washington, D.C.

Schwartz, J. R. & Tallal, P. (1980). Rate of acoustic change may underlie hemispheric specialization for speech perception. *Science, 207,* 1380–1381.

Sergent, J. (1982). The cerebral balance of power: Confrontation or cooperation. *Journal of Experimental Psychology: Human Perception and Performance, 8,* 253–272.

Sergent, J. (1983). Role of input in visual hemispheric asymmetries. *Psychological Bulletin, 93,* 481–512.

Sergent, J. (1985). Influence of input and task factors in hemispheric involvement in face processing. *Journal of Experimental Psychology: Human Perception & Performance, 11,* 846–861.

Sergent, J. (1986). Methodological constraints on neuropsychological studies of face perception in normals. In R. Bruyer (Ed.), *The neuropsychology of face perception and facial expression.* Hillsdale, N.J.: Lawrence Erlbaum & Associates.

Sergent, J. (1991). Judgments of relative position and distance in representations of spatial relations. *Journal of Experimental Psychology: Human Perception and Performance, 17,* 762–780.

Sergent, J. (1993). Music, the brain and Ravel. *Trends in Neuroscience, 16,* 168–172.

Sergent, J. & Hellige, J. B. (1986). Role of input factors in visual-field asymmetries. *Brain and Cognition, 5,* 174–199.

Shankweiler, D. (1966). Effects of temporal-lobe damage on perception of dichotically presented melodies. *Journal of Comparative Psychology, 62,* 115–119.

Shankweiler, D. & Studdert-Kennedy, M. (1967). Identification of consonants and vowels presented to left and right ears. *Quarterly Journal of Experimental Psychology, 19,* 59–63.

Shapiro, B. E. & Danly, M. (1985). The role of right hemisphere in the control of speech prosody in propositional and affective contexts. *Brain and Language, 25,* 19–36.

Shapley, R. (1985). Spatial frequency analysis in the visual system. *Annual Review of Neuroscience, 8,* 447–483.

Shettleworth, S. J. (1983). Memory in food-hoarding birds. *Scientific American, 248,* 102–110.

Shipley-Brown, F., Dingwall, W. O., Berlin, C. I., Yeni-Komshian, G., & Gordon-Salant, S. (1988). Hemispheric processing of affective and linguistic intonation contours in normal subjects. *Brain and Language, 33,* 16–26.

Shulman, G. L., Sullivan, M. A., Gish, K., & Sakoda, W. J. (1986). The role of spatial frequency channels in the perception of local and global structure. *Perception, 15,* 259–273.

Shulman, G. L. & Wilson, J. (1987). Spatial frequency and selective attention to local and global information. *Perception, 16,* 89–101.

Sidtis, J. J. (1980). On the nature of the cortical function underlying right hemisphere auditory perception. *Neuropsychologia, 18,* 321–330.

Sidtis, J. J. (1981). The complex tone test: Implications for the assessment of auditory laterality effects. *Neuropsychologia, 19,* 103–112.

Sidtis, J. J. (1988). Dichotic listening after commisurotomy. In K. Hugdahl (Ed.), *Handbook of dichotic listening: Theory, methods, and research* (pp. 161–184). New York: John Wiley & Sons.

Sidtis, J. J. & Volpe, B. T. (1988). Selective loss of complex-pitch or speech discrimination after unilateral lesion. *Brain and Language, 34,* 235–245.

Smith, M. E. & Oscar-Berman, M. (1991). Attention, apperception and alcoholism. Paper presented at symposium of International Neuropsychological Society, San Antonio, Texas.

Sparks, R. & Geschwind, N. (1968). Dichotic listening in man after section of neocortical commissures. *Cortex, 4,* 3–16.

Sperry, R. W. (1968). Hemisphere disconnection and unity in conscious awareness. *American Psychologist, 23,* 723–733.

Sperry, R. W. (1993). The impact and promise of the cognitive revolution. *American Psychologist, 48,* 878–891.

Spinelli, D. & Zoccolotti, P. (1992). Perception of moving and stationary gratings in brain damaged patients with unilateral spatial neglect. *Neuropsychologia, 30,* 393–401.

Sprague, J. M. (1991). The role of the superior colliculus in facilitating visual attention and form perception. *Proceedings of the National Academy of Sciences, 88,* 1286–1290.

Springer, S. P. & Deutsch, G. (1981). *Left brain, right brain.* San Francisco: W. H. Freeman.

Stein, D. G., Brailowsky, S., & Will, B. (1995). *Brain repair.* New York: Oxford University Press.

Stevens, K. N. & Blumstein, S. E. (1981). The search for invariant acoustic correlates of phonetic features. In P. D. Eimas & J. L. Miller (Eds.), *Perspectives on the study of speech.* Hillsdale, N.J.: Erlbaum & Associates.

Stevens, K. N. & Klatt, D. H. (1974). Role of formant transitions in the voiced-voiceless distinction for stops. *Journal of the Acoustic Society of America, 55,* 653–659.

Studdert-Kennedy, M. & Mody, M. (1995). Auditory temporal perception deficits in the reading-impaired: A critical review of the evidence. *Psychonomic Bulletin and Review, 2,* 508–514.

Studdert-Kennedy, M. & Shankweiler, S. (1970). Hemispheric specialization for speech perception. *Journal of Acoustical Society of America, 48,* 579–594.

Summerfield, A. Q. & Haggard, M. P. (1974). Perceptual processing of multiple cues and contexts: Effects of following vowel upon stop consonant voicing. *Journal of Phonetics, 2,* 279–295.

Szelag, E., Budohoska, W., & Koltuska, B. (1987). Hemispheric differences in the perception of gratings. *Bulletin of the Psychonomic Society, 25,* 95–98.

Tallal, P. (1980). Auditory temporal perception, phonics, and reading disabilities. *Brain and Language, 9,* 182–198.

Tallal, P., Miller, S. L., Bedi, G., Byma, G., Wang, X., Nagarajan, S. S., Schreiner, C., Jenkins, W., & Merzenich, M. M. (1996). Language comprehension in language-learning impaired children improved with acoustically modified speech. *Science, 271,* 81–84.

Tallal, P., Miller, S., & Fitch, R. H. (1993). Neurobiological basis of speech: A case for the preeminence of temporal processing. *Annals of the New York Academy of Sciences, 682,* 27–47.

Tallal, P. & Newcombe, F. (1978). Impairment of auditory perception and language comprehension in dysphasia. *Brain and Language, 5,* 13–24.

Tallal, P. & Piercy, M. (1973). Defects of non-verbal auditory perception in children with developmental aphasia. *Nature, 241,* 468–469.

Tallal, P. & Piercy, M. (1975). Developmental aphasia: The perception of brief vowels and extended stop consonants. *Neuropsychologia, 13,* 69–74.

Tallal, P., Stark, R., Kallman, C., & Mellits, D. (1981). A reexamination of some nonverbal perceptual abilities of language-impaired and normal children as a function of age and sensory modality. *Journal of Speech and Hearing Research, 24*, 351–357.

Tanguay, P., Taub, J., Doubleday, C., & Clarkson, D. (1977). An interhemispheric comparison of auditory evoked responses to consonant-vowel stimuli. *Neuropsychologia, 15*, 123–131.

Tayler, A. T. & Hellige, J. B. (1987). Effects of retinal size on visual laterality. *Bulletin of the Psychonomic Society, 25*, 444–446.

Tootell, R. B., Silverman, M. J., Switkes, E., & De Valois, R. L. (1982). Deoxyglucose analysis of retinotopic organization in primary striate cortex. *Science, 218*, 902–904.

Treisman, A. (1969). Strategies and models of selective attention. *Psychological Review, 76*, 282–299.

Treisman, A. (1988). Features and objects: The fourteenth Barlett memorial lecture. *Quarterly Journal of Experimental Psychology, 40A*, 201–237.

Treisman, A. & Gelade, G. (1980). A feature integration theory of attention. *Cognitive Psychology, 12*, 97–136.

Tucker, D. M., Watson, R. T., & Heilman, K. M. (1977). Discrimination and evocation of affectively intoned speech in patients with right parietal disease. *Neurology, 27*, 947–950.

Tucker, D. M. & Williamson, P. A. (1984). Asymmetric neural control systems in human self-regulation. *Psychological Review, 91*, 185–215.

Turkewitz, G. (1988). A prenatal source for the development of hemispheric specialization. In D. L. Molfese and S. J. Segalowitz (Eds.), *Brain Lateralization in Children: Developmental Implications* (pp. 73–81). New York: Guilford Press.

Tyler, H. R. (1968). Abnormalities of perception with defective eye movements (Balint's syndrome). *Cortex, 4*, 154–171.

Ungerleider, L. G. & Mishkin, M. (1982). Two cortical visual systems. In D. J. Ingle, M. A. Goodale, & R. J. W. Mansfield (Eds.), *Analysis of visual behavior.* Cambridge, Mass.: MIT Press.

Ungerleider, L. G. & Mishkin, M. (1994). "What" and "where" in the human brain. *Current Opinion in Neurobiology, 4*, 157–165.

van den Brink, G. (1996). Experiments on binaural diplacusis and tone perception. In R. Plomp & G. F. Smoorenburg (Eds.), *Frequency analysis and periodicity detection in hearing* (pp. 362–374). The Netherlands: Driebergen.

Van Kleeck, M. H. (1989). Hemispheric differences in global versus local processing of hierarchical visual stimuli by normal subjects: New data and a meta-analysis of previous data. *Neuropsychologia, 27*, 1165–1178.

Van Lancker, D. & Fromkin, V. A. (1973). Hemispheric specialization for pitch and "tone": Evidence from Thai. *Journal of Phonetics, 1*, 101–109.

Van Lancker, D. R., Kreiman, J., & Cummings, J. (1989). Voice perception deficits: Neuroanatomical correlates of phonagnosia. *Journal of Clinical and Experimental Neuropsychology, 11*, 665–674.

Wang, W. S. Y. (1976). Language change. *Annals of the New York Academy of Sciences, 280*, 61–72.

Ward, W. D. (1957). Hearing of naval aircraft personnel. *The Journal of the Acoustical Society of America, 29*, 1289–1301.

Ward, L. M. (1982). Determinants of attention to local and global features of visual forms. *Journal of Experimental Psychology: Human Perception & Performance, 8,* 562–581.

Warrington, E. K. (1985). Agnosia: The impairment of object recognition. In P. J. Vinken, G. W. Bruyn, & H. L. Klawans (Eds.), *Handbook of clinical neurology* (pp. 333–349). New York: Elsevier Science Publishing.

Warrington, E. & James, M. (1967). An experimental investigation of facial recognition in patients with unilateral cerebral lesions. *Cortex, 3,* 317–326.

Watt, R. J. (1988). *Visual processing: Computational psychophysical and cognitive research.* Hillsdale, N.J.: Lawrence Erlbaum & Associates.

Weiller, C., Isensee, C., Rijntjes, M., Huber, W., Muller, S., Bier, D., Durschka, K., Woods, R. P., Noth, J., & Diener, H. C. (1995). Recovery from Wernicke's aphasia: A positron emission tomographic study. *Annals of Neurology, 37,* 723–732.

Weinberger, D. R., Berman, K. F., & Zec, R. F. (1986). Physiological dysfunction of dorsolateral prefrontal cortex in schizophrenia: I. Regional cerebral blood flow evidence. *Archives of General Psychiatry, 43,* 114–125.

Wernicke, K. (1874). Der aphasische Symptomenkomplex. Breslau. (Translated in *Boston Studies of Philosophy of Science, 4,* 34–97).

Wertheimer, M. (1938). The general theoretical situation. In W. D. Ellis (Ed.), *A source book of Gestalt psychology.* London: Kegan Paul, Trench, Trubner. (Originally published in 1923).

Whitehouse, P. J. (1986). The concept of subcortical and cortical dementia: Another look. *Annals of Neurology, 19,* 1–6.

Wolfe, J. M., Cave, K. R., & Franzel, S. L. (1989). Guided search: An alternative to the feature integration model for visual search. *Journal of Experimental Psychology: Human Perception and Performance, 15,* 419–433.

Wood, C. C., Goff, S. R., & Day, R. S. (1971). Auditory evoked potentials during speech perception. *Science, 173,* 1248–1251.

Yund, E. W., Efron, R., & Nichols, D. R. (1990). Detectability gradients as a function of target location. *Brain & Cognition, 12,* 1–16.

Zaidel, E. (1975). A technique for presenting lateralized visual input with prolonged exposure. *Vision Research, 15,* 283–289.

Zaidel, E. (1978). Auditory language comprehension in the right hemisphere following cerebral commissuotomy and hemispherectomy: A comparison with child language and apahseia. In A. Caramazza & E. B. Zurif (Eds.), *Language acquisition and language breakdown: Parallels and divergencies* (pp. 229–275). Baltimore: Johns Hopkins University Press.

Zaidel, E., Clarke, J. M., & Suyenobu, B. (1990). Hemispheric independence: A paradigm case for cognitive neuroscience. In A. B. Scheibel & A. F. Wechsler (Eds.), *Neurobiology of higher cognitive function* (pp. 297–355). New York: Guilford.

Zani, A. & Proverbio, A. M. (1995). ERP signs of early selective attention effects to check size. *Electroencephalography and Clinical Neurophysiology, 95,* 277–292.

Zatorre, R. (1979). Recognition of dichotic melodies by musicians and non-musicians. *Neuropsychologia, 17,* 607–617.

Zatorre, R. J. (1984). Musical perception and cerebral function: A critical review:. *Music Perception, 2,* 196–221.

Zatorre, R. J. (1988). Pitch perception of complex tones and human temporal-lobe function. *Journal of the Acoustical Society of America, 84,* 566–572.

Zatorre, R. J. (1989). Effects of temporal neocortical excisions on musical processing. *Contemporary Musical Review, 4,* 265–277.

Zatorre, R. J., Blumstein, S. E., & Oscar-Berman, M. (1987). Lack of laterality effect for monaural categorization of VOT. *Brain and Language, 30,* 1–7.

Zatorre, R. J., Evans, A. C., & Meyer, E. (1994). Neural mechanisms underlying melodic perception and memory for pitch. *Journal of Neuroscience, 14,* 1908–1919.

Zatorre, R. J., Evans, A. C., Meyer, E., & Gjedde, A. (1992). Lateralization of phonetic and pitch discrimination in speech processing. *Science, 256,* 846–849.

Zatorre, R. J. & Samson, S. (1988). Melodic and harmonic discrimination following unilateral cerebral excision. *Brain and Cognition, 7,* 348–360.

Zatorre, R. J., & Samson, S. (1991). Role of the right temporal neocortex in retention of pitch in auditory short-term memory. *Brain, 114,* 2403–2417.

Zeki, S. (1993). *A vision of the brain.* Oxford: Blackwell Scientific Publications.

Author Index

Subject Index

Left hemisphere specialization. *See also* Cerebral asymmetry; Right hemisphere specialization
  and hierarchical pattern perception, 83–86, 137–145
  and language, 3–6, 169, 193–199, 202–207, 214–224
  and pitch perception, 46–50, 64–71, 175–188, 199–200
  and spatial cognition, 129–133, 145–151
  and time perception, 170, 202–207
  and visual spatial frequency, 52, 57–59, 67–68, 78–82, 133

Music. *See also* Dichotic listening, Double filtering by frequency theory; Frequency; Pitch perception; Right hemisphere specialization
  effects of practice, 189–190
  left ear advantage, 169, 180–184, 189
  missing fundamental illusion, 177–178, 182–184
  octave illusion, 185–187
  scale illusion, 187–188
  temporal lobes, 182–184, 200

Neurological patients
  neural reorganization in, 29
  selection of, 93–96
  as a source of converging evidence, 29

Part/whole processing. *See* Hierarchical visual patterns
Pitch perception. *See also* Dichotic listening; Double filtering by frequency theory; Frequency; Language; Music
  and attention, 60–64
  cerebral asymmetry, 47–50, 175–188, 199–200

Receptive fields
  auditory, 38
  visual, 38–39
Rey-Osterrieth test, 10
Right hemisphere specialization. *See also* Cerebral asymmetry; Left hemisphere specialization
  and apraxia, 9–11
  and emotion, 195–199, 200–204
  and face perception, 116–120
  and hierarchical pattern perception, 83–86, 137–145
  and language, 3–6, 169, 193–199, 202–207, 214–224

and music, 169, 180–184, 189
and pitch perception, 46–50, 64–71, 175–188, 199–200
and time perception, 202–204
and unilateral neglect, 7–9, 126, 156–162
and visual spatial frequency, 52, 57–59, 67–68, 78–82, 133

Schizophrenia
  attentional deficits, 262–263
  perceptual deficits, 263–264
  relation to deficits in frequency-based processing, 264–265
Spatial cognition. *See also* Attention; Unilateral neglect; Balint's syndrome
  and frames of reference, 151–156
  objects vs. locations, 129–133, 145–151
  spatial resolution, 124–129, 133–139
Spatial frequency. *See* Frequency
Speech perception. *See* Language
Split-brain research (callosotomy), 14–20

Time perception, in language
  phonological processing, 170, 202–207
  prosody, 202–204

Unilateral neglect, 7–9, 18, 126, 148–165
  and attention, 148–151, 160–161, 162–164
  cerebral asymmetry, 7–9, 126, 156–162
  and frame of reference, 151–154
  and hierarchical visual patterns, 157–159
  and internal representation of space, 154–156
  and spatial frequency, 159–160

Visual system organization, 15–16